ORGANIZATIONS, COMMUNICATION, AND HEALTH

Organizations, Communication, and Health focuses on theories and constructs of organizational communication and their relationship to health. The goal of the volume is to offer a current picture of organizational and organizing processes and practices related to health.

Research in the area of health communication has expanded in recent years, and this research has advanced understandings of campaigns, patient–provider interactions, and social support. However, a gap in the area of health, organizations, and organizing processes emerged—a niche this volume fills. It does so by having chapters identify an organizational theory or organizing process and how aspects of that theory relate to health. Chapters discuss how to marry theory to practice and the other factors (e.g., organizational structure, role, occupation, industry, or environment) that need to be considered in the process of utilizing the theory in organizations.

This volume, aimed at advanced undergraduate and graduate students studying health communication, as well as health professionals, provides useful theory and practice related to organizations and health, and issues a call for further theorizing on the practice of health communication in organizations.

Tyler R. Harrison (PhD, University of Arizona) is a professor of Communication Studies and a member of the Center for Communication, Culture, and Change at the University of Miami. His research focuses on the design, implementation, and evaluation of communication systems for organizational, health, and conflict processes.

Elizabeth A. Williams (PhD, Purdue University) is an assistant professor of Communication Studies at Colorado State University and an affiliate faculty member in the Colorado School of Public Health. Her current work examines the intersections among identification, leadership, training initiatives, and policy implementation in a variety of organizational contexts.

ORGANIZATIONS, COMMUNICATION, AND HEALTH

Edited by Tyler R. Harrison and
Elizabeth A. Williams

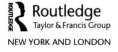
Routledge
Taylor & Francis Group

NEW YORK AND LONDON

First published 2016
by Routledge
711 Third Avenue, New York, NY 10017

and by Routledge
2 Park Square, Milton Park, Abingdon, Oxon, OX14 4RN

Routledge is an imprint of the Taylor & Francis Group, an informa business

Library of Congress Cataloging in Publication Data
Organizations, communication, and health / Tyler R. Harrison,
Elizabeth A. Williams.
pages cm
Includes bibliographical references and index.
1. Communication in public health. 2. Communication in medicine.
3. Communication in organizations. 4. Health services administration.
I. Harrison, Tyler R., editor.
RA423.2.O74 2016
362.1—dc23
2015021688

ISBN: 978-1-138-85308-9 (hbk)
ISBN: 978-1-138-85309-6 (pbk)
ISBN: 978-1-315-72302-0 (ebk)

Typeset in Bembo
by Swales & Willis Ltd, Exeter, Devon, UK

Printed and bound in the United States of America by Publishers Graphics,
LLC on sustainably sourced paper.

This book is dedicated to Susan, who knew this was the book I had to write years before I was ready. Your constant love, support, and encouragement made this possible.

Tyler R. Harrison

To my Dad and Mom—for all the lessons you taught me, the opportunities you gave me, and the love you showed me. And to Mark, Grace, and Laura—you remind me every day of the important things in life.

Elizabeth A. Williams

CONTENTS

FIGURES

TABLES

PREFACE

This book has as its genesis a statement made by Calvin Morrill to me (Tyler) as a graduate student studying organizational communication and conflict. By training, Cal was an organizational sociologist working in the Department of Communication at the University of Arizona. He and Dave Buller had just received a large federal grant for cancer prevention. The project used network analysis to select and develop peer educators to promote five-a-day fruits and vegetables consumption in over 90 workgroups in Arizona. This was in the early 1990s—health communication was in its nascent days in the discipline and grant funding was becoming more of a priority for social scientists. While I was working on the research team doing network analysis, Cal made a simple statement, somewhat in jest that, "eventually we all become health communication scholars." Despite being married to a health communication scholar and being surrounded by people working on health communication projects and grants, I stayed away from the area for a number of years until I was able to find a project that let me also ask questions about organizations. Since then I have worked on numerous interventions in organizational contexts to improve organ donation campaigns. I have also had the chance to bring numerous students of organizational communication onto these projects and I have repeated the conversation I had with Cal—eventually we all become health communication scholars. It was on one of these projects that I first had the chance to work with my co-editor, Elizabeth Williams.

I (Elizabeth) was a first-year Master's student studying organizational communication and applied to be a Research Assistant for one of Tyler's grant-funded projects. The project interested me, not because I had a desire to study health communication (admittedly, I did not even know the sub-discipline existed before arriving at Purdue), but because a family member had recently been on the organ donation waiting list and I wanted desperately to give back. Through the years as

I worked on various projects with Tyler and Susan Morgan, and eventually began designing my own projects, it became clear to me that theories from organizational and health communication could greatly inform one another. Indeed, I realized, like many of the scholars who have contributed to this volume, that by putting the sub-disciplines into conversation we can improve two areas which are ubiquitous in our lives—our health and our membership in a variety of organizations.

Since those early days, research in the area of health communication has burgeoned. This research has advanced our understandings of campaigns, patient–provider interactions, social support, and many other areas as well. Despite the growth in health communication research, one area that has not advanced as rapidly as others is the area of health, organizations, and organizing processes. Research for our proposal confirmed what we suspected, that there were few sources related to organizations, communication, and health. There are a few chapters in the *Handbook of Health Communication*, some books on communication in health care organizations, and a small body of journal articles. We realized that this gave us a great opportunity to push the boundaries and move the area forward. As we developed our ideas for the book and approached authors, we wanted to move away from a traditional handbook type of volume and focus as much as possible on generating new approaches and creating new nexuses of organizations, organizing, communication, and health. We wanted a book that would help scholars go out and use these theories in new ways.

In order to do this, this volume focuses on theories and constructs of organizational communication and their relationship to health. Our goal is to offer a current picture of organizational and organizing processes and practices related to health, and to issue a call for further theorizing on the practice in this area. "Organization," for this volume, is broadly defined, and draws on notions of organizations as being constituted by communication. As such, we look beyond the traditional bricks and mortar (container) metaphors of organizations and view organizations and organizing processes as symbolically created.

Authors in this volume fall into three categories. First, there are those who have already been working at the intersections of these areas. For most authors in this category, contributing to this book was a no-brainer. Even those who initially had some resistance became enthusiastic as they heard the details. One author later shared that when her co-author approached her to see if she would participate; her response was, "Why do I need another book chapter?" But, after hearing the project's vision she thought it made perfect sense and enthusiastically contributed an excellent chapter. A second group of authors in this volume are more traditional organizational communication scholars who do less direct work with health. However, we saw their areas of research as being directly relevant, and asked them to extend their theorizing into the area of health. Finally, we have more traditional health communication scholars whose work we saw as having strong organizational implications. We pushed these scholars to consider how their work influences and is influenced by organizing and organizations.

To create a volume that would spur a new generation of scholars and advance practice in this area, we asked authors to develop their chapters around a series of guiding questions:

1. Identify the organizational theory or organizing process under consideration, as well as the specific components and relationships of the theory in relation to health.
2. Discuss the unique contributions of the approach to health and discuss the contexts in which it has been used, to what effect, and with which audiences.
3. Talk about how the theory could be effectively translated into practice in organizations, and where possible, identify each of the constructs of the theory that can be operationalized into message features, actual messages, interactions, or other organizing and communication strategies.
4. Given the different levels of theorizing and organizing, focus on other factors (e.g., organizational structure, role, occupation, industry, environment) that need to be considered in the process of utilizing the theory in organizations.
5. Write about potential pitfalls that need to be avoided in the process of implanting theory into practice; discuss how to avoid those pitfalls; and identify areas of future theorizing, research, and utilization of their approach. While our goal is always to improve health, we need to be aware of the unintended consequences and challenges associated with our work.
6. Where applicable, focus on a specific project and use that project to illustrate the elements and processes of theorizing and research.

We hope this volume generates new ideas and provides guidance on using these theories for implementing interventions, designing systems, or producing new research and knowledge. We see both theoretical and practical relevance for health and organizational communication scholars, those involved in medical and interprofessional education, leaders and administrators in both health care organizations and non-health care organizations, nonprofits seeking to expand their collaborative abilities, and those interested in changing systems and practices of health and well-being.

ACKNOWLEDGMENTS

While the origins of a book like this start during discussions with one or two friends and colleagues, the creation of the book is the result of the hard work, cooperation, and engagement with many people. The authors in this volume have all been enthusiastic, engaged, and responsive, even to our often tight deadlines. Thank you all for seeing the contributions we hoped the book would make, and for using your creative and intellectual powers to produce stimulating chapters, and for being willing to push your work in new directions. Because of you, this book represents a collective vision of how we can engage organizations, communication, and health. We also wish to thank our editor at Routledge, Linda Bathgate, for seeing the value in advancing a new set of perspectives about organizing and health communication, and her support and advice in developing the project and helping us see it through to completion.

Thank you also to our editorial assistant, Ross Wagenhofer, who helped us navigate the challenges of managing and organizing all of the details and guiding us through the publication process. We also thank our three reviewers who provided guidance and suggestions as we developed the project. Your insights helped strengthen the project. Finally, thank you to our families, many friends, and colleagues who engaged in discussions about our vision over wine and wonderful dinners, provided advice on structuring chapters, and shared their experiences in book publishing. Your advice, humor, and support made the process fun and manageable.

ABOUT THE CONTRIBUTORS

Mark Aakhus (PhD, University of Arizona) is a professor at the School of Communication and Information at Rutgers University. He investigates the use of language, argumentation, and social interaction in professional practice, organizational processes, and information systems. His research articulates the competence and creativity involved in managing complex situations through communication and design. His current projects focus on collaborative governance and open innovation in multi-sector, multi-stakeholder enterprises and methods for mapping controversy over business practice in global production networks.

Joshua B. Barbour (PhD, University of Illinois) is an assistant professor in the Department of Communication Studies and affiliate faulty in the Center for Health Communication in the Moody College of Communication at The University of Texas at Austin. He studies the communicative, organizational, and macromorphic problems that recur in the conduct of knowledge-intensive work. His research seeks to make individuals and organizations more effective, to make them safer, and to make organizations more conducive to human health and well-being.

Ryan S. Bisel (PhD, University of Kansas) is an associate professor of Organizational Communication at the University of Oklahoma. His research interests include leadership communication, organizational culture, and behavioral ethics. His research is published in outlets such *as Management Communication Quarterly, Human Relations, Small Group Research*, and the *Leadership Quarterly*.

Heather E. Canary (PhD, Arizona State University) is an associate professor in the Department of Communication at the University of Utah. Her primary research focus is communication across lay and professional groups, particularly processes of knowledge construction and decision-making in contexts of public policies, health, and disability. She has published articles in *The American Journal of Public Health*, *Communication Theory*, and *Management Communication Quarterly*, among other scholarly journals. Her work appears in several books, including *Communication and Organizational Knowledge: Contemporary Issues for Theory and Practice*.

Nick Carcioppolo (PhD, Purdue University) is an assistant professor of Communication Studies and director of the Cancer Communication Lab at the University of Miami. His research focuses on persuasion and health communication largely in the context of cancer prevention and screening. His research has been published in refereed outlets such as *Health Communication*, *Public Understanding of Science*, and the *Journal of Communication*.

Lisa V. Chewning (PhD, Rutgers University) is an assistant professor of Corporate Communication at Penn State University, Abington. Her research interests include social networks, crisis communication, public relations, and information and communication technology (ICT). Her research has been published in outlets such as the *Management Communication Quarterly*, *Communication Monographs*, *Public Relations Review*, the *Journal of Communication*, and *Human Communication Research*.

Marleah Dean (PhD, Texas A&M University) is an assistant professor in the Department of Communication at the University of South Florida. She studies patient–provider communication in health communication and is currently examining genetics and risk communication in hereditary cancer. Her research has been published in *Health Communication*, *Academic Medicine*, *Patient Education & Counseling*, *Journal of Health and Mass Communication*, and *Qualitative Research in Organizations and Management*.

Marya L. Doerfel (PhD, University at Buffalo) is an associate professor at the School of Communication and Information at Rutgers University. Her research focuses on networked forms of organizing with a particular interest in disrupted networks and community resilience. She has been funded by the National Science Foundation and has published her research in journals such as *Communication Monographs*, *Management Communication Quarterly*, *Human Communication Research*, the *Journal for the Association for Information Science and Technology*, *New Media & Society*, *Voluntas*, and *The Public Relations Review*.

Thomas Hugh Feeley is the professor and chair of Communication at University at Buffalo, The State University of New York. Professor Feeley recently authored a book entitled *Research from the Inside-Out: Lessons learned from exemplary studies in communication* (Routledge). Dr. Feeley's research in organizational communication examines the role of social networks in employee assimilation and turnover. His work in this area has appeared in *Human Communication Research* and the *Journal of Applied Communication Research*.

Bernadette M. Gailliard (PhD, University of California Santa Barbara) is an assistant professor at the School of Communication and Information at Rutgers University. Her research examines processes of career socialization and member-ship negotiation in organizations, with particular attention to identity and the inter-sections of race, gender, and class. Her research has been published in *Management Communication Quarterly*, *Human Relations*, and *Communication Yearbook*.

Patricia Geist-Martin received her PhD in Communication from Purdue University in 1985. She is a professor in the School of Communication at San Diego State University where she teaches organizational communication, health communication, ethnographic research methods, and gendering organizational communication. Her research interests focus on narrative and negotiating iden-tity, voice, ideology, and control in organizations, particularly in health and ill-ness. She has published three books, *Communicating Health: Personal, Political, and Cultural Complexities* (2004) (with Eileen Berlin Ray and Barbara Sharf), *Courage of Conviction: Women's Words, Women's Wisdom* (1997) (with Linda A. M. Perry), and *Negotiating the Crisis: DRGs and the Transformation of Hospitals* (1992) (with Monica Hardesty). She has published over 60 articles and book chapters cover-ing a wide range of topics related to gender, health, and negotiating identities. Her forthcoming edited book is *Storied Health and Illness: Communicating Personal, Cultural, and Political Complexities* (with Jill Yamasaki and Barbara Sharf).

Rebecca Gill (PhD, University of Utah) is a senior lecturer in the School of Management and School of Communication, Journalism and Marketing at Massey University in New Zealand. She is interested in occupational identity, place and work, with particular attention to gender and difference. She is currently focused on understanding the regional construction of entrepreneurship and innovation. Her research has been published in *Human Relations*, *Communication Monographs*, *Organization*, *Management Communication Quarterly*, and the *Journal of Applied Communication Research*, among other outlets.

Tyler R. Harrison (PhD, University of Arizona) is the professor of Communication Studies and a member of the Center for Communication, Culture, and Change at the University of Miami. His research focuses on the design, implementation, and evalu-ation of communication systems for organizational, health, and conflict processes. He has received multiple HRSA-funded grants to support his research, which includes the implementation of organ donation campaigns in different organizational contexts. He also has certificates in mediation and negotiation from Harvard University and has worked as an arbitrator for the Better Business Bureau. He is currently working on the prevention of commercial sexual exploitation of children with the Colombian National Police and cancer prevention with firefighters in Florida.

Paula Hopeck (PhD, Purdue University) is an assistant professor in the Department of Languages, Cultures, and Communication at Stephen F. Austin

State University. Her work has been published in the *Management Communication Quarterly*, the *International Journal of Conflict Management*, and *Health Communication*. In addition to conflict management, she studies how individuals and organizations manage end-of-life issues.

Michael L. Kent is a professor in the School of Advertising, and Public Relations at the University of Tennessee, Knoxville. His research focuses on new technology, social media, dialogic public relations, and international public relations. Kent's work has been published in *Public Relations Review*, *The Journal of Public Relations Research*, *Management Communication Quarterly*, *Atlantic Journal of Communication*, *Communication Studies*, *Critical Studies in Media Communication*, *Gazette*, and other sources.

Natalie J. Lambert (MA) is a PhD student in the Department of Communication at the University of Illinois at Urbana-Champaign. Her research applies computational methods in health, small group, and online contexts in order to develop organizational theory that is informed by large-scale empirical data. Her work has appeared and is forthcoming in *Communication Research*, *Organizational Research Methods*, and the *Encyclopedia of Health Communication*.

John C. Lammers (PhD, University of California-Davis) is a professor in the Department of Communication and director of the Health Communication Online Masters of Science Program at the University of Illinois at Urbana-Champaign. His research applies institutional theory to communication among health professionals and organizations. His work has appeared in *The Academy of Management Review*, *Management Communication Quarterly*, *Communication Theory*, *Health Communication*, *Annals of Internal Medicine*, and the *Annals of Emergency Medicine*.

Steven K. May (PhD, University of Utah) is an associate professor in the Department of Communication at the University of North Carolina at Chapel Hill. His research interests include organizational ethics and corporate social responsibility. His books include *The Handbook of Communication Ethics*, *The Handbook of Communication and Corporate Social Responsibility*, *The Debate Over Corporate Social Responsibility*, *Case Studies in Organizational Communication: Ethical Perspectives and Practices* and *Engaging Organizational Communication Theory and Research: Multiple Perspectives*, each of which has won a top book award from national and international associations. His current book projects include *Corporate Social Responsibility: Virtue or Vice?* and *Working Identities*.

Susan E. Morgan (PhD, University of Arizona) is a professor of Communication Studies as well as the director of the Center for Communication, Culture, and Change at the University of Miami. Her research focuses on message design to promote improved positive social and behavioral change in health communication contexts. She has received major federal funding from NIDA, NIOSH, and HRSA to support this research and the findings of her research have been published in medical and social science journals.

Ashton Mouton is a doctoral candidate at Purdue University where she is currently exploring the intersections of health communication, organizational communication, and gender. Her work focuses on two specific types of organizations: health care and academic. Her research on health care organizations, specifically, examines how communication and the practice of organizing impacts patient care, but also how people interact with(in) the organization and the outcomes of those interactions.

Karen K. Myers (PhD, Arizona State University) is an associate professor in the Department of Communication at the University of California, Santa Barbara. Her current research includes membership negotiation (socialization, assimilation); vocational anticipatory socialization; workplace flexibility and work–life balance issues; organizational identification; and interaction between generational cohorts in the workplace. Her work has appeared in *Management Communication Quarterly*, *Human Communication Research*, the *Journal of Applied Communication Research*, *Communication Monographs*, the *Communication Yearbook*, *Human Relations* and elsewhere.

Anne M. Nicotera (PhD, Ohio University) is a professor and chair in the Department of Communication at George Mason University, where she teaches courses in organizational and interpersonal communication. Her research is grounded in a constitutive perspective and focuses on culture and conflict, diversity, race and gender, and aggressive communication, with a particular interest in health care organization and nursing communication. She has published her research in numerous national journals. She has also published five books and several chapters.

Aisha K. O'Mally is a PhD student at University at Buffalo, The State of University of New York. Her area of focus is health communication. Specifically, she is interested in organ donation message effects, and medical adherence among transplant patients. Fascinatingly, Aisha's research is closely related to her experience as a heart transplant recipient. Through her research she hopes to help post transplanted patients better adhere to their medical regime and decrease re-hospitalization.

Marshall Scott Poole (PhD, University of Wisconsin, 1980) is a David L. Swanson professor in the Department of Communication, senior research scientist at the National Center for Supercomputing Applications, and director of the Institute of Computing in the Humanities, Arts, and Social Sciences at the Department of Communication at the University of Illinois at Urbana-Champaign.

Jeffrey D. Proulx (MA, Michigan State University) is a doctoral student in the Department of Communication at the University of Illinois at Urbana-Champaign. His research focuses on how institutional factors impact the role of profession in the behavioral health industry. His work attempts to inform institutional, evolutionary, and structuration theories through the use of network approaches to communication research.

Kevin Real (PhD, 2002, Texas A&M University) is an associate professor of Communication in the Department of Communication at the University of Kentucky. He is interested in how communication theory and research can provide opportunities for improving everyday life for organizational stakeholders. His work has been published in the *Handbook of Health Communication*, *American Journal of Infection Control, Journal of Business and Psychology, Health Communication, Management Communication Quarterly*, and *Journal of Applied Communication Research*.

Torsten Reimer (PhD, Free University of Berlin/Germany, 1996) is an associate professor of Communication and Psychology at Purdue University. His research focuses on the role of communication in decision-making and aims to understand the functionality of heuristic information processing in group and organizational decision-making. His research program has the overarching goal of exploring how communication principles facilitate decision-making by guiding information processing and reducing information overload. Applied topics include the design of persuasive messages and risk communication.

Christopher Roland is a Master's student at Purdue in the Brian Lamb School of Communication. His research interests concern persuasion and decision-making. In particular, his work adopts a decision-making perspective on argument design to explore the effects of persuasive message strategies on individual and group choice behavior.

Tillman Russell (PhD, Purdue University) is an assistant professor of advertising and public relations at the University of Southern Indiana. His research explores the relationship between communication and cognition, specifically the role of semantic networks in persuasion and group decision-making.

Jennifer A. Scarduzio (PhD, Arizona State University) is an assistant professor in the Department of Communication at the University of Kentucky. Her research examines the intersections of emotion, violence, and wellness in a variety of organizational and health settings. She has published in journals such as *Communication Monographs, Management Communication Quarterly*, and *Journal of Interpersonal Violence*, among others.

Kami Silk (PhD, University of Georgia) is an associate dean for Academic Programs in the College of Communication Arts and Sciences and professor in the Department of Communication and AgBioResearch at Michigan State University. A health communication scholar, her research focuses on how to communicate effectively to promote positive health outcomes among the lay public. Her most recent projects, breast cancer risk reduction among adolescents and healthy infant feeding practices, are funded by the NIH.

Sandi W. Smith is the director of the Health and Risk Communication Center and professor in the Department of Communication at Michigan State University. Her work has been funded by NSF, HRSA, NCI, NIEHS, and the U.S. Dept. of Education. It centers on the impact of communication on health behavior such as the prevention of breast cancer, enrolling on state organ donor registries and encouraging family discussion about organ donation, and persuading college students to consume alcohol moderately.

Keri K. Stephens is an associate professor at The University of Texas at Austin and the associate director of the UT Center for Health Communication where she studies Organizational Communication and Technology. She has published over 40 peer-reviewed articles and book chapters, and a co-authored book. Her research examines how organizations are entwined with technology, health, and safety communication. She is interested in redundant communication, brevity, and the complexities involved when multiple communication technologies are present.

Maureen Taylor is the professor and director of the School of Advertising and Public Relations at the University of Tennessee, Knoxville. Taylor's research interest is in international public relations, nation building and civil society campaigns. Her work has appeared in the *Journal of Public Relations Research*, *Public Relations Review*, *Communication Monographs*, *Communication Theory*, *Human Communication Research*, *Journal of Communication*, *Management Communication Quarterly*, *Gazette*, and *Atlantic Journal of Communication*.

Lien Tran is an assistant professor of Interactive Media at the University of Miami where she specializes in game, web, and interaction design for social good. She is an award-winning game designer who creates social impact games that help nonprofits and humanitarian organizations communicate critical messages in an accessible and engaging manner. Her game partnerships include: Open Society Foundations, United Nations, World Bank, National Police of Colombia, and the International Federation of Red Cross and Red Crescent Societies.

Jessica Wendorf is a doctoral student in the School of Communication at the University of Miami. Her research focuses on information dissemination and social change through the use of serious games. She has received funding from Open Society Foundations, Consortium for Latin American Studies, and the Tinker Foundation, among others, to support this research. Current projects include *Jugando a lo Seguro*, an experiential dengue prevention campaign, and *Por Estas Calles*, a role-playing game aimed at increasing reporting of sexual exploitation.

Elizabeth A. Williams (PhD, Purdue University) is an assistant professor in the Department of Communication Studies at Colorado State University and an affiliate faculty member in the Colorado School of Public Health. Her current work examines the intersections among identification, leadership, training initiatives, and policy implementation in a variety of organizational contexts. Her work has been published in *Journal of Communication*, *Journal of Applied Communication Research*, *Communication Studies*, *Journal of Health Communication*, *Health Communication*, and various edited volumes.

Kevin B. Wright (PhD, University of Oklahoma) is a professor in the Department of Communication at George Mason University. His main research interests include new technologies and health information-seeking, social support and health outcomes, and stress and burnout among health care workers. In addition, his research examines the links between conflict and stress as well as work–life balance issues within health care organizations.

Alaina C. Zanin (PhD, University of Oklahoma) is an assistant professor in the Department of Management at the University of Central Missouri. She researches leadership communication and organizational communication in unique organizational contexts. She specializes in structuration, sensemaking and framing theories as well as issues surrounding power, control, resistance, gender, and body work. Her dissertation is on the structuring processes of resistance and control within an athletic health care organization.

Yaguang Zhu (MA, The University of Texas at Austin) is a doctoral student in the Department of Communication Studies at The University of Texas at Austin. He studies organizational health communication and has produced research on topics such as workplace health promotion, social media use to constrain adolescent smoking behaviors, crisis communication, and multiple communication technology use.

1

INTRODUCTION TO ORGANIZATIONS, COMMUNICATION, AND HEALTH

Exploring Intersections for Theory, Practice, and Change

Tyler R. Harrison and Elizabeth A. Williams

Communication in and by organizations, and as an organizing process, has profound implications for the health of individuals, organizations, and society as a whole. While there are numerous books about health care organizations, no volume explores broader processes of organizing and organizational contexts. This volume intends to fill that gap, investigating processes and contexts in three key areas: (a) organizing and communication issues and processes in health care organizations and professions, (b) work and organizations' effect on individuals' health, and (c) collaboration, systems design, and interorganizational efforts at improving health.

Organizing and Communication Issues and Processes in Health Care Organizations and Professions

While most of the extant research bridging organizational and health communication focuses on health care organizations—a hugely important area—this section departs from earlier work by directly applying organizational theories in order to improve our understanding of these issues. Indeed, the processes and issues of communication in health care organizations are different from issues in other organizations, as communication is often directly concerned with health decisions for non-organizational members. Issues of assimilation and socialization into the organization influence how health-related work is accomplished. Additionally, doing the work of health care creates different stresses and tensions for both the individual and the workplace. In this section, these issues are discussed in relation to teams, conflict, decision-making, and wrongdoing.

We begin the book with Lammers and Proulx's chapter on professions and professional logic, which are put forth as a counterpoint to organizations as a way in which work occurs. The concept of profession plays an important role in the organization and delivery of health services in the United States, and it is strongly implicated in health communication. Profession concerns the motivations and socialization of providers (including physicians, nurses, and others), their identities, social status, autonomy, and authority at work, and their social power in communication with patients, managers, and other providers. Lammers and Proulx explore these concepts by examining the changing nature of medicine as exemplified by issues related to eHealth. This chapter sets the stage for more in-depth discussion of many chapters in the first section of the book. They address professions in 4 realms: (a) the personal realm, which focuses on identity and socialization, an issue explored in more depth by Myers and Galliard; (b) the interaction realm, which concerns interaction between professionals and patients, an area further explored in chapters by Morgan and Mouton as it relates to patient recruiting and clinical trial accrual, Barbour, Gill, and Dean as they explore gender, space and role in emergency departments, and Hopeck as she explores the role of health care organization members in their interactions with patients and families at end of life; (c) the organization realm, which focuses on communication between professionals, an area explored by Reimer, Russell, and Roland in their chapter on how medical teams make health care decisions; and (d) the institutional realm, which focuses on groups, associations, coordination, and systems, an area explored by Real and Poole in their chapter on a systems approach to health care teams. Concepts from the institutional realm also carry over into the next section, in which Wright and Nicotera explore conflict in health care organizations from a more structural and systems perspective.

While Lammers and Proulx create a space of intersection, we have organized chapters in the first section so they move from broad principles to specific instances. The next chapter, by Myers and Galliard, examines literature on entry, socialization, and assimilation into health care organizations. They make the argument that individuals in these organizations experience these processes differently because of their professional identities. Specifically, this chapter looks at how these processes can influence how individuals get to know their coworkers and are acculturated, how they are recognized within their team, and how they deal with stress and emotions, as well as how the processes can be influenced by these relationships.

In their examination of how communication inputs in teams influence processes and outcomes of health care, Real and Poole bring a systems perspective to the focus of teams. They argue that there is not one best structure or set of communication inputs, but rather that the structure needs to be adaptive to the culture, context, and set of tasks to be accomplished. Additionally, their systems approach to teams acknowledges the larger contexts in which health care occurs, exploring implications at the societal, organizational, clinical, and team levels.

Reimer, Russell, and Roland focus on specific elements of team processes as they relate to health care decision-making. Using the case of Jesica Santillan, who had a failed organ transplantation, they situate team functioning in terms of task environments, implicit and explicit coordination, and team structure and composition as they relate to time, space, expertise, and team interaction. They advance the argument that no single decision-making process or group structure is best, but that groups and teams need to be adaptive as they engage in processes related to the specific functions of the group.

With Morgan and Mouton's chapter we move to a more specific focus related to the design of patient recruitment and accrual systems for clinical trials while simultaneously taking a broad view of systems design. Their chapter delineates systems problems that have broad implications for how we manage health processes, and also presents patient barriers derived from their sensemaking and interaction with health care processes. They present a model of patient accrual to clinical trials that identifies points of entry for engagement with communication design to improve the system, which should increase patient participation in clinical trials and create more opportunities for improving patient care and treatments.

Barbour, Gill, and Dean also focus on a specific type of health care organization, examining how space can be conceptualized and designed in an emergency department to challenge traditional d/Discourses that reify gender and racial norms in medical occupations. The chapter draws from their study of EmergiCare and makes suggestions for how a communication design perspective can open up space for challenging discursive constructions that create separation and conflict between nurses and physicians.

Continuing on the theme of power and how it influences discourses, Bisel and Zanin explore the concept of moral dissent in health care organizations. Their chapter highlights power differentials which likely influence the "moral mum"—the propensity of individuals to resist labeling the actions of others as unethical. The chapter also highlights how a biomedical approach combined with managed care creates a discourse that is inherently unethical—all patients are treated the same, but not all patients have the same needs, medically or psychosocially.

Hopeck's chapter on health care employees' involvement in end-of-life conflicts concludes the first section. She focuses on conflict among family members and how such conflicts might impact how health care workers do their jobs as they intervene to help families during this difficult time. She identifies five key strategies that health care workers use in their attempts to resolve family conflicts and relates these strategies to two models of conflict management. The chapter highlights how an effective system might alleviate the conflicts that exist during patient care, resulting in both a better (or at least less traumatic) experience for the patient/family and a decreased chance of negative outcomes (i.e., lawsuits, dissatisfaction) for the health care organization.

A recurring theme through all these chapters is the tensions that are experienced in health care organizations, largely stemming from issues related to professions and the inherent power differences, and the structural barriers they create. Different theoretical approaches to communication provide opportunities for invention and change to overcome these challenges and improve patient care, organizational member interactions, and the communication design of health care organizations.

Work and Organizations' Effects on Individuals' Health

The second section of this book addresses issues related to how work and organizations affect individuals' health. The process of work itself has implications for health, and non-health-care organizations have become increasingly involved in health and health decisions. Organizations engage in targeted health campaigns, general wellness campaigns, and use incentives (or punishments) to help us engage in desirable health activities (e.g., exercising or quitting smoking). Additionally, organizations and work are sources of stress, burnout, and decisions about safety that have consequences in and out of the workplace. Organizations put forward policies, create messages and images about social responsibility and health, implement conflict intervention strategies, and design workplaces to encourage healthy behavior. This section of the book addresses those processes by which organizations become directly involved in members' health.

Wright and Nicotera begin the section with a chapter that highlights the negative effects of conflict in the workplace: burnout and stress, including the attendant health consequences and ways those effects and consequences can be mediated by social support. They provide a bridge to broader organizational contexts by distinguishing between health care organizations and non-health care organizations and how these issues of stress and burnout affect employee health in all organizations. They advance two ways that organizations can approach conflict: competence-based approaches (training in conflict competencies); and structurational divergence approaches (focusing on structural issues that lead to conflict).

Scarduzio and Geist-Martin shift to organizations taking a more direct and planned approach to employee health, focusing on workplace wellness programs. They expand the concept of health beyond the physical to also include the psychological, social, and spiritual. In their chapter, they advocate for a whole-person approach to workplace wellness campaigns, and argue that such an approach is beneficial not only for the employees but the organization as well. They also show how organizational and managerial practices, such as supportive supervision, challenging work, skill development, and empowerment increase happiness and psychological well-being.

May also examines organizations' attempts to address employee health. Where the previous chapter points out all positive ways organizations can affect health, he reminds us that in these settings fraught with power imbalances, we must question motivations. May approaches employee assistance programs (EAPs) through the lens of corporate social responsibility and shifts the focus to internal stakeholders—employees. EAPs began with a problem-based orientation focused on helping people with marital, drug, alcohol, financial, and other problems as well as helping to reduce turnover and increase profits. But, these EAPs can also be used as a source of control, creating a situation where the body has become a site to be examined, studied, understood, and managed by the corporation.

Stephens and Zhu examine the role that organizations play in technology-infused health communication practices. Using the theoretical lenses of Social Identity Theory (SIT) and Organizational Identification (OI), Stephens and Zhu begin to explain the role of organizations in disseminating health messages and why some organizations are better at this process than others. They present a model that connects variables related to SIT and OI to message influence, and suggest that SIT may influence variables associated with persuasion such as message salience.

Harrison also examines message dissemination and draws on theories of diffusion to offer a model of interaction environments for health interventions in organizations. Drawing from communication design and experiences with several campaigns, he theorizes about the various elements that influence how health messages are diffused and accepted (or rejected) in organizations. The chapter presents opportunities both for empirically testing claims of the model and for practitioners to put the knowledge to use in current health campaigns. Whereas Harrison focuses more on the structural features of organizations, and the nature and materiality of work, Stephens and Zhu focus on the connection between workers and the organization to explain the positive effects of conversation.

Carcioppolo, Wendorf, and Tran provide an innovative focus on serious games (games for change) and their relationship to health and organizations. This chapter makes the argument that serious games can mimic and encourage organizing processes resulting in specific organizational and health outcomes, using a very different type of intervention than we commonly think of for worksite campaigns. Using several games as examples, the chapter highlights various theoretical frameworks that have been used to explore games as learning tools and then theorizes how this translates into an instance of organizing for health outcomes. They take a multilayered approach and show that games are organizing structures, but also that games can help individuals assimilate and learn organizational practices. At the more macro level, games can help organize communities to action.

Canary moves away from the idea of interventions and highlights the ways that processes and practices of organizational knowledge construction influence health and well-being at a variety of organizational levels and contexts, including for organizational members, between organizations and clients or patients, and at the level of public policy and health. She uses knowledge transfer and exchange (KTE) to show that information and knowledge creation is a two-way process. But, organizational culture influences how KTE occurs. She argues knowledge is social, and that no one size fits all. Ultimately, Canary contends we must move toward the measurement of health outcomes, not just knowledge creation processes.

The section concludes with a chapter by Lammers and Lambert on institutional theory and health. In this chapter, institutional theory is used to examine areas of stability and instability in health care. Using the four "tools" of institutional theory, they specifically look at patient–provider communication, organizational communication, and mass mediated communication (through eHealth) to see how institutional theory informs and generates further research on these areas. This macro approach moves beyond individual organizations and helps frame the broader role of organizations and institutions as they relate to health.

The chapters in this second section work together to encourage us to think about both the impact organizations have on the health of their members, and the potential for further promotion of health by organizations. We see how formal programs (i.e., EAPs), communication systems (i.e., technology and the overarching interaction environment), and larger institutional forces provide ways of influencing the health of organizational members. They further remind us that there is no simple answer, that our approaches must recognize unique organizational contexts, and that we must be mindful of unanticipated and unintended consequences when organizations involve themselves in individuals' health and well-being.

Collaboration, Systems Design, and Interorganizational Efforts at Improving Health

The third section addresses large-scale organizing for health. Organizations often cooperate with other organizations, engage with nonprofits and communities, and design systems to improve health and achieve an overall goal of wellness. Chapters in this section move beyond work constituted by a particular organization to demonstrate how we organize leaders, transdisciplinary health research collaborations, networks, and organizations themselves in order to improve health processes and outcomes in a variety of contexts. Several of the contributions in this section draw upon long-term research projects to explore issues of social networks, the role of social capital and interorganizational cooperation, and the design of complex health systems.

We begin the final section of our book with a chapter by Silk and Smith, who show us how organizing processes are important for addressing transdisciplinary research processes to help improve health from a variety of disciplines and perspectives. They approach transdisciplinary teams as learning organizations using the Four Flows Model of membership negotiation, self-structuring, activity coordination, and institutional positioning. They use the transdisciplinary Breast Cancer and Environment Research Center/Program (BCERC/P) to illustrate how learning organization principles helped them build a cohesive team, which includes members from epidemiology, biology, community outreach and translation, and health advocates, to address both epidemiological issues about breast cancer, and community translation of those findings into health messages for women and girls. This model provides a forum to bring together a range of stakeholders to research the same problem while maximizing the knowledge network of the team, hopefully generating new approaches and ideas.

Feeley and O'Mally also focus on processes of collaboration, but they shift the focus to linking nonprofits with other organizations to advance specific public health goals. They identify six types of collaborative relationships, such as cause-related marketing and joint-issue promotion, and discuss the motivations organizations have for engaging in those collaborations. Using organ donation as an exemplar, the authors highlight the various types of collaborations that might exist and how these collaborations can be mutually beneficial for both parties and for the larger goal of public health. The chapter proposes a model of the communicative relationship that exists between the various stakeholders in these collaborative relations.

While the first two chapters in this section focus on team and organizational collaboration, the next three chapters focus on core processes that can help these collaborations occur. To begin, Williams merges two theoretical frameworks, multi-team systems, and exchange theories of leadership, to situate coordination between organizational leaders as central to the success of large-scale health collaborations. Using the 2014/2015 West Africa Ebola crisis as an exemplar, this chapter explores how relationships between leaders can facilitate or constrain organizing processes and goal achievement in interorganizational health collaborations. Specifically, work on leader–leader exchange theory is offered as a way to understand the influence of these high-level relationships on organizational partnerships, and consequently on the success of health initiatives

In her chapter, Chewning offers the citizen-stakeholder model which establishes "how communication, social capital, and organizations can intersect to create better health outcomes." The chapter makes the argument that connections enabled by technology actually strengthen possibilities for citizenship. Several current examples of this model are given which illustrate the potential connections between the organization and the individual, and how these connections can build and effectively utilize social capital for improved health outcomes.

Doerfel's chapter highlights how networked forms of organizing can help reestablish healthy communities following a disaster. She frames disaster and disaster recovery as a public health issue. Looking at networked and hierarchical organizational forms, this chapter draws on examples from post-Hurricane Katrina New Orleans to explore how organizations can be flexible, and therefore resilient after disasters. Specifically, the chapter frames a robust/flexible network as a health asset that organizations and communities should cultivate. This health asset approach focuses on building communities and capacities, particularly when it comes to creating conditions for wellness rather than the prevention of disease.

Taylor and Kent advance a formal theory of community acceptance that operates from the assumption that we can change structures, community, and capacity by building individual capacities that enhance community engagement and involvement. During the recent Ebola outbreak in Liberia, the Peer Education in Neglected Health Issues Project trained vulnerable Liberian youth as peer educators to combat Ebola. The youth developed capacity as innovators, addressed a critical health issue, and acquired social empowerment for themselves and their communities, allowing them to choose medical options that might previously have been subject to community disapproval. This social empowerment creates future opportunities for these youth to also become community leaders, carrying on social change. The project demonstrates how a bottom-up approach to health knowledge and organizing can lead to societal change around a health issue.

We conclude the book with a chapter by Aakhus and Harrison that draws together many of the themes of the previous chapters. The authors focus on two "health entrepreneurs," Sir Harry Burns, the former Chief Medical Officer of Scotland who worked to re-design the Scottish Health System based on principles of health assets and salutogenesis, and Dr. Jeffery Brenner, who developed the concept of "hotspotting." Their efforts change the way we conceptualize the delivery of health and wellness. Their design thinking is illustrated through discussions of their approaches to systemic change and illustrates how communication as design and design thinking can make meaningful change to health systems. Central to the approach of both Burns and Brenner is the role of changing communication practices as a way to build health within communities.

These chapters demonstrate that it is through thoughtful, well-designed collaboration that we can impact health. Indeed, the chapters in this section leave us with the hope that by organizing various stakeholders in different ways and paying attention to the communication processes between these stakeholders, we can enact changes that lead to improved health at the individual, community, and global level.

Healthy People 2020

With its focus on these key areas, this volume addresses three objectives presented in Healthy People 2020 (HealthyPeople.gov): social determinants of health, the use of health communication to improve health outcomes, and a focus on educational and community-based programs. Each of these issues has direct links to the role of organizations and health communication as ways to improve health processes and health outcomes. First, issues related to social determinants of health are addressed through chapters that focus on creating social and physical environments that promote good health for all. Next, the use of health communication and health information technology to improve population health outcomes and health care quality is a theme that is addressed throughout the volume. At the organizational level of health communication interventions, this includes a focus on building social support networks, providing sound principles in the design of programs and interventions that result in healthier behavior, and providing opportunities to connect with culturally diverse and hard-to-reach populations. At the individual level this includes chapters on medical decision-making, health care teams, and many other areas.

The third area of Healthy People 2020, educational and community-based programs, focuses on preventing injury and disease, improving health, and enhancing quality of life by reaching people outside of traditional health care settings, including organizations. This issue is addressed in multiple areas of the volume, including in chapters on wellness and health campaigns, engineering healthy work environments, and organizing processes to bring diverse groups together for health change. Additionally, we explore processes associated with organizing non-traditional settings where health communication processes occur by examining issues such as organizing NGOs, processes of collaboration, network development, leadership, and coalition building.

Suggestions for Reading This Book

The organization of this book went through several iterations and as such we believe that there are many different ways you could approach reading this book. You could read it from front cover to back cover, moving through organizational contexts and levels of organizational processes. However, you could also read the book based on theoretical approaches. For example, there are four chapters that utilize communication design (Barbour, Gill, & Dean; Morgan & Mouton; Harrison; and Harrison & Aakhus), each operating at different levels of organizing, and as such are in conversation with each other. Chapters by Myers and Galliard, Canary, and Silk and Smith provide another example of readings crossing contexts and levels; these chapters share complementary approaches as they explore organizational learning and knowledge and their relationship to health. Our hope is that as you read the book you will see further connections in the work that will help create your own ideas about research and practice.

We have also provided a few tools to encourage future examination of these concepts and to generate discussion among readers, especially in educational contexts. First, at the end of each chapter you will find suggested readings. These are pieces that the authors have identified as being central to the ideas presented in their work. Second, each chapter ends with a series of discussion questions. These questions take different forms—some ask you to reflect on your experience, some ask you to connect various concepts in the chapter, and some ask you to take a stance on a particular issue. It is our hope that these chapters inspire you to further explore and join the conversations occurring at the intersections of organizations/organizing, health, and communication.

PART I

Organizing and Communication Issues and Processes in Health Care Organizations and Professions

2

THE ROLE OF PROFESSIONAL LOGIC IN COMMUNICATION IN HEALTH CARE ORGANIZATIONS

John C. Lammers and Jeffrey D. Proulx

Profession is one of the most studied concepts in social science. As early as the 1890s, Emile Durkheim (1996), one of the fathers of sociology, considered profession to be elemental in the division of labor in society and a critical aspect of modernity. Across the 20th century the medical profession was the subject of many theories and debates (see Hafferty & Castellani, 2010; see also Freidson, 1970; McKinlay & Arches, 1985; Parsons, 1939, 1963). Thus it is difficult to overstate the role profession plays in the organization and delivery of health services in the United States. Profession concerns the motivations and socialization of providers (including physicians, nurses, and others), their identities, social status, autonomy, and their social power in communication with patients, managers, and other providers. Profession determines the legitimacy of health messages and the conditions under which health care is provided. Thus profession works at both a micro-interactional level as well as at a macro-social level. As such, it is strongly implicated in health communication. In health communication, our analytical understanding of profession is weak, however, despite recent forays into the subject by organizational communication scholars (Cheney & Ashcraft, 2007; Lammers & Garcia, 2009). This chapter takes initial steps to develop a general analytic approach to communication and profession with a specific focus on professionalized occupations in health care (see also Barbour, Gill, & Dean, this volume).

A starting point for developing a communicative theory of profession is to recognize its pervasive and taken-for-granted character. Cheney and Ashcraft (2007) took the field of organizational communication to task for uncritically accepting the term: "In spheres ranging from popular culture to the home to the workplace, we refer and react to the professional like a social reflex" (p. 146).

While Cheney and Ashcraft critiqued the term "professional" in broad terms, health communication scholars likewise have not studied profession or professionalism in its own right. A search of titles and abstracts of our flagship journal, *Health Communication,* identified only three articles in its 26-year history dealing directly with a health profession as their foci (Ellingson, 2011; Lowrey & Anderson, 2006; Patterson & Patterson, 2010). The *Journal of Health Communication* fared no better, and neither the 2003 nor the 2011 *Handbook of Health Communication* (Thompson, Dorsey, Miller, & Parrot, 2003; Thompson, Parrott, & Nussbaum, 2011) featured any special focus on profession in health care as a topic *sui generis.* The *Journal of Interprofessional Care* has published several articles exploring the meaning of profession (Evetts, 1999; Hall, 2005; Kvarnström, 2008), but none investigated the concept communicatively. Communication scholars generally have accepted profession as the assumed characteristics of communicators with unique or important responsibilities in interactions with other health care providers (for example Apker et al., 2010), with patients (for example, Sharf & Street, 1997; Lambert et al., 1997), or with their families and social groups (for example, Brashers, 2001). Over twenty years ago Sharf (1993) raised this issue in the context of health communication, arguing "it is insufficient and perhaps misleading to examine clinical communication as if all doctors, patients, and settings are essentially comparable" (p. 37). Given the profound influence of the role of professions in the context of health communication, it seems appropriate to investigate its communicative constitution.

A challenge in unpacking the communicative constitution of profession is that the phenomenon is manifest across the personal, interactional, organizational, and institutional realms of communicative behavior. (We use "realms" here rather than "levels" to denote the quasi-independence but interpenetration of communication across these areas, and to avoid the implication that we view the arrangement as hierarchical.) In the personal realm, profession involves the motives and identities of individuals—typically physicians, nurses, and others of particular occupational status (Lammers & Barbour, 2009; Barbour & Lammers, 2015). The interactional realm has received considerable attention with respect to patient–provider communication, but much less attention with respect to interactions among physicians or between physicians and others (notable exceptions include Eisenberg, Baglia, & Pynes, 2006; Faraj & Xiao, 2006; and Apker et al., 2010). Profession manifests in the organizational realm as management draws on, organizes, and contests the power of professionalized occupations, and as they push back (Hafferty & Castellani, 2010). This realm has received little or no attention from health communication scholars. The institutional realm of profession is manifest in the enduring, widespread, obligatory, and relatively salient beliefs and practices shared by professionalized occupations, their peers, and clients across governmental and nongovernmental audiences. Health communication scholars are absent from this area as well—a search of our leading journals finds no studies of health reform rhetoric or policy making. Each of these realms overlaps and implicates the others, confounding the effort to show coherently how they are communicatively linked.

One approach to show how the realms are linked is suggested by recent work on institutional logics (Friedland & Alford, 1991; Thornton & Ocasio, 2008; Thornton, Ocasio, & Lounsbury, 2012). Institutional logics were first suggested by Friedland and Alford (1991) as sets "of material practices and symbolic constructions—which constitutes [their] organizing principles and which [are] available to organizations and individuals to elaborate" (p. 248). A number of scholars have developed the idea of logics, mostly in general institutional studies (Thornton, 2004), to a considerable extent in health care studies (e.g., Scott, Ruef, Mendel, & Caronna, 2000; van den Broek, Boselie, & Paauwe, 2014), but hardly at all in health communication (although see Lemire, Sicotte, & Pare, 2008; Barbour & Lammers, 2015). In the remainder of this chapter we develop a communicative conception of professional logic with particular reference to health care. In order to do this we briefly review definitional elements of profession. Then we consider the general idea of institutional logic, arguing that it has been underspecified in communicative terms. We suggest that a communicative understanding of institutional logic can be applied usefully to the case of health professions. Considering the case of eHealth, we draw on a sample of relevant research from each of the aforementioned realms to explore the implication of medical professional logic. Finally we suggest possible avenues for future research employing the idea of professional logic.

The Definition(s) of Profession

Profession as a General Category

It is useful to see profession as an institutionalized occupation (Abbott, 1988). Inasmuch as institutions are "constellations of established practices guided by formalized, rational beliefs that transcend particular organizations and situations" (Lammers & Barbour, 2006, p. 364), profession may be seen as "occupations characterized by formalized beliefs that specify and emerge from established practices transcending particular workplaces" (Lammers & Garcia, 2009, p. 358). Profession also plays a profound role in institutional stability (Scott, 2008), generating homophily, and contributing to the legitimacy of established beliefs and practices. We also know, however, that as a form of institution and institutionalization, profession is an ongoing process, the outcome of which is never entirely certain (Suddaby & Viale, 2011). In other words, it is useful to see profession as fluid despite its role in institutional persistence (Leicht & Fennel, 2001).

Recognized Features of Professions

Carr-Saunders (1966) defined profession as an occupation characterized by limited special knowledge, long and intense training and socialization periods, affect neutrality, internalized motives, self-control, and intra-professional norms of conduct. More communicatively, in a field study of veterinarians, Lammers and Garcia (2009) observed that profession meant "(a) knowledge providing, seeking, and sharing; (b) self-management of behavior, emotions, and productivity; (c) internal sources of motivation; (d) a service orientation; (e) the invocation of field standards; and (f) participation in a knowledge community beyond the workplace" (p. 357). A number of observers have been reluctant to embrace a single list of traits or behaviors of professions (Evetts, 1999), instead emphasizing that profession has a dual and somewhat self-contradictory nature: it serves society on the one hand but limits access to special knowledge for its own economic benefit on the other (Evetts, 1999; see also Cheney & Ashcraft, 2007).

Profession, Professionalization, and Professionalism

A considerable amount of scholarship has worked to identify the process by which an occupation might become professionalized. In the last century, this was thought to be an orderly sequence: "the emergence of a full-time occupation, the founding of a training school, a university school, a local association, a national association, the passing of state-level licensing laws, and the establishment of codes of professional ethics" (Evetts, 1999, p. 121). The fact that a number of occupations have gone through these steps and not obtained the status or autonomy of the classical professions of law or medicine has not discouraged incumbents from trying, although it has made researchers more wary of the process of professionalization.

In everyday parlance, the idea of professionalism means doing work well, doing a good job, or being a competent person (Evetts, 1999). For example, Dugdale, Siegler, and Rubin (2008) argued that medical professionalism means:

> commitment to providing patients with the best possible care . . . commitments to the fundamental principles of medical ethics . . . a strong commitment to the welfare and safety of their patients. . . . function as a good steward of society's medical resources . . . support policy initiatives designed to decrease health disparities and improve access to care. . . . [and] a commitment to developing and maintaining strong and effective doctor–patient relationships.
>
> *(pp. 550–551)*

While these statements may sound like slogans or moralisms, they should be taken seriously as claims to a privileged social status which has been the subject of hot debate and considerable discussion within the medical community (Hafferty & Castellani, 2010).

Hafferty and Castellani (2010) charted the emergence on the part of organized medicine in the United States of a concerted campaign to re-assert its social importance, beginning in the 1990s and continuing to the present day.

They identified a series of editorials, reports, and commentaries denouncing "'corporate medicine' [and] 'commercialism' . . . as 'corrosive', and 'antithetical' to professionalism" (p. 208). The campaign to re-assert the social value of medical professionalism was organized:

> Led by the ABIM [American Board of Internal Medicine] Foundation, early writers first sought to "outline the problem," followed by formal efforts to define and then measure medical professionalism . . . [and] Various professional societies (e.g., oncology, orthopedics, pathology, etc.) began to publish articles on the "problem of professionalism" and the need for physicians and organized medicine to "rediscover their professional roots."
>
> *(p. 208)*

The upshot of these developments is that organized medicine in the U.S., in the form of the American Medical Association, the American Association of Medical Colleges, the boards of the various specialties, and the Accreditation Council of Graduate Medical Education (the board that governs admission to residency programs) to name just a few, have become self-consciously deliberate in specifying just what medical professionalism means, right down to measures of its characteristics in individuals (Stern, 2006). In other words, medicine as an institution is working to defend, sustain, and recreate itself.

Profession and Organization

From an organization's point of view, professionals come and go; from professionals' points of view, organizations rise and fall while professions endure. Any particular organization is but one site in which the professional worker can function. The professional may therefore be seen as a guest, working semi-autonomously on behalf of the principles of the profession (Scott, 1965). Hospitals might be seen as hosts to the medical profession, while the profession may be seen as an *inquiline* within the hospital. However, the relationship is symbiotic, as both the profession and the host hospital mutually benefit from their imbricative arrangement. Nevertheless, professionalized workplaces have also been recognized as places where struggle for control over work, status, and autonomy are worked out in daily interactions (Freidson, 2001; Cheney & Ashcraft, 2007).

Thus organization and profession are analytically distinguishable and actually constitute alternative arrangements for accomplishing work. The profession tends to be flatter and characterized by horizontal, internalized, and concertive forms of control (Barker, 1993); the organization by contrast is typically hierarchical and characterized by formal positions and impersonal relations (Weber, 1947). Therefore the stability and endurance of the organization is rivaled by that of the profession. There are implications of this view for interaction among professionals and other workers. In addition to executing discrete tasks, some of the work of the profession is in defending itself; professional workers may be observed resisting control by management, or actually joining management to share control. Conversely, organizations work to control professions, rationalize their work, and seek human and technological alternatives to professionals.

Various authors (Scott, 2008; Freidson, 1986, 2001) have suggested that as a form of control over work, profession stands in contrast to the market, in which consumers' demands for efficiency and effectiveness sort out who does what at what price. Profession stands in contrast to administration as well, where bureaucratic rules and regulations are enforced by functionaries. In contrast, the profession is seen as a "third logic" (Freidson, 2001) that advances expertise and client welfare as guiding (and sometimes conflicting) elements of control over work. Even though Freidson (2001) used the term *logic* in the title of his book on professionalism, he did not actually employ it conceptually in his articulation of professionalism. The identification of profession as a form of institutional logic offers communication scholars an opportunity to make a contribution to the understanding of profession.

Putting Communication in Institutional (and Professional) Logics

The development of institutional logics scholarship has proceeded without insights from the discipline of communication, and without particular attention to professional communication in health care. Friedland and Alford (1991) referred to symbolic constructions in their original articulation of institutional logics, but did little to connect large-scale institutions like markets to the individual level of interaction, discourse, or interpretation. Later, DiMaggio (1997) identified logics of action as "interdependent set[s] of representations or constraints that influence action in a given domain" (p. 227). DiMaggio also found a common thread in Boltanski and Thevenot's (1991/2006) "modes of justification . . . institutionally linked discourses embodying specific orientations toward action and evaluation" (cited in DiMaggio, 1997, p. 227), but was similarly vague with respect to specific interactions, messages, or utterances. More recently, Thornton, Ocasio, and Lounsbury (2012) have linked institutional logics to schemas and narratives, implicating cognitive processes, but tending to leave out human interaction. Barbour and Lammers (2015) based a notion of physicians' professional identities on the institutional logics perspective, arguing that professional identity is composed of the psychological phenomena of feelings of attachment, belonging, and beliefs particular to an occupation, such as medicine. Each of these efforts to extend and develop the institutional logics perspective illuminates the connections between action, organizations, and institutions, but has not been developed from a specifically communicative point of view.

In order to develop a more communicatively nuanced view of the institutional logics perspective, we must view the idea of logic—nominally, a particular way of thinking about something—itself as communication. Lammers (2011) suggested that institutional logics were carried by *institutional messages*, "collations of thoughts that take on lives independent of senders and recipients" (p. 157). Relatedly, Lammers and Garcia (2009) argued that professions are "characterized by formalized beliefs that specify and emerge from established practices transcending particular workplaces" (p. 358). This idea has been advanced in general terms by Ocasio, Loewenstein, and Nigam (2015). They argued that "specific processes of communication such as coordinating, sensegiving, translating, and theorizing demarcate cognitive categories of understanding, help individuals form collective bonds or relationships around those categories, and link those categories to specific practices and experiences" (cited in Cornelissen, Durand, Fiss, Lammers, & Vaara, 2015, p. 18). Here we similarly suggest that profession is usefully understood communicatively as a set of arguments or propositions about the world. Such arguments may be composed of common rhetorical elements such as claims, grounds, warrants, and backings (Toulmin, Rieke, & Janik, 1979).

In the case of medical professionals, specifically physicians, professional reasoning is characterized by two broad claims: 1) medical knowledge is the province of a community of experts, not a single individual; and 2) non-experts cannot understand or evaluate medical reasoning. Generally it is useful to think of logics as the characteristic ways that a belief, message, or practice is defended. Within each of the realms of communication, however, medical professionals operate from a small number of related arguments. Within the personal realm of communication, physicians' identity is cultivated through the long period of training and socialization that sets one apart from others and cultivates a belief in one's personal authority and responsibility. In the interactional realm, the argument that forms perhaps the core of medical professionalism recognizes that physicians work alongside others in a community of experts, do not give orders to other physicians, and must lead non-experts, including patients. In the organizational realm, the underlying argument is that medical work is unusual and valuable, and cannot be completely understood by management. In the institutional realm, the representatives of the profession advocate for these arguments, and advance the additional argument that the profession exists for, and is indispensable in, the betterment of society.

Within these broad and more realm-specific claims, contradictions are also apparent. Despite the emphasis on a community of experts, most physicians work in a one-to-one relationship with patients, so they deliver their expertise in semi-private circumstances. And even though non-experts are not qualified to judge medical expertise, physicians must gain non-experts' trust and cooperation in order to work and be remunerated. Moreover, probing the contradictions in the arguments offers clues to the tensions and likely alterations in the arguments underlying professional logic. Notwithstanding the contradictions, taken together, we argue, these arguments amount to a professional logic. In the next section we consider how medical professionals use professional logic in reacting to developments in electronic media, also known as eHealth.

Applying the Idea of Professional Logic: Professions and the Advent of eHealth

The ways that health professions confront the advent of communication technologies and internet connectivity offer an opportunity to illustrate how professional logic works in each of the personal, interactional, organizational, and institutional realms of communication (and how these realms overlap). The term "eHealth" first appeared in academic literature in 1999 (Eysenbach, 2001). Over the following 15 years, literature on eHealth has grown substantially. Although eHealth may now be commonly used to denote the use of technology to improve care outcomes, few common definitions have been proposed (Hernandez, 2014). An inspection of these definitions reveals the themes of 'health' and 'technology' as universal. Six sub-themes of "commerce, activities, stakeholders, outcomes, place, and perspectives" are also present across most definitions (Oh, Rizo, Enkin, & Jadad, 2005, Data Synthesis section). From an organizational communication perspective the following definition is used:

> [eHealth is] an emerging field in the intersection of medical informatics, public health, and business, referring to health services and information delivered or enhanced through the Internet and related technologies
> *(Eysenbach, 2001, Introduction section, para. 3)*

The development of eHealth technologies and infrastructure is cited as a primary impetus for change in health care delivery (Wilson & Tulu, 2010). In this development, the logic of market forces is written into the technology infrastructure of health care. Concurrently, an increase in internet access has led to changes in communicative logics for patients and providers (Healthcare Information and Management Systems Society, 2014). Although some commonality exists, these logics are not the same as those traditionally codified by the medical profession. The field of eHealth creates a frontier where the dynamic between technology systems and the traditional profession interact.

Profession and eHealth in the Personal Realm

The personal realm of communication concerns individual-level processes such as socialization and identity formation (see Meyers & Gaillard, this volume). Socialization is an institutional mechanism that establishes identities of the members of a profession. One means by which a profession maintains its integrity is its members' strong identification, or sense of oneness, attachment to, or belief in the precepts of the profession as a social object (Barbour & Lammers, 2015). Aside from the well-recognized principles of the Hippocratic Oath, members of the medical professions also recognize a duty to care that moves beyond self-interest. This bundle of identifications and motivations is intrinsic to a profession, not necessarily the particular organization in which the professional works.

E-professionalism is an area of study focused on the intersection of professional behaviors and social technologies. The use of social technologies among health professionals creates a space where personal identity and professional identity collide. In this space, the professional identity is inherently bound to conservative expression due to ethical guidelines and confidentiality restrictions (Jain, 2009; Aase, 2010). Scanlon (2011) argued that becoming a professional is a lifelong process that constructs an identity through formal education, workplace interactions, and even popular culture in an age of globalization and technologically assisted consumerism.

With changes in the technologies that health professionals encounter in the workplace, educational programs may act as resistance mechanisms to buffer change in an effort to preserve profession (Apker & Eggly, 2004). In this sense, the socialization process may be seen as an evolving communicative logic where practitioners who once worked to acquire and maintain the identity of the profession now actively work to maintain the integrity of the profession through the acceptance or rejection of technological change. This process of challenging the work–identity relationship as a means to enrich the identity of the medical profession is demonstrated empirically as a pattern of identity formation and enrichment (Pratt, Rockmann, & Kaufmann, 2006). Once the identity of profession has been established by the individual, potential threats to this identity may further dichotomize providers into those who feel their profession is threatened by technology and those who feel their profession is enhanced (Abhay Nath, Catherine, & Agarwal, 2012). For example, these mechanisms act to preserve the identity of traditional health professionals, and the use of eHealth technologies has also been found to also enhance the credibility of naturopathic medical practitioners to stakeholders (Walden, 2013).

Profession and eHealth in the Interactional Realm

The interactional realm of communication for professions concerns communication between professionals and their patients. The influence of the eHealth technologies has profoundly altered the communicative experience and demands of the health care professional (Katz & Moyer, 2004; Ball & Lillis, 2001; Klein, 2007). Although uptake of online patient and provider communication has been shown to be positively viewed by those using the technology, health professionals cite a need for additional patient education to ensure continued appropriate use (Katz, Nissan & Moyer, 2004; Kittler et al., 2004). These concerns may indicate a point of friction for professionals attempting to broker the relationship between a new technology and their current professional identity. More than ever, patients enter the offices of providers already having sought information online. Some providers may feel threatened by a new accessibility of information to patients (McMullan, 2006). This change in identity can also be seen in an increasing trend of patient-asserted autonomy and a relative decrease in the control or beneficence once held by health professionals (Gray, 2011).

The professionalism of patient–provider interaction can be characterized by the amount of social distance the provider grants for the enhancement of medical service delivery (Jain, 2009). To help enforce the communicative enactment of profession in e-professionalism, providers are urged to refer to accredited professional guidelines of conduct when engaging through eHealth technologies (Gorrindo, Gorrindo & Groves, 2008). Adhering to a set of professional guidelines is credited as being one way in which the profession can distinguish itself by delivering online health delivery (Miller & Derse, 2002).

Profession and eHealth in the Organizational Realm

The organizational realm concerns the interactions among professionals and other workers. The manner by which interorganizational communication takes place in the eHealth era may have profound implications for the profession. With a shift toward value-based care and adoption of electronic health records, the communicative environment within organizations has changed.

Value-based care can be defined as the practice of "rewarding those who improve patient outcomes and do so at lower costs. The ultimate destination is a more efficient, higher-quality, consumer-focused health care system—one firmly anchored in value" (Ernst & Young, 2014). This change in the logic of care affects providers as the "triple aim" of achieving "improved care, better health for populations, and reduced health care costs," and is sought by health organizations' managements and policy makers (Alper & Grossmann, 2014; Ernst & Young, 2014). In this model providers are positioned as working in opposition to managed care if patient outcomes at comparatively lower costs do not become part of their professional identities.

In an effort to transfer medical information within and across organizational borders, electronic health records (EHRs) are an example of a specific technology that influences the profession. Use of EHR technologies is promoted for improved patient outcomes and greater cost efficacy (Shachak & Reis, 2009). This motivation is however offset by the relatively low adoption rates of EHRs by providers. Providers cite financial, organization and change processes as being the primary barriers to implementation (Boonstra & Broekhuis, 2010). Resistance by physicians and difficulty in achieving uptake of EHR functions that may impact clinical productivity have also been found as a rationale for the refusal to adopt (Ilie, Courtney, & Van Slyke, 2007; Jha et al., 2009).

Profession and eHealth in the Institutional Realm

The institutional realm includes what Finet (2001) called the institutional rhetoric of professions—their groups', associations', and public pronouncements *vis-à-vis*

other organizations in the health care environment such as hospitals, other associations, or governments. Under the Affordable Care Act (ACA) of 2010, the logic
of professional medicine is challenged on several fronts. First, the act encourages
the use of EHRs through penalties to hospitals and medical practices that do not
meaningfully use EHRs, so despite their reluctance physicians in practices large
and small are finding EHRs mandatory and well-established ways of doing work.
Second, the ACA and other acts before it have encouraged the development
of a "medical home" for every patient. The medical home is a model of care
that emphasizes increased patient-centered, integrated access for patients. One
of its principles is that "the personal physician lead[s] a team of individuals at the
practice level who *collectively* take responsibility for the ongoing care of patients"
(Rittenhouse et al., 2011 emphasis added). Moreover, despite its promise, the
use of "eVisits" in facilitating the medical home for patients has proved to be
uneven and problematic (Hickson, Talbert, Thornbury, Perin, & Goodin, 2014).
Ironically the medical home approach was initially supported by primary care
medical specialty societies. However, as a focus on professional logic might lead
us to expect, the idea has not had much uptake in small and medium medical
practices. Rittenhouse and colleagues (2011) found that on average, practices
used just one fifth of the patient-centered medical home processes measured
as part of this study. Third, both the ACA and movements within the health
care community have for a number of years emphasized "evidence-based" care.
The EHR is implicated in evidence-based care because it is linked to computerized decision support systems, which physicians are increasingly encouraged to
use (Romano & Stafford, 2011). Thus far, the hoped-for improvements in care
resulting from computerized, evidence-based decision support systems are not
proven, and physicians' support is mixed. In each of these cases, the professional
logic of medicine is involved, submitting to management rules for recording
clinical work, coordinating care instead of simply providing it on a one-to-one
basis, and relying on a computerized database for clinical decision-making instead
of the physician as expert.

Summary and Conclusions

In this chapter we have argued that profession as a concept has been underdeveloped in health communication literature. To address this gap, we have
reviewed its importance in four realms of communication, outlined common
definitional elements, and discussed how profession may be understood as a
type of institutional logic. We then applied this set of ideas briefly to the case
of the medical profession response to eHealth, outlining how the logic of the
medical profession is challenged by eHealth developments, and describing
briefly how it is reacting. Given the breadth and depth of eHealth developments, only a cursory examination of its impact on the profession was possible
here. There is little question, however, that new technologies are changing the

face of professional work. The physician is more accountable, less independent, and more of a team member.

Considerable work remains to develop the notion of professional logic in communicative terms. We find the general framework of logic-as-communication appealing, but we acknowledge that the question of whether a formal set of communicative acts or forms might properly constitute logic is problematic. Nominations for such forms include but would not be limited to coordinating, sensegiving, translating, theorizing, and framing. As well, formal aspects of arguments (claims, grounds, warrants, and backings), and rhetorical devices such as tropes also may be viewed as characterizing the arguments that constitute logics. In our discussion we more commonly resorted to describing the characteristic way that practices and beliefs in health care are defended as composing the logic of the profession.

We also recognize the continuing tension between the profession as a self-interested social entity and one that serves a clientele, in this case patients. In preserving its independence, autonomy, and control over work, the profession must also change to meet the needs and requirements of a patient community. That patient community has changed via communication technologies we have discussed, but it has also evolved as chronic diseases, requiring more team management, have replaced the acute conditions to which the expert has historically and heroically applied esoteric knowledge and skill.

These observations suggest several issues for communication scholars to investigate. First, what is the relationship between professional workers and their organizational hosts? What characterizes the patterns of communication between management and professional workers? Second, what are the features of inter-professional communication? What makes it particularly effective, satisfying, or problematic? Finally what does professionalism look like to the patient? Is it likely that patients might get what they want in the nature of medical care from unprofessional but well-managed services?

The larger purpose of this chapter is to draw health communication scholars' attention to profession as a relevant topic in its own right. Ignoring the distinction between profession and organization overlooks important aspects of health communication. Regardless of our views of the merits of profession versus those of organization, replacing profession with managed employment relations is likely to deprive health care workers of a valuable source of applied expertise, motivation, and attachment, and imperil the duty to care. Taking account of profession alters our understanding of identification, interaction, employment relations, and institutional change. Physicians' primary identification is not with the organizations in which they work. Their interactions with patients and others are deeply colored by views of authority and legitimacy. Their relationship to organization is symbiotic and never entirely integrated. Profession connects the individual physician with multiple realms of communication that ultimately help us see in part why the health care system is so difficult to change.

DISCUSSION QUESTIONS

1. Consider what *profession* or *professional* means to you by thinking of as many synonyms as possible. What is the larger meaning of the term? What parts of it do we take for granted?
2. Think about what profession means communicatively. Is there any way that you might distinguish professional communication from management communication? Can you distinguish specifically professional communication from just good communication?
3. What is the value of professionalism in health care? What value is added by having a physician as compared to, for example, a vending machine (like a *Redbox* at a grocery store) that dispenses health care?
4. One staple of hospital dramas is conflict between managers and physicians (see the movie *John Q*). Why is that tension common?
5. Professions such as medicine have traditionally been associated with high social status. Has that changed? Why or why not?

Suggested Reading

Apker, J. & Eggly, S. (2004). Communicating professional identity in medical socialization: Considering the ideological discourse of morning report. *Qualitative Health Research, 14*, 411–429.

Eisenberg, E., Baglia, J., & Pynes, J. (2006). Transforming emergency medicine through narrative: Qualitative action research at a community hospital. *Health Communication, 19*, 197–208.

Author Note

The authors gratefully acknowledge Professor Sally Jackson for guidance and support.

References

Aase, S. (2010). Toward e-professionalism: Thinking through the implications of navigating the digital world. *Journal of the American Dietetic Association, 110*, 1442–1449.

Abbott, A. (1988). *The system of professions: An essay on the division of expert labor.* Chicago, IL: University of Chicago Press.

Abhay Nath, M., Catherine, A., & Agarwal, R. (2012). Electronic health records assimilation and physician identity evolution: An identity theory perspective. *Information Systems Research, 23*, 738–760.

Alper, J. & Grossmann, C. (2014). Integrating research and practice: Health system leaders working toward high-value care: Workshop summary. *IOM Routable on Value & Science-Driven Health Care.* Retrieved from: http://books.nap.edu/openbook.php?record_id=18945&page=1.

Apker, J. & Eggly, S. (2004). Communicating professional identity in medical socialization: Considering the ideological discourse of morning report. *Qualitative Health Research, 14*, 411–429.

Apker, J., Mallak, L. A., Applegate, B. A., Gibson, S. C., Ham, J. J., Johnson, N., & Street, R. L., Jr. (2010). Exploring emergency physician-hospitalist handoff interactions: Development and use of the handoff communication assessment. *Annals of Emergency Medicine, 55*, 161–170.

Ball, M. J. & Lillis, J. (2001). E-health: Transforming the physician/patient relationship. *International Journal of Medical Informatics, 61*, 1–10.

Barbour, J. B. & Lammers, J. C. (2015). Measuring professional identity: A review of the literature and a multilevel confirmatory factor analysis of professional identity constructs. *Journal of Professions and Organizations, 2*, 38–60.

Barker, J. R. (1993). Tightening the iron cage: Concertive control in self-managing teams. *Administrative Science Quarterly, 38*, 408–437.

Boltanski, L. & Thevenot, L. (2006). *De la justification*. Paris: Gallimard, 1991. English translation, *On justification*. Princeton: Princeton University Press. Original work published in 1991.

Boonstra, A. & Broekhuis, M. (2010). Barriers to the acceptance of electronic medical records by physicians from systematic review to taxonomy and interventions. *BMC Health Services Research, 10*, 231.

Brashers, D. E. (2001). Communication and uncertainty management. *Journal of Communication, 51*, 477–497.

Carr-Saunders, A. M. (1966). Professionalization in the historical perspective. In H. M. Vollmer & D. L. Mills (Eds.), *Professionalization* (pp. 2–9). Englewood Cliffs, NJ: Prentice Hall.

Cheney, G. & Ashcraft, K. L. (2007). Considering "the professional" in communication studies: Implications for theory and research within and beyond the boundaries of organizational communication. *Communication Theory, 17*, 146–175.

Cornelissen, J. P., Durand, R., Fiss, P., Lammers, J. C., & Vaara, E. (2015). Putting communication front and center in institutional theory and analysis. *Academy of Management Review, 4*, 10–27.

DiMaggio, P. (1997). Culture and cognition. *Annual Review of Sociology, 23*, 263–87.

Dugdale, L. S., Siegler, M., & Rubin, D. T. (2008). Medical professionalism and the doctor-patient relationship. *Perspectives in Biology and Medicine, 51*, 547–553.

Durkheim, E. (1996). *Professional ethics and civic morals*. London: Routledge.

Eisenberg, E., Baglia, J., & Pynes, J. (2006). Transforming emergency medicine through narrative: Qualitative action research at a community hospital. *Health Communication, 19*, 197–208.

Ellingson, L. (2011). The Poetics of Professionalism among Dialysis Technicians. *Health Communication, 26*, 1–12.

Ernst & Young (2014). *Health Care Industry Report 2014: New horizons-Voyage to value.* (Ernst & Young Publication). Retrieved from: http://www.ey.com/Publication/vwLUAssets/ey-new-horizons-health-care-industry-report-2014/$FILE/ey-new-horizons-health-care-industry-report-2014.pdf.

Evetts, J. (1999). Professionalization and professionalism: Issues for interprofessional care. *Journal of Interprofessional Care, 13*, 119–28.

Eysenbach, G. (2001). What is e-health? *Journal of Medical Internet Research, 3*(2), e20.

Faraj, S. A. & Xiao, Y. (2006). Coordination in fast-response organizations. *Management Science, 52*, 1155–1169.

Finet, D. (2001). Sociopolitical environments and issues. In F. M. Jablin & L. Putnam (Eds.), *The new handbook of organizational communication: Advances in theory, research, and methods* (pp. 270–290). Thousand Oaks, CA: SAGE.

Freidson, E. (1970). *Profession of medicine: A study of the sociology of applied knowledge.* New York: Harper and Row.

Freidson, E. (1986). *Professional powers: A study in the institutionalization of formal knowledge.* Chicago, IL: University of Chicago Press.

Freidson, E. (2001). *Professionalism: The third logic.* Chicago, IL: University of Chicago Press.

Friedland, R. & Alford, R. (1991). Bringing society back in: Symbols, practices, and institutional contradictions. In W. W. Powell & P. J. DiMaggio (Eds.), *The new institutionalism in organizational analysis* (pp. 232–266). Chicago, IL: University of Chicago Press.

Gorrindo, T., Gorrindo, P., & Groves, J. (2008). Intersection of online social networking with medical professionalism: Can medicine police the Facebook boom? *JGIM: Journal of General Internal Medicine, 23,* 2155.

Gray, J. (2011). From "directing them" to "it's up to them": The physician's perceived professional role in the physician-patient relationship. *Journal of Communication in Healthcare, 4,* 280–287.

Hafferty, F. W. & Castellani, B. (2010). Two cultures: Two ships: The rise of a professionalism movement within modern medicine and medical sociology's disappearance from the professionalism debate. In B. A. Pescosolido, J. Martin, J. McLeod, & A. Rogers (Eds.), *Handbook of the sociology of health, illness, and healing: A blueprint for the 21st Century* (pp. 201–220). New York: Springer.

Hall, P. (2005). Interprofessional teamwork: Professional cultures as barriers. *Journal of Interprofessional Care, 19* (Suppl. 1), 188–196.

Harter, L. M. & Krone, K. J. (2001). Exploring the identities of future physicians: Toward an understanding of the ideological socialization of osteopathic medical students. *Southern Journal of Communication, 67,* 66–84.

Healthcare Information and Management Systems Society (2014). *The state of patient engagement and health IT.* (HIMSS Publication). Retrieved from: http://himss.files. cms-plus.com/FileDownloads/The%20State%20of%20Patient%20Engagement%20 and%20Health%20IT%20%28HIMSS%29.pdf.

Hernandez, L. M. (2014). Health Literacy, eHealth, and Communication: Putting the Consumer First: Workshop Summary. *Roundtable on Health Literacy: Board on Population Health and Public Health Practice-Institute of Medicine of the National Academies.* Retrieved from: http://www.nap.edu/openbook.php?record_id=12474&page=R1.

Hickson, R., Talbert, J., Thornbury, W. C., Perin, N. R., & Goodin A. J. (2014). Online medical care: The current state of "eVisits" in acute primary care delivery telemedicine and e-Health. *Telemedicine and eHealth.* Published online ahead of print December 4, 2014. Doi:10.1089/tmj.2014.0022.

Ilie, V., Courtney, J. F., & Van Slyke, C. (2007). *Paper versus electronic: Challenges associated with physicians' usage of electronic medical records.* Proceedings of the 40th Hawaii International Conference on System Sciences. Waikoloa, HI: IEEE Computer Society.

Jain, S. H. (2009). Practicing medicine in the age of Facebook. *New England Journal of Medicine, 361,* 649–651.

Jha, A. K., DesRoches, C. M., Campbell, E. G., Donelan, K., Rao, S. R., Ferris, T. G., . . . & Blumenthal, D. (2009). Use of electronic health records in US hospitals. *New England Journal of Medicine, 360,* 1628–1638.

Katz, S. J. & Moyer, C. A. (2004). The emerging role of online communication between patients and their providers. *JGIM: Journal of General Internal Medicine, 19,* 978–983.

Katz, S. J., Nissan, N., & Moyer, C. A. (2004). Crossing the digital divide: Evaluating online communication between patients and their providers. *American Journal of Managed Care, 10,* 593–598.

Kittler, A. F., Wald, J. S., Volk, L. A., Pizziferri, L. L., Jagannath, Y. Y., Harris, C. C., & . . . Bates, D. W. (2004). The role of primary care non-physician clinic staff in e-mail communication with patients. *International Journal of Medical Informatics, 73*, 333–340.

Klein, R. (2007). An empirical examination of patient-physician portal acceptance. *European Journal of Information Systems, 16*, 751–760.

Kvarnström, S. (2008). Difficulties in collaboration: A critical incident study of interprofessional healthcare teamwork. *Journal of Interprofessional Care, 22*, 191–203.

Lambert, B., Street, R. L., Jr., Cegala, D. J., Smith, D. H., Kurtz, S., & Schofield, T. (1997). Provider-patient communication, patient-centered care, and the mangle of practice. *Health Communication, 9*, 27–44.

Lammers, J. C. (2011). How institutions communicate: Institutional messages, institutional logics, and organizational communication. *Management Communication Quarterly, 25*, 154–182.

Lammers, J. C. & Barbour, J. B. (2006). An institutional theory of organizational communication. *Communication Theory, 16*, 356–377.

Lammers, J. C. & Barbour, J. B. (2009). Exploring the institutional context of physicians' work: Professional and organizational differences in physician satisfaction. In D. Goldsmith & D. Brashers (Eds.). *Managing health and illness: Communication, relationships, and identity* (pp. 91–112). Mahwah, NJ: Erlbaum.

Lammers, J. C. & Garcia, M. (2009). Exploring the concept of 'profession' for organizational communication research: Institutional influences in a veterinary organization. *Management Communication Quarterly, 22*, 357–384.

Landman, M. P., Shelton, J., Kauffmann, R. M., & Dattilo, J. B. (2010). Guidelines for maintaining a professional compass in the era of social networking. *Journal of Surgical Education, 67*, 381–386.

Leicht, K. & Fennel, M. (2001). *Professional work: A sociological approach.* Malden, MA: Blackwell.

Lemire, M., Sicotte, C., & Paré, G. (2008). Internet use and the logics of personal empowerment in health. *Health Policy, 88*, 130–140.

Lowrey, W. & Anderson, W. B. (2006). The impact of internet use on the public perception of physicians: A perspective from the sociology of professions literature. *Health Communication, 19*, 125–131.

Maheu, M. M., Pulier, M. L., Wilhelm, F. H., McMenamin, J.P., Brown-Connolly, N. E. (2005). *The mental health professional and the new technologies: A handbook for practice today.* Mahwah, NJ: Erlbaum.

McKinlay, J. B. & Arches, J. (1985). Towards the proletarianization of physicians. *International Journal of Health Services, 15*, 161–195.

McMullan, M. (2006). Patients using the Internet to obtain health information: How this affects the patient–health professional relationship. *Patient Education and Counseling, 63*, 24–28.

Miller, T. E. & Derse, A. R. (2002). Between strangers: The practice of medicine online. *Health Affairs, 21*, 168–179.

Ocasio, W., Loewenstein, J., & Nigam, A. 2015. How streams of communication reproduce and change institutional logics: The role of categories. *Academy of Management Review, 40*, 28–48.

Oh, H., Rizo, C., Enkin, M., & Jadad, A. (2005). What is eHealth (3): A systematic review of published definitions. *Journal of Medical Internet Research, 7*, N.PAG.

Parsons, T. (1939). The professions and social structure. *Social Forces, 17*, 457–467.

Parsons, T. (1963). Social change and medical organization in the United States: A sociological perspective. *Annals of the American Academy of Political and Social Science, 346,* 21–33.

Patterson, S. & Patterson, K. (2010). (Re)Storying the profession of dentistry. *Health Communication, 25,* 383–385.

Pratt, M. G., Rockmann, K. W., & Kaufmann, J. B. (2006). Constructing professional identity: The role of work and identity learning cycles in the customization of identity among medical residents. *Academy of Management Journal, 49,* 235–262.

Rittenhouse, D. R., Casalino, L. P., Shortell, S. M., McClellan, S. R., Gillies, R. R., Alexander, J., A., & Drum, M. L. (2011). Small and medium-size physician practices use few patient-centered medical home processes. *Health Affairs, 30,* 1–10.

Romano, M. J. & Stafford, R. S. (2011). Electronic health records and clinical decision support systems impact on national ambulatory care quality. *Archives of Internal Medicine, 171,* 897–903.

Scanlon, L. (Ed.) (2011). *"Becoming" a professional: An interdisciplinary study of professional learning.* Dordrecht, Netherlands: Springer.

Scott, W. R. (1965). Reactions to supervision in a heteronomous professional organization. *Administrative Science Quarterly, 10,* 65–81.

Scott, W. R. (2008). Lords of the dance: Professionals as institutional agents. *Organization Studies, 29,* 219–238.

Scott, W. R., Ruef, M., Mendel, M. and Caronna, G. (2000). *Institutional change and healthcare organizations: From professional dominance to managed care.* Chicago, IL: University of Chicago Press.

Shachak, A. & Reis, S. (2009). The impact of electronic medical records on patient–doctor communication during consultation: A narrative literature review. *Journal of Evaluation in Clinical Practice, 15,* 641–649.

Sharf, B. F. (1993). Reading the vital signs: Research in health care communication. *Communication Monographs, 60,* 35–41.

Sharf, B. F. & Street, R. L., Jr. (1997). The patient as a central construct: Shifting the emphasis. *Health Communication, 9,* 1–12.

Stern, D. T. (Ed.). (2006). *Measuring medical professionalism.* New York: Oxford University Press.

Suddaby, R. & Viale, T. (2011). Professionals and field-level change: Institutional work and the professional project. *Current Sociology, 59,* 423–442.

Thompson, T., Dorsey, A., Miller, K., & Parrot, R. (Eds.) (2003). *Handbook of health communication.* Mahwah, NJ: Lawrence Erlbaum Associates.

Thompson, T. L., Parrott, R., & Nussbaum, J. F. (2011). *The Routledge handbook of health communication (Routledge Communication Series).* Routledge: New York.

Thornton, P. (2004). *Markets from culture: Institutional logics and organizational decisions in higher education publishing.* Stanford, CA: Stanford University Press.

Thornton, P. H. & Ocasio, W. (2008). Institutional logics. In R. Greenwood, C. Oliver, R. Suddaby, & K. Sahlin-Andersson (Eds.), *The handbook of organizational institutionalism* (pp. 99–129). Thousand Oaks, CA: Sage.

Thornton, P. H., Ocasio, W., & Lounsbury, M. (2012). *The institutional logics perspective: A new approach to culture, structure and process.* Oxford: Oxford University Press.

Toulmin, S. E., Rieke, R., & Janik, A. (1979). *An introduction to reasoning.* New York: Macmillan.

van den Broek, J. J. C., Boselie, J. P. P. E. F., & Paauwe, J. (2014). Multiple institutional logics in health care: Productive ward: 'Releasing time to care.' *Public Management Review, 16,* 1–20.

Walden, J. (2013). A medical profession in transition: Exploring naturopathic physician blogging behaviors. *Health Communication, 28,* 237–247.

Weber, M. (1947). *The theory of social and economic organization.* (A. M. Henderson & T. Parsons, Trans.). London: Collier Macmillan Publishers.

Wilson, E. V. & Tulu, B. (2010). The rise of a health-IT academic focus. *Communications of the ACM, 53,* 147–150.

3

ORGANIZATIONAL ENTRY, SOCIALIZATION, AND ASSIMILATION IN HEALTH CARE ORGANIZATIONS

Karen K. Myers and Bernadette M. Gailliard

Health care workers have long dealt with illness and death while also serving the seemingly endless physical and emotional needs of patients and their loved ones. Today's health care workers also face added challenges due to the changing health care environment, including rapidly changing and increasingly complex technology, an increasingly litigious society, and an aging population. These changes now require most health care workers to attain more advanced education and training to become competent health care professionals (Ares, 2014). As part of that training, physicians and other medical personnel adopt the traditional voice of medical professionalism to distance themselves from patients and assert their power in the social hierarchy (MacLeod, 2011). Then, when they join organizations, employers also must socialize workers of all types—from physicians and nurses to receptionists and morgue workers— to the particulars of the organization's facilities, people, procedures, and rules. This socialization enables them to perform their duties, coordinate with coworkers and, hopefully, develop attachment to the organization. Thus, management socializes and trains workers to develop their job competencies and also facilitates their identities as organizational members.

Through organizational socialization and assimilation individuals are introduced and trained to the various elements of organizations, workgroups, and jobs (Jablin, 1987; Jablin & Sias, 2001; Kramer, 2010). Over the years and across multiple disciplines, scholars have referred to these processes using various terms. In this chapter, we adopt the terminology and definitions used by Jablin, whom many consider the patriarch of this line of research in the field of communication. Thus, *organizational socialization* (OS) includes efforts on behalf of the organization and newcomers themselves to familiarize the newcomer with the organization, coworkers, tasks, and rules (Jablin, 1987). He described *organizational assimilation* (OA) as the process of individuals becoming integrated into an organization (Jablin, 2001). Both OS and OA are foundational in organizational research providing practical guidance to management to acculturate new members and to foster their development as productive organizational members. This research can also assist organizational newcomers themselves to help them better understand their own and their colleagues' integration and membership experiences. Importantly, while many may consider OS and OA to include only the period immediately following organizational entry, learning about the organization and coworkers and adapting to one's role are long term, often occurring until organizational exit (Davis & Myers, 2012; Kramer, 2010).

Research on newcomers' organizational entry has revealed many communicative behaviors and other activities related to processes of OA (Gailliard, Myers, & Seibold, 2010; Myers & Oetzel, 2003), content areas of OS (Chao, O'Leary-Kelly, Wolf, Klein, & Gardner, 1994), the effect of realistic job previews (Wanous, 1992; Wanous, Poland, Premack, & Davis, 1992), the importance of organizational and job fit (Kim, Cable, & Kim, 2005), newcomer information seeking (V. Miller & Jablin, 1991), and the memorable messages newcomers receive that affect settling into the organization (Knapp, Stohl, & Reardon, 1981; Stohl, 1986).

We draw on social identity theory (SIT) to examine and discuss issues of OS and OA. According to SIT, organizational membership and the perceptions individuals have about themselves and the perceptions others have about them, strongly affect the individual's personal and social identity (Ashforth & Mael, 1989). An individual's *identity* plays an important role in members' receptiveness to socialization and one's motivation and ability to assimilate (Ashforth, 2001; Myers, 2005). Closely linked to an individual's identity is organizational identification (Gibson & Papa, 2000). Organizational identification describes the link between one's organizational membership and his or her global identity (Cheney, 1991; Sluss & Ashforth, 2007).

OS and OA in health care contexts are different than in many other industries. Context affects the nature and goals of organizational roles; hierarchical structures including working relationships, contact and relationships with clients, and physical locations; and has a strong affect on newcomers' transitions. Health care organizations share some commonalities (see Lammers and Lambert, this volume, for a discussion of institutional processes that lead to these similarities). One important and overriding contextual factor is that health care organizations, such as medical centers, surgical centers, and even physicians' offices, are high reliability organizations (HROs). Health care workers in HROs must perform with high efficiency, in stressful situations for the patients and their families, all the while avoiding accidents or oversights that can have major negative consequences for patients.

In this chapter, we examine the unique nature of OS and OA in health care organizations (see Figure 3.1 for a visual representation). First, we introduce

Vocational Anticipatory Socialization	Organizational Entry and Assimilation	Effects on Personal and Professional Identity

• Communication from family, educators, peers, media, and part-time jobs influence interest in (and perceptions of) particular careers
 	
• VAS messages provide details about potential careers and encourage personal fulfillment
 	
• Medical education and training communicates the expectations of the profession (emphasizing specialization)
 	
• Individuals begin to develop identities as future medical professionals
	• Organizational assimilation processes:
	  ○ Getting to know coworkers
	  ○ Acculturation
	  ○ Feeling recognized
	
	• Workgroups and teams train new members on task-related procedures and communication systems
	
	• Organizational routines (such as the morning report, rounds, the weekly morbidity and mortality conference, etc.) establish role expectations across multiple situations
	
	• Norms for work impact relationship development among colleagues and patients (e.g., use of eHealth systems to maintain patient information, conventions for passing information between shifts)
		• Health care professionals develop professional identity (and expectations) through VAS messages as well as medical education and training
		
		• Employees are more likely to identify with medical facilities and leaders who reflect their personal beliefs and values
		
		• Workers often experience role conflict when their roles in patient care, particularly in team-based environments, do not align with professional expectations
		
		• Specialized training and weak interpersonal relationships can weaken interprofessional identity and collaboration
		
		• Health care workers learn to maintain a professional distance and to portray particular emotions for the benefit of patients and/or the organization

FIGURE 3.1   Visual Representation of Organizational Socialization and Assimilation.

organizational identity and identification and their tie to OA. Second, we discuss vocational anticipatory socialization (VAS) that includes communication and other exposure generating interest in particular careers and causes individuals to begin to develop related professional identities. VAS may be especially significant for future health care workers who often must enter science-intensive educational tracks before they enter post-secondary school. In addition, during medical training, they are exposed to *the hidden curriculum* which instills the values, norms and traditions of the medical profession (Hafferty & Franks, 1994). Third, we discuss entry and adjustment into health care organizations and focus our attention on three aspects of OA—getting to know coworkers, acculturating, and feeling recognized. We link these processes to professional and personal identities and the dynamic environment of health care organizations. We conclude the chapter with issues and questions that may be examined in future research.

Professional Identity and Organizational Identification

Individuals assimilate into organizational roles influenced by their previous and simultaneous physical, psychological, work, and social identities such that individuals strive to align their past, present, and future identities to avoid internal and external role conflict (Alvesson, Ashcraft, & Thomas, 2008). Health care workers who have undergone extensive training to acquire knowledge and skills also learn about and begin to adopt attitudes and behaviors of the profession's identity (Zorn & Gregory, 2005). However, at times professional identity conflicts with organizational roles (Johnson, Morgeson, Ilgen, Meyer, & Lloyd, 2006) as seen when individuals enter into organizations ready to occupy *occupational* roles that may not align with *organizational* roles. For example, in many health care situations members must perform their duties in interdependent teams comprised of individuals who occupy a variety of occupations and backgrounds (see Real and Poole, as well as Reimer, Russell, and Roland, this volume, for further discussion of team processes). Some may feel that their extensive education and role as a physician or other medical professional entitles them to autonomous or leadership roles (see also Lammers and Proulx, this volume). In fact, often their medical training emphasizes the importance of their dominating conversations to reinforce their authority (Apker & Eggly, 2004). Thus, they may resist the interdependency that goes along with teamwork. Also, as individuals rhetorically position themselves, and others position them, it affects the identity and effective role they assume in their organization and workgroup (Davies & Harre, 1990; Harter & Krone, 2001).

Many have argued that traditional training—focused only on the duties and perspectives of one profession, *uni-professional socialization*—is flawed because it is limited to imparting the knowledge and skills of a particular profession with little regard for others providing patient care (Khalili, Orchard, Spence Laschinger, & Farah, 2013; Reeves, Perrier, Goldman, Freeth, & Zwarenstein, 2013; World Health Organization, 2010). Critics contend that in contemporary health care, medical personnel rarely work independently and, instead, perform their duties in conjunction with medical workers in a variety of roles. Therefore, socialization should provide interprofessional training in which students learn about how their knowledge and skills can be used to better collaborate with other health care professionals creating a more holistic approach to patient care. Another implication is that while uni-professional socialization strengthens professional identity and in-group relationships, it also creates barriers between the students and those in other medical professions. In interprofessional socialization, students are brought together with medical workers from a variety of professions to learn about each other's roles, thereby increasing understanding and trust between professions (Khalili et al., 2013). Although interprofessional training may lessen strong intra-group professional identity, this may strengthen identification with their employer.

Membership in organizations is linked to organizational identification such that the success of OS is often tied to newcomers' feelings of identification toward the organization (Bullis & Bach, 1989; Klein & Weaver, 2000). According to Scott and Myers (2010), OA is a membership negotiation process between newcomers, organizational incumbents, and the organization in which organizational identification is a medium in which the negotiation occurs "because it aids attempts to resolve tensions between individual needs for identity and collective organizational interests" (p. 95). While organizational identification has direct effects on their desire to assimilate, for many health care roles, *occupational* or *professional identities* are foundational and frequently prioritized. In the next section, we introduce vocational anticipatory socialization (VAS), a process through which individuals destined for careers in health care often begin to develop professional identities.

Vocational Anticipatory Socialization: Learning About and Adopting a Professional Identity

Long before health care workers begin their careers, they are subject to the effects of VAS. In general, VAS includes communication from family, educators, peers, media, and part-time jobs that can influence adolescents' interest in particular careers (Jablin, 1985; Vangelisti, 1988) and "explains how individuals learn about and develop interests in educational and eventual career pursuits" (Myers, Jahn, Gailliard, & Stoltzfus, 2011, p. 88). Adolescents report two types of messages that affect their career interests—messages that provide details about particular careers and messages that encourage adolescents to pursue careers that will give personal fulfillment (Jahn & Myers, 2014). VAS has particular implications for science, technology, engineering, and mathematics (STEM) industries— including health care fields—that have experienced labor shortages, and especially low numbers of women and ethnic minorities. It is estimated that 78% of college students majoring in STEM areas made the choice to study STEM in high school or earlier, and one in five (21%) decided to enter STEM-based studies in middle school or earlier (Harris Interactive, 2011). Their early decisions may be necessary given the early and extensive educational requirements for many medical professionals. Because of crucial labor shortages and lack of diversity in the STEM workforce, numerous educational efforts have aimed to attract females and ethnic minorities to STEM-based academic programs and careers. These socialization efforts appear to have some effects. As of 2012, women make up nearly half of all students graduating from medical schools compared to only 9.2% in 1970 (Association of American Medical Colleges, 2014).

In addition to educating and training future medical professionals about technical aspects of their roles, medical schools simultaneously introduce the normative attitudes and behaviors of the profession (Hafferty & Franks, 1994; Harter & Krone, 2001; Zorn & Gregory, 2005). For example, medical students learn about the human body and practice performing medical techniques with cadavers, treating the bodies not as deceased individuals, but as objects of study (Hafferty, 1988). This training prepares them for encounters with patients in which they must mentally and discursively distance themselves to retain control and objectivity (Geist & Dreyer, 1993). Similarly, more advanced medical students often are trained by means of problem-based learning (PBL) in which students read patient cases and attempt to diagnose or problem-solve the issue. PBL is widely acclaimed as an effective approach to give students opportunities to independently scrutinize patient symptoms towards a diagnosis (Wood, 2003). However, critics argue that the written cases used in PBL take an overly *scientific*, rather than a *patient-centered* approach by focusing on *disease* rather than *illness*, and on *detecting* the disease rather than *curing* the patient (MacLeod, 2011).

These and other activities in medical school allow students to anticipate entering the profession and begin to adopt the associated identity (Myers, 2005). This may be useful because the medical professional identity can motivate medical students to endure through extensive and difficult training, solidifying their commitment toward achieving their goals (Jahn & Myers, 2014). However, adopting a prestigious professional identity also may later inhibit their ability to assimilate into some organizations when they prioritize the values they perceive are associated with the profession above those prioritized by their organization (Beyer & Hannah, 2002). This topic will be explored in the next section as we discuss health care workers' organizational entry.

Organizational Encounter: Learning About the Organization's Culture, People and Procedures

Once newcomers enter the organization, management's primary objectives are to introduce newcomers to the organization and facilitate their acquiring task knowledge and skills (see Canary, this volume, for a discussion on organizational knowledge processes). Gailliard et al. (2010) identified seven processes that newcomers experience as they assimilate. Here, we discuss OA by health care workers framed by three of those processes that are directly involved in adopting and managing one's professional identity: becoming familiar with coworkers, acculturation, and recognition. Because getting to know coworkers is an important part of acculturating into organizations, we discuss these assimilation processes in unison.

Getting to Know Coworkers and Acculturation

Getting to know coworkers is foundational for OA. Myers and Oetzel (2003) described this aspect of OA as becoming comfortable interacting with coworkers in dyads or in meetings, feeling supportive of one another, and generally feeling a part of the community. Getting to know coworkers improves functioning, in part, because it can improve communication between workers facilitating the exchange of information—crucial in health care settings and especially health care teams (Sias, 2005). Newcomers must also acculturate, which involves learning about how to function in the organization's culture (Gailliard et al., 2010; Myers & Oetzel, 2003). Learning about the organizational culture—the explicit and implied values and beliefs communicated through norms, rituals, language, stories, and artifacts (Pacanowsky & O'Donnell-Trujillo, 1983)—helps members to know what are and are not acceptable behaviors in the organization. Organizational form and structure have a strong effect on organizational culture and this is especially true in the health care industry in which workers can be employed in a wide range of organizations including inner-city medical centers to suburban surgical centers to small-town private practice physicians' offices.

Larger medical centers or hospitals feature a multitude of departments, centers, and specialties each with their own cultures affecting the realm of tasks, workers' interactions with coworkers and patients, and identification with the medical center and its leaders. Although health care workers are socialized and to some extent, assimilated into the larger organization, they receive a great deal of their socialization from their immediate department or workgroup (Moreland & Levine, 2001). Those closest to them—fellow workgroup members—introduce newcomers to the environment, often provide hands-on training, and draw them into productive working relationships (Anderson, Riddle, & Martin, 1999). This localized source is important because the various workgroups of the organization may have differing norms, values, and objectives. Each workgroup's membership, goals, or context create a unique set of demands for learning and for adjustment and may influence member assimilation more than the broader socialization of the organization (Cini, Moreland, & Levine, 1993; Hennessy & West, 1999). The influence of workgroups on newcomer assimilation may be particularly strong in *interdependent* teams. In health care, team members must learn to coordinate and rely on each other in order to perform their jobs, all the while taking precautions to avoid accidents and deliver quality care (Riddle, Anderson, & Martin, 2000). Although these have always been foundational objectives, they may be even more crucial to the long-term health of the organization in the current litigious environment.

In addition to size and type of facility, other factors contribute to and shape the culture of a medical setting, including profit or nonprofit status, religious or non-religious missions, and the surrounding community. These factors can have greater or lesser effects depending on the workers' identification with the organization. For example, OA may be facilitated when an individual supports the religious mission of his employer because it fits within his social identity. Thus, newcomers are eager to become contributing members when they believe membership in the organization positively affirms their personal and professional identity.

Recognition and Teamwork

Recognition is another aspect of OA with implications for medical workers and their organizational and professional identities. According to Gailliard et al. (2010, p. 556), "being recognized as valuable and feeling one's work is important to the organization" is a foundational aspect of OA. The link to social identity is apparent—when individuals feel that they are important contributors and recognized by supervisors and coworkers they are inclined to become more invested and more identified with the organization and workgroups. Because they are in professions dedicated to saving lives and the well-being of others, health care workers are apt to take pride in their professional identities (Ashcraft, 2007; Lammers & Garcia, 2009).

When individuals are newcomers, especially as part of health care teams, the recognition they need to feel assimilated can be particularly difficult to attain. Their perceptions about the recognition they should receive in their roles may not mesh with those of their teammates. For example, consider a new interning physician who is part of a health care team comprised of other physicians, nurses, and technicians. As a physician, she may be disinclined to see other members of a health care team whose education levels may be considerably lower than her own, as equal contributors. She may be unwilling to take their advice and may attempt to rhetorically position herself above others. Teammates may see her as overly authoritarian and be unwilling to cooperate with her directives. Identity issues also can emerge with team members who are more senior and are unwilling to comply with the wishes of a younger colleague. Team members who are not accustomed to taking orders from women also may reject her attempts at leadership (see Barbour, Gill, and Dean, this volume, for discussion of gender in health care organizations).

Identity issues can also affect receptivity to OS. Consider, for example, a new registered nurse who enters into his first hospital setting. He may be unreceptive to the orientation sessions designed to introduce general hospital policies. He may be more concerned about applying and learning his trade than following hospital policies that he may perceive are focused on profitability. Thus, in order to assimilate into his organization, he may need to better identify with the needs and objectives of the hospital. At first he may feel as though he is not performing as a registered nurse should, but, eventually, he may reconcile his nurse and organizational member identities so that his roles are not in conflict.

Conversely, some health care workers have social identities that lack prestige. Medical workers who perform tasks such as bathing patients, transporting hazardous materials, or handling bodies in the morgue may even be considered dirty workers. *Dirty workers* are individuals who perform work that many might consider dirty or disgusting because it is either physically, socially, or morally tainted (Ashforth & Kreiner, 1999). This does not mean that their work is not considered important or valuable; often the opposite is true. Few would discount the value of orderlies who change bed linen and clean bedpans. However, many dirty workers claim that coworkers may view them as *dirty* or somehow tainted. Although colleagues value their work, they may be less inclined to befriend them or facilitate their social inclusion.

Learning to Cope With Stress and Emotions

Working in HROs such as hospitals, surgical centers, or other medical facilities demands that workers perform their tasks quickly and effectively, and are attentive to the accuracy of their work and to system anomalies that can affect the well-being of their patients (Perrow, 1984; Roberts, 1990). This is especially relevant for newcomers who must perform their work reliably from day one. Errors are not only embarrassing, but they can invite litigation and even be deadly for patients under their care. Through socialization, newcomers learn that one means of reducing accidents is through procedures that ensure mindfulness (C. W. Scott & Myers, 2005). Members must double-check work through the use of checklists, questions to patients, and redundancy (Langer, 1989). Performing work under these conditions can be taxing for workers because constantly ensuring high standards of performance can be exhausting, and checking and rechecking oneself and coworkers can be mind-numbing (Langer, 1989).

Many health care workers deal with the stress of caring for seriously ill or injured patients and also dealing with their families. In doing so, they must perform *emotional labor* (Hochschild, 1983) by managing their emotions according to the expectations of their employer, patients, and others in their profession (Hafferty, 1988; Smith & Kleinman, 1989), or at times they may also be required to perform double face emotion management (C. W. Scott & Myers, 2005; Tracy & Tracy, 1998) in which workers manage their own emotions in order to manage the emotions of patients or family members. Even those workers who do not have direct contact with patients interact with colleagues who are subject to these pressures, thus the communication may be rushed or strained. Other working conditions also can make their OA more difficult. Because medical centers must operate around the clock, they may be required to continually or at least occasionally adjust their shift times. This can mean that individuals often work with rotating coworkers and are not afforded the ability to develop trust and interdependent working relationships with teammates (Myers & McPhee, 2006).

In another context, physicians or nurses who join private practices or other small medical offices often have more traditional schedules, making aspects of the environment more predictable. The medical personnel are more apt to see patients in non-crisis situations, making the environment less frantic and chaotic. Personnel also are more likely to interact with patients over time, affording them the opportunity to establish relationships, and interactions can be more personable and enduring. However, entry into private practices and other small offices can mean dealing with demanding patients who may frequently access medical care, seemingly mundane medical situations can quickly escalate into larger medical emergencies, and, like in many organizations, working with the same colleagues day in and day out, especially when relations between coworkers are strained, can tax the emotions of organizational members.

Workers who give daily empathy and instrumental support to distressed patients can experience considerable stress and burnout (K. Miller, Stiff, & Ellis, 1988; Morgan & Krone, 2001). However, the long-term negative impact is related to how the workers manage their emotional empathy. Health care workers who have empathetic concern for clients are well suited to be communicatively responsive. Conversely, health care workers who are so concerned with patients *that they themselves experience their patients' feelings* are less capable of effective communicative response (K. Miller et al., 1988). Thus, developing emotions such that one actually feels the emotions of another—emotional contagion—makes him or her less capable of lending support and more prone to burnout (Maslach, 1982). With this in mind, to be most beneficial, OS must teach workers how to effectively manage their emotions in order to be effective.

As health care organizations become more reliant on technology, this can provide another potential source of stress. Health care is a highly collaborative field that depends on individuals with strong professional identities and long-established hierarchical relationships to engage in routinized practices that reify these structures. Technology becomes a stressor particularly when it is integrated into established workflows and routines (Goh, Mein Gao, & Agarwal, 2011). Not only does it take time to learn the new systems, but employees also have to rebuild and reconfigure routines to adapt to the technology. This is particularly stressful in fast-paced and unpredictable environments such as emergency departments and trauma units. With more technology, organizations also risk having weaker interpersonal connections among colleagues (Flanagin & Waldeck, 2004). As interactions occur less in face-to-face formats and more information is relayed through eHealth systems, it can inhibit coworker relationships that are necessary for working in team atmospheres.

On the other hand, eHealth systems can potentially relieve stress as well. Technology can improve the accuracy and efficiency of information processing. It keeps much of a patient's information in a central location that is easily accessible by multiple staff members who may be providing services. This makes it much easier to coordinate care. Once new routines become normalized, they often are more efficient as well. For example, carts on wheels allow attending physicians and residents to have simultaneous access to a patient's medical information, thus facilitating the education of newer physicians in the OS process without having to go through longer, more redundant information-sharing routines while at the patient's bedside. So, an important part of OS for health care organizations is also to help newcomers understand the benefits and costs of an increasingly technological workplace and to ensure that all members are adequately trained on the eHealth systems while also maintaining strong coworker relationships.

Future Research

As health care organizations seek to intake greater numbers of professionals to meet the growing demand for health care, it will be important for organizational leaders to have a better understanding of the complexities involved in the socialization and assimilation processes. In this chapter, we discussed implications that emerge from the extant literature on OS and OA. However, more research and theorizing should be done regarding OS and OA in the unique context of health care organizations. We conclude with some directions for future research in this area to help expand theory and influence organizational practices.

From a theoretical perspective, scholars first need to understand how the health care context is evolving. Fewer services are being provided in hospitals, patient stays are being shortened, and medical resources and staffing are being consolidated (Apker, 2001; Kaboli et al., 2012). Meanwhile, as individuals live longer, the population is getting older and patients are requiring more varied types of medical resources from a shrinking number of providers. Some statistics suggest that many health professions will not be able to sustain the increased demand for health care services by the year 2020 (CDC, 2004). Thus, an initial empirical question is why are young adults not pursuing these health professions? What about the Millennial generation makes them not want to pursue careers that have the appeal of high prestige and lucrative salaries? Research in VAS may provide some insights and even remedies. According to VAS research, adolescents receive messages that encourage and even discourage their pursuit of STEM careers (Myers et al., 2011). Future studies could involve current health care workers and explore messages that may have had a significant positive influence on their choice to enter their profession. However, negative messages are also of consequence. Do health care workers recall receiving messages that might have dissuaded them from these careers? Were there negative perceptions about the work that is involved in being a health care professional? Are there ways of helping youth understand the tremendous value and intrinsic rewards associated with health care professions? Bunderson and Thompson (2009) reported some individuals think of their careers as a "calling" and view their work as a central aspect of their personal identity. Many health care professionals often describe their work as something they have wanted to do since childhood and they have long had expectations about what it will be like to be a doctor, nurse or other specialized health care worker (Pitkala & Mantyranta, 2003). Researchers should further investigate these connections between identity and meaningful work of health care professionals to reveal better ways of fostering young adults' interest and motivation for pursuing these careers.

Scholars also must examine issues of identity in relation to the increasing diversity of identities being represented in health care. According to SIT, social categories based on age, socio-economic status, and professions are relevant when individuals join organizations, perform tasks, and interact with others in the workplace. Ethnicity affects values, perspectives, and behaviors and it is a common categorizing factor that can create barriers to developing relationships. On this basis, some individuals may choose to change their communication and behaviors in order to avoid some forms of categorization. For example, new African-American male physicians often alter their communication practices to better fit in with their colleagues and patients (Beaumont, 2012). Given the evolving nature of health care professions, researchers should examine how the presence of more diverse identities impacts OS and OA. As health care workers experience the various processes of socialization and assimilation, social identities may affect the types of relationships they develop and the quality of their relationships with others in their workgroups. Researchers should investigate these questions in health care contexts, similar to research done in business and educational contexts, in order to understand the benefits of diversity within health care organizations and to propose ways to leverage these differences into better health care for the changing patient population.

More scholarship should also attend to the multiple identifications of health care professionals. These workers often belong to multiple organizations that compete for resources (e.g., funding, patients), and some rotate teams so group memberships are continually in flux. They also have strong professional identities that, when taken together, lead to having multiple targets of identification with potentially conflicting goals and priorities (C. R. Scott, 1997). These identity conflicts have implications for how assimilated or identified they may feel with the workgroup, organization, or profession. Moreover, Lammers et al. (Lammers, Atouba, & Carlson, 2013) have discussed how professional workers may experience different kinds of attachments to their multiple identities which may influence, and perhaps inoculate against, the feelings of stress and burnout that are common in health care professionals. Thus, scholars should pursue questions about the nuanced relationship between professions and different kinds of identification in order to unpack these relationships and understand the implications for how work is done in health care organizations.

Practical Implications

From a practice perspective, organizational leaders should understand that health care jobs are becoming more specialized and requiring longer periods of role socialization—for example, as nursing becomes more professionalized and degree requirements increase, it takes longer for individuals to become practicing professionals. Additionally, advances in medicine and more specialization can require them to return to school after years in their career (Ares, 2014). An implication is that nurses develop a stronger professional identity as a nurse, but they are less clear about their role as an organizational member. Human resource departments and even workgroup leaders need to focus on implementing strong OS programs and training to orient incoming members to their workgroups and teams as well as how to effectively assimilate into the organization. As Chao et al. (1994) discuss, newcomers not only need to learn about the skills necessary for the job (performance proficiency) and professional language, but also about organizational goals and values, history, politics, and people. Likewise, successful assimilation occurs when newcomers develop productive relationships with coworkers, receive recognition for their work, and learn how to effectively manage the stress that comes with the job. Given that these processes take time, health care organizations should treat OA as a long-term process and recognize that it may not be enough to conduct orientation sessions during the first weeks in an organization. In addition to standard continuing education courses, organizations should offer courses and training that will help workers assimilate over time on topics such as use of new technologies, emotion management, conflict resolution, teamwork, leadership, and building effective relationships with coworkers and patients.

Like researchers, organizational leaders also need to attend to the shrinking numbers of potential employees for the fast-growing field. While scholars address the messages and motivations of the workforce, organizational leaders should be more cognizant of the changing needs of their workers. With more dual-career households, more support is needed for managing families. As the workforce shortage grows and all employees have to work longer hours in chronically stressful environments, more attention must be given to ways to alleviate and prevent burnout. Moreover, as the health care-seeking population ages, more training must be provided for physicians, nurses, and other direct care providers on how to bridge intergenerational differences and attend to the needs of the older patients. This includes providing more formal geriatric training and even changing the financial structures within the medical field to reflect the increased need for geriatric care (CDC, 2004).

Conclusion

In conclusion, OS and OA are important areas of consideration for members of health care organizations. Just as individuals are socialized into their professions and professional identities beginning with VAS, they also should be socialized to develop strong identities as organizational members. Upon organizational encounter, new members should be introduced to the organization's culture, values, and procedures. They also should build relationships with coworkers and strive to understand workgroup norms. However, the particular health care context affects these issues, and especially how they interact with and develop relationships with coworkers.

Theoretically, the discussion points to the importance of social identity in workers and how workers' identities affect their socialization and assimilation. Practically, this discussion can provide guidance to health care managers whose objective is to create and maintain teams that are effective in providing care and also meeting organizational goals. It can also give insight to workers about how to develop relationships with others in their workgroup and better understand their own feelings and responses to socialization and organizational membership. In summary, understanding the dynamics that operate during these intake and integration processes is important for better preparing health care workers to navigate the current and future health care environment.

DISCUSSION QUESTIONS

1. How can health care employers socialize workers to better ensure that members of health care teams effectively communicate to coordinate and to provide the best patient care?
2. How can strong professional identities affect workers' performance?
3. How can the health care industry better ensure that they will have an adequate supply of physicians, nurses, and other health care workers in the future?
4. What are other contextual factors of the health care field that might affect organizational members' assimilation, socialization, and/or identification processes?

Suggested Reading

Gailliard, B., Myers, K. K., & Seibold, D. R. (2010). Organizational assimilation: A multidimensional reconceptualization and measure. *Management Communication Quarterly, 24*, 552–578.

Myers, K. K. (2005). A burning desire: Assimilation into a fire department. *Management Communication Quarterly, 18*, 344–384.

Rink, F., Kane, A. A., Ellemers, N., & Van der Vegt, G. (2013). Team receptivity to newcomers: Five decades of evidence and future research themes. *The Academy of Management Annals, 7*(1), 245–291.

References

Alvesson, M., Ashcraft, K. L., & Thomas, R. (2008). Identity matters: Reflections on the construction of identity scholarship in organization studies. *Organization, 15*(1), 5–28.

Anderson, C. M., Riddle, B. L., & Martin, M. M. (1999). Socialization processes in groups. In L. R. Frey, D. S. Gouran, & M. S. Poole (Eds.), *The handbook of group communication theory and research* (pp. 139–166). Thousand Oaks, CA: SAGE.

Apker, J. (2001). Role development in the managed care era: A case of hospital-based nursing. *Journal of Applied Communication Research, 29*(2), 117–136. Doi: 10.1080/00909880128106.

Apker, J. & Eggly, S. (2004). Communicating professional identity in medical socialization: Considering the ideological discourse of morning report. *Qualitative Health Research, 14*(3), 411–429.

Ares, T. L. (2014). Professional socialization of students in clinical nurse specialist programs. *Journal of Nursing Education, 53*(11), 631–640.

Ashcraft, K. L. (2007). Appreciating the "work" of discourse: Occupational identity and difference as organizing mechanisms in the case of commercial airline pilots. *Discourse & Communication, 1*, 9–36.

Ashforth, B. E. (2001). *Role transitions in organizational life: An identity perspective.* Mahwah, NJ: Lawrence Erlbaum Associates.

Ashforth, B. E. & Kreiner, G. (1999). "How can you do it?" Dirty work and the challenge of constructing a positive identity. *Academy of Management Review, 24*, 413–434.

Ashforth, B. E. & Mael, F. (1989). Social identity theory and the organization. *The Academy of Management Review, 14*(1), 20–39.

Association of American Medical Colleges (2014). Women in Academic Medicine Statistics and Medical School Benchmarking 2010–2011. In S. Y. MEDICAL STUDENTS, 1965–2012 (Ed.). Retrieved from https://www.aamc.org/members/gwims/statistics/.

Beaumont, C. G. (2012). *Exploring the experiences of racial identity and stereotype threat in African American male medical doctors.* (Doctoral dissertation). Seton Hall University, New Jersey. Available from *Counseling Psychology Commons.* http://scholarship.shu.edu/dissertations/1841/.

Beyer, J. M. & Hannah, D. R. (2002). Building on the past: Enacting established personal identities in a new work setting. *Organization Science, 13*, 636–652.

Bullis, C. & Bach, B. W. (1989). Socialization turning points: An examination of change in organizational identification. *Western Journal of Speech Communication, 53*, 273–293.

Bunderson, J. S., & Thompson, J. A. (2009). The call of the wild: Zookeepers, callings, and the double-edge sword of deeply meaningful work. *Administrative Science Quarterly, 54*, 32–57.

Centers for Disease Control (CDC) (2004). The state of aging and health in America, 2004. Retrieved from: http://www.cdc.gov/aging/pdf/ (State_of_Aging_and_Health_in_America_2004.pdf).

Chao, G. T., O'Leary-Kelly, A. M., Wolf, S., Klein, H. J., & Gardner, P. D. (1994). Organizational socialization: Its content and consequences. *Journal of Applied Psychology, 79*(5), 730–743.

Cheney, G. (1991). *Rhetoric in an organizational society: Managing multiple identities.* Columbia, SC: University of South Carolina Press.

Cini, M., Moreland, R. L., & Levine, J. M. (1993). Group staffing levels and responses to prospective and new group members. *Journal of Personality and Social Psychology, 65*, 723–734.

Davies, B., & Harre, R. (1990). Positioning: The discursive productive of selves. *Journal for Theory of Social Behaviour, 20*, 43–63.

Davis, C. W. & Myers, K. K. (2012). Communication and member disengagement in planned organizational exit. *Western Journal of Communication, 76*, 194–216.

Flanagin, A. J. & Waldeck, J. H. (2004). Technology use and organizational newcomer socialization. *Journal of Business Communication, 41*(2), 137–165.

Gailliard, B. M., Myers, K. K., & Seibold, D. R. (2010). Organizational assimilation: A multidimensional reconceptualization and measure. *Management Communication Quarterly, 24*(4), 552–578.

Geist, P. & Dreyer, J. (1993). The demise of dialogue: A critique of medical encounter ideology. *Western Journal of Communication, 57,* 233–246.

Gibson, M. K. & Papa, M. J. (2000). The mud, the blood, and the beer guys: Organizational osmosis in blue-collar work groups. *Journal of Applied Communication Research, 28*(1), 68–88.

Hafferty, F. W. (1988). Cadaver stories and the emotional socialization of medical students. *Journal of Health and Social Behavior, 29,* 344–356.

Hafferty, F. W. & Franks, R. (1994). The hidden curriculum, ethics teaching, and the structure of medical education. *Academic Medicine, 69,* 861–871.

Harris Interactive (2011). *STEM perceptions: Student & parent study. Parents and students weigh in on how to inspire the next generation of doctors, scientists, software developers and engineers.* Study commissioned by Microsoft, Corp. Available at: http://www.microsoft.com/en-us/Search/result.aspx?form=MSHOME&mkt=en-us&setlang=en-us&q=STEM%20Perceptions%3A%20Student%20%26%20Parent%20Study%202011

Harter, L. M. & Krone, K. J. (2001). Exploring the emergent identities of future physicians: Toward an understanding of ideological socialization of osteopathic medical students. *Southern Communication Journal, 67,* 66–83.

Hennessy, J. & West, M. A. (1999). Intergroup behavior in organizations: A field test of social identity theory. *Small Group Research, 30,* 361–382.

Hochschild, A. R. (1983). *The managed heart.* Berkeley, CA: University of California Press.

Jablin, F. M. (1985). An exploratory study of vocational organizational communication socialization. *Southern Speech Communication Journal, 50,* 261–282.

Jablin, F. M. (1987). Organizational entry, assimilation, and exit. In F. M. Jablin, L. L. Putnam, K. H. Roberts, & L. W. Porter (Eds.), *Handbook of organizational communication: An interdisciplinary perspective* (pp. 679–740). Thousand Oaks, CA: Sage.

Jablin, F. M. (2001). Organizational entry, assimilation, and disengagement/exit. In F. M. Jablin & L. L. Putnam (Eds.), *The new handbook of organizational communication: Advances in theory, research, and methods* (pp. 732–818). Thousand Oaks, CA: Sage.

Jablin, F. M. & Sias, P. M. (2001). Communication competence. In F. M. Jablin & L. L. Putnam (Eds.), *The new handbook of organizational communication: Advances in theory, research, and methods* (pp. 819–864). Thousand Oaks, CA: Sage.

Jahn, J. L. S., & Myers, K. K. (2014). Vocational anticipatory socialization of adolescents: Messages, sources and frameworks that influence interest in STEM careers. *Journal of Applied Communication Research, 42,* 85–106.

Johnson, M. D., Morgeson, F. P., Ilgen, D. R., Meyer, C. J., & Lloyd, J. W. (2006). Multiple professional identities: Examining differences in identification across work-related targets. *Journal of Applied Psychology, 91,* 498–506.

Kaboli, P. J., Go, J. T., Hockenberry, J., Glasgow, J. M., Johnson, S. R., Rosenthal, G. E., Jones, M. P., & Vaughan-Sarrazin, M. (2012). Associations between reduced hospital length of stay and 30-day readmission rate and mortality: 14-year experience in 129 veteran's affairs hospitals. *Annals of Internal Medicine, 157*(12), 837–845.

Khalili, H., Orchard, C., Spence Laschinger, H. K., & Farah, R. (2013). An interprofessional socialization framework for developing an interprofessional identity among health professions students. *Journal of Interprofessional Care, 27*(6), 448–453.

Kim, T. Y., Cable, D. M., & Kim, S. P. (2005). Socialization Tactics, Employee Proactivity, and Person-Organization Fit. *Journal of Applied Psychology, 90*(2), 232–241.

Klein, H. J. & Weaver, N. A. (2000). The effectiveness of an organization-level orientation training program in the socialization of new hires. *Personnel Psychology, 53*, 47–66.

Knapp, M. L., Stohl, C., & Reardon, K. K. (1981). "Memorable" Messages. *Journal of Communication, 31*(4), 27–41.

Kramer, M. W. (2010). *Organizational socialization: Joining and leaving organizations.* Cambridge: Polity.

Lammers, J. C., Atouba, Y. L., & Carlson, E. J. (2013). Which identities matter? A mixed-method study of group, organizational, and professional identities and their relationship to burnout. *Management Communication Quarterly, 27*(4), 503–536.

Lammers, J. C. & Garcia, M. A. (2009). Exploring the concept of "profession" for organizational communication research: Institutional influences in a veterinary organization. *Management Communication Quarterly, 22*(3), 357–384.

Langer, E. (1989). Minding matters: The consequences of mindlessness-mindfulness. In L. Berkowitz (Ed.), *Advances in experimental social psychology* (Vol. 22, pp. 137–173). San Diego, CA: Academic Press.

MacLeod, A. (2011). Six ways problem-based learning cases can sabotage patient-centered medical education. *Academic Medicine, 86*, 818–825.

Maslach, C. (1982). *Burnout: The cost of caring.* New York: Prentice Hall.

Mein Goh, J., Gao, G., & Agarwal, R. (2011). Evolving work routines: Adaptive routinization of information technology in healthcare. *Information Systems Research, 22*(3), 565–585. Doi: 10.1287/isre.1110.0365.

Miller, K. I., Stiff, J. B., & Ellis, B. H. (1988). Communication and empathy as precursors to burnout among human service workers. *Communiation Monographs, 55*, 250–265.

Miller, V. D. & Jablin, F. M. (1991). Information seeking during organizational entry: Influences, tactics, and a model of the process. *Academy of Management Review, 16*(1), 92–120.

Moreland, R. L. & Levine, J. M. (2001). Socialization in organizations and work groups. In M. E. Turner (Ed.), *Groups at work: Theory and research* (pp. 69–112). Mahwah, NJ: Lawrence Erlbaum.

Morgan, J. M. & Krone, K. J. (2001). Bending the rules of "professional" display: Emotional improvisation in caregiver performances. *Journal of Applied Communication Research, 29*, 317–340.

Myers, K. K. (2005). A burning desire. *Management Communication Quarterly, 18*(3), 344–384.

Myers, K. K., Jahn, J. L. S., Gailliard, B. M., & Stoltzfus, K. (2011). Vocational anticipatory socialization (VAS): A communicative model of adolescents' interests in STEM. *Management Communication Quarterly, 25*(1), 87–120.

Myers, K. K. & McPhee, R. D. (2006). Influences on Member Assimilation in Workgroups in High Reliability Organizations: A Multilevel Analysis. *Human Communication Research, 32*(4), 440–468.

Myers, K. K. & Oetzel, J. G. (2003). Exploring the dimensions of organizational assimilation: Creating and validating a measure. *Communication Quarterly, 51*(4), 438–457.

Pacanowsky, M. E. & O'Donnell-Trujillo, N. (1983). Organizational communication as cultural performance. *Communication Monographs, 50*(2), 126–147.

Pitkala, K. H. & Mantyranta T. (2003). Professional socialization revised: Medical students' own conceptions related to adoption of the future physician's role–a qualitative study. *Medical Teacher, 25*(2), 155–160. Doi: 10.1080/0142159031000092544.

Perrow, C. (1984). *Normal accidents: Living with high-risk technologies.* New York: Basic Books.

Reeves, S., Perrier, L., Goldman, J., Freeth, D., & Zwarenstein, M. (2013). Interprofessional education: Effects on professional practice and health care outcomes. *Cochrane Database of Systematic Reviews, 3, CD002213.* Retrieved from http://www.ncbi.nlm.nih.gov/pubmed/23543515.

Riddle, B., L., Anderson, C. M., & Martin, M. M. (2000). Small group socialization scale: Development and validity. *Small Group Research, 31,* 554–572.

Roberts, K. H. (1990). Managing high reliability organizations. *California Management Review, 32,* 101–113.

Scott, C. R. (1997). Identification with multiple targets in a geographically dispersed organization. *Management Communication Quarterly, 10,* 491–522.

Scott, C. W. & Myers, K. K. (2005). The socialization of emotion: Learning emotion management at the fire station. *Journal of Applied Communication Research, 33*(1), 67–92.

Scott, C. W. & Myers, K. K. (2010). Toward an integrative theoretical perspective on organizational membership negotiations: Socialization, assimilation, and the duality of structure. *Communication Theory, 20*(1), 79–105.

Sias, P. M. (2005). Workplace relationship quality and employee information experiences. *Communication Studies, 56*(4), 375–395.

Sluss, D. M. & Ashforth, B. E. (2007). Relational identity and identification: Defining ourselves through work relationships. *Academy of Management Review, 32,* 9–32.

Smith, A. C. III & Kleinman, S. (1989). Managing emotions in medical school: Students' contacts with the living and the dead. *Social Psychology Quarterly, 52,* 56–69.

Stohl, C. (1986). The role of memorable messages in the process of organizational socialization. *Communication Quarterly, 34*(3), 231–249.

Tracy, S. J. & Tracy, K. (1998). Emotion labor at 911: A case study and theoretical critique. *Journal of Applied Communication Research, 26,* 390–411.

Vangelisti, A. L. (1988). Adolescent Socialization into the Workplace: A Synthesis and Critique of Current Literature. *Youth and Society, 19*(4), 460–484.

Wanous, J. P. (1992). *Organizational entry: Recruitment, selection, orientation, and socialization of newcomers.* Reading, MA: Addison Wesley.

Wanous, J. P., Poland, T. D., Premack, S. L., & Davis, K. S. (1992). The effects of met expectations on newcomer attitudes and behaviors: A review and meta-analysis. *Journal of Applied Psychology, 77*(3), 288–297.

Wood., D. F. (2003). ABC of learning and teaching in medicine: Problem based learning. *BMJ, 326.*

World Health Organization (2010). *Framework for action on interprofessional education & collaborative practice.* Health Professions Networks. Geneva: WHO.

Zorn, T. E. & Gregory, K. W. (2005). Learning the ropes together: Assimilation and friendship development among first-year male medical students. *Health Communication, 17,* 211–232.

4

A SYSTEMS FRAMEWORK FOR HEALTH CARE TEAM COMMUNICATION

Kevin Real and Marshall Scott Poole

Health Care Teams

Patients in the University of Kentucky's cardiothoracic and vascular intensive care unit (CTVICU), which treats patients with severe heart/cardiac-related conditions, are cared for by registered nurses (RNs) such as Katie Burns, who trained in that unit in 2012. "All around me I saw the innovation, the teamwork, the sense of professionalism, and the fast pace. I knew right away that I wanted to work in an intensive care unit," Burns stated (University of Kentucky News, 2014). Dr. Hassan Reda, a cardiothoracic surgeon, said that nurses are "with the patient constantly. They provide care, they educate, they nurture, they are the voice of the patient, and that makes them an integral part of the care team" (University of Kentucky News, 2014). In today's health care system, the care of patients is in the hands of many different health care practitioners. For example, in a typical CTVICU, patients will see physicians (MDs), RNs, respiratory, physical and occupational therapists, pharmacists, dieticians, patient care facilitators, social workers, and pastoral care personnel. Scholars have estimated that in a typical 4-day hospital stay, patients may interact with 50 different employees from various occupations, educational levels, and professions (O'Daniel & Rosenstein, 2008; Baker, Gustafson, Beaubien, Salas, & Barach, 2005).

Health care organizations increasingly rely upon health care teams (HCTs) for the delivery of patient care. This is particularly so since the publication of *To Err is Human* (Institute of Medicine, 2000), the groundbreaking report on medical errors and patient safety in health care. This report estimated that between 15,000 and 44,000 patients die each year in U.S. hospitals from preventable medical errors, many of which were attributed to communication problems. The evidence suggests that when health care professionals do not communicate well, patients are at risk. Examples of communication problems are misunderstanding messages, lack of crucial information, problems interpreting clinical information due to channel issues (not correctly hearing phone messages, jumbled text messages, etc.), problems coordinating different disciplines, and much more (Joint Commission, 2005; O'Daniel & Rosenstein, 2005). Communication problems have been linked to patient safety, medical errors, and other adverse events (Baker et al., 2005; Institute of Medicine, 2000). The Institute's 2000 report recommended that health care organizations implement team-based care.

There is substantial research that indicates health care teams are successful when communication processes work well (Lemieux-Charles & McGuire, 2006; Lingard et al., 2008; Poole & Real, 2003). Researchers have suggested that the internal processes of teams are primarily communicative and that team processes ensure team effectiveness (McGrath, 1984; Salas, Sims, & Burke, 2005). Teams play a vital role in health care organizations and when they are ineffective (often due to poor communication) they can have outputs such as delayed patient care, lack of coordinated care, inefficiencies, bad outcomes for patients, and more (Salas et al., 2005; Lingard et al., 2008; Ramanujam & Rousseau, 2006). When teams have good communication processes they are likely to be more effective, thus contributing to better patient outcomes and organizational performance.

Our goal in this chapter is to describe theory and research in health care team communication processes within health care organizations. We utilize a systems framework (Poole, 2014) that traces inputs, processes, and outputs to examine how team structures foster (or inhibit) communication in health care teams. To do this, first, we introduce the systems model and discuss how systems theory provides a general frame for understanding health care organizations. Second, we focus specifically on health care teams and discuss how systems theory translates to that level. Third, we introduce a typology of health care teams, each of which has particular configurations of inputs and structure and requires different communication processes in order to be effective. Fourth, we expand our discussion to consider multi-team systems in health care, a perspective on "teams of teams." Following this, we examine contextual factors that affect health care team processes and outcomes. We wrap up the chapter with a discussion of challenges that need to be addressed in understanding the practice of team dynamics and communication in health care organizations.

Systems Theory for Health Care Organizations

Health care is a complex system composed of distinct sub-systems that are connected and interdependent. Systems theory helps us understand how health care organizations are both components of a larger system (e.g., the U.S. health care system) as well as systems in their own right. A hospital contains a number of sub-systems, such as trauma, intensive care, laundry, pastoral care, food services, emergency department, radiology, information technology, and more. Each of these sub-systems often has sub-components, many of which are teams. A systems theory approach that has been very influential in health care is Donabedian's (1966) structure-process-outcome model, which describes the manner in which patient care is delivered across a variety of settings. In this model, structure refers to the context in which patient care is delivered. It involves organizational (hospital, clinics in Walmart, etc.), clinical (surgery, pediatrics, emergency department), building design, staff, resources, equipment, and technology components. Process describes patient care procedures such as diagnoses, treatment, and patient education as well as communication and quality improvement processes. Outcomes denote the effect of inputs and processes on patient care and are typically concerned with patient morbidity and mortality but can also include patient safety and patient and staff satisfaction.

This model is very general, but where it can be specified in some detail, it is useful for understanding and adapting organizational practices. For example, it is clear that communication and information are important to the coordination and care of patients. If a pediatric unit within a large health care organization uses paper medical records (structure) to coordinate care and exchange information between physicians and staff (process), but this slower method has created problems for referrals and billing (outcomes), then it may consider changing to electronic health records (a new structure) as a way of improving its processes and outcomes. Systems theory provides both a conceptual and applied framework for understanding the internal operations of health care organizations.

Addressing Patient Care Using Health Care Teams

To appreciate how teams work using systems theory, let's examine the classic input-process-output (IPO) model (McGrath, 1984; Hackman, 1987), which is related to Donabedian's Model, but at the team level. Salas et al. (2005) have suggested that the IPO framework is the dominant model underlying many theories of team performance. Although it has been subjected to criticism and revisions have been offered (Mathieu, Marks & Zaccaro, 2001), the IPO framework remains the most commonly used model in health care team research (Salas, Cooke & Rosen, 2008). Medical scholars believe it remains useful for understanding of how health care teams function (Fernandez, Kozlowski, Shapiro, & Salas, 2008).

In an earlier paper, we used the IPO framework as a basis for applying how health care practitioners utilize communication inputs and processes and how these shape health care team outputs (see Real & Poole, 2011). In this approach, we indicate specific communication inputs (or structures) that influence team communication processes. These include formal team meetings and briefings, structured communication checklists, channels for routine information exchange (such as electronic health records, or the older but more stable paper charts), channels for face-to-face interaction, locations where informal interactions occur (hallways, patient rooms, etc.), and informal networks.

Processes of communication include what people do when they communicate, such as exchanging information, asking for help, acknowledging others' communication, communication failures (miscommunication, misinterpretation, missed communication, etc.), feedback, addressing team conflict, voice, nonverbal communication, informal talk, and backstage communication. Note that these kinds of processes can be formal or informal. Many health care professionals have told us of the importance of informal conversations in the hallway or other places that are crucial to patient outcomes. Ellingson's (2003) study is a good example of how informal sites such as hallways (inputs) provide the setting for important informal talk between providers (processes) that impact what they do in patient care (outputs) (see also Barbour, Gill, and Dean, this volume, for their focus on space as a key issue in discourse between physicians, nurses and patients).

Outputs of communication inputs and processes can be positive or negative and include quality of care, delays in care, wasted time, adverse events, procedural errors, efficiency, team cohesion, morale, retention, improved communication, and patient satisfaction. This communication-related IPO framework advanced by Real and Poole (2011) is useful because it shows how communicative elements of teamwork are connected and provides a means for facilitating team improvement. Studies have shown how the development of communication inputs such as checklists and team briefings have improved team processes and patient care outcomes (Haynes et al., 2009; Lingard et al., 2008). This systemic catalog of inputs, processes, and outputs can be related to how teams are structured, which affects within-team communication and coordination with other health care teams. We address these issues in the following section, where we operationalize systems theory into health care team communication structures and practices.

Translating Theory Into Practice: A Typology of Health Care Teams

In an earlier review of the health care team literature, we described six generic types of health care teams based on structural and organizational factors such as boundedness, centralization, diversity, interdependence, and nature of collaboration among disciplines (Poole & Real, 2003). We shall briefly describe them here but, for an extended treatment of these issues, we refer the reader to the 2003 review. *Ad hoc* teams are created to address a specific issue for a limited period of time and disband when the work has been accomplished. An example of an ad hoc group would be a team formed to address central line infections within the neo-natal intensive care unit. A central line is the long tube inserted into patients that carries medicine and nutrients into their body. Central line infections are very serious and result in thousands of deaths each year and billions of dollars in added costs to the U.S. health care system (CDC, 2012). An ad hoc team to address this issue might be composed of a physician, a nurse, an infection specialist, a lab technician, and a mid-level hospital manager. It would be charged with identifying major causes of infections in the hospital and developing measures to prevent them.

Nominal care groups are groups, not teams, because members do not set goals, plan, or carry out activities together. Instead a single physician coordinates care, working primarily with her/his assistants and staff and bringing in specialists as needed. They are "nominal" because caregivers work independently and care is coordinated by the primary physician. *Unidisciplinary* teams are composed of a single discipline, such as physical therapy teams. These professionals may work with other specialists but are tightly linked within their own team. Their work with others is episodic and peripheral compared to what they do within their team.

These teams are best suited to cases where extended care is required, such as a hospital ward or when there is a complex yet narrowly defined problem, such as spinal surgery or physical therapy. Members of these teams come from the same discipline, though they may specialize in different aspects of the discipline. An example of this could be a team of physical therapists who have deep experience rehabilitating different parts of the body. While there may be differences among them in terms of expertise, members of unidisciplinary teams view themselves as belonging to a single, common discipline.

Unidisciplinary teams often work in concert with other teams in order to accomplish broader patient care goals. This alignment of team goals with larger system goals is the core of multiteam systems (MTS) theory (Mathieu et al., 2001). Mathieu et al. describe how unidisciplinary teams coordinate activities around an accident: the fire department extracts a patient from a car crash, the emergency medical team keeps the patient stable while delivering him to the hospital, where the emergency room doctors take over. These teams are linked together through sequential input-process-output interdependencies (this will be described in more detail in the section on multiteam systems further on in this chapter). A status briefing is critical during handoffs between teams in these situations. A key problem in these cases is that each discipline emphasizes different types of information and may not notice or collect information that the next team in the chain needs. Careful planning beforehand, as well as exercises in which the teams practice handoffs, can forestall these problems, as can forms, briefings, and checklists.

The next three teams require greater interdependence and collaboration as the tasks they address grow increasingly more complex. The types of teams that address multifaceted patient care issues are multidisciplinary, interdisciplinary, and transdisciplinary. *Multidisciplinary* teams are providers who work in conjunction with each other but function autonomously, such as various professionals involved in the treatment of a single cancer patient. In these teams there is a division of labor according to discipline; with each handling its specialty and keeping the other members posted concerning information they should know.

Interdisciplinary teams are composed of providers from two or more disciplines who work interdependently in the same setting; their members coordinate so that they develop shared routines and common responsibilities and make care decisions together. Hospice care teams, often consisting of physicians, nurses, social workers, pastoral care and more will work together in providing end-of-life care for patients. Accurate transactive memory structures (Hollingshead, Gupta, Yoon, & Brandon, 2011), where the group, rather than any one individual, is responsible for its division of labor, skills, knowledge and information, contribute to interdisciplinary team effectiveness. Understanding sources of expertise within the team enables members to identify who handles specific care issues, problems or emergencies.

Transdisciplinary teams are those groups which take interdisciplinary care to a greater level of trust, mutual confidence, and collaboration. While not as common as interdisciplinary teams, transdisciplinary teams are often found in long-term care facilities, where the same patients are provided for by the same team of providers over time. In these settings, members actively seek to break down the boundaries among disciplines through learning and taking on functions and roles of other disciplines (see Silk and Smith, this volume, on coordinating transdisciplinary research). Extensive cross-training enables team members to handle routine functions in multiple disciplines and manage difficult cases.

No type of team is necessarily better than any other; which is best depends on the team's tasks, the health care issues involved, the current standard of practice in health care, and the organizational context—in other words, on the purpose and function of the team system and its environment. One important environmental influence is the culture or tradition of the organization in which the team is embedded, which often gives preference to certain types of teams; for example, multi-physician specialty practices often prefer unidisciplinary teams, and community health care organizations tend to favor interdisciplinary approaches (Poole & Real, 2003). Culture and tradition are not always adaptive, however—preferred team types may not necessarily be the best if standards of practice change in response to scientific, medical, and technological advances. Ideally, the team should be tailored to the demands of the situation.

In Table 4.1, we illustrate how each team type is manifested in health care with a focus on particular elements that represent communication in health care teams. We provide an example context for each team type and suggest particular advantages and challenges specific to each one. We then locate communication structures and practices derived from Real and Poole (2011) which focused on how communication inputs (formal meetings, briefings, checklists, routine channels for information exchange, ongoing formal interaction, formal handoffs, and sites for informal interaction) influence the processes and outcomes of care. Team leadership is also considered in the table, as it is an important feature that establishes the extent to which these structures function effectively within each team (see Williams, this volume, for more on leadership in multiteam systems). These communication structures and leadership practices constitute a set of "building blocks" that can be employed in the design and management of teams. As seen in Table 4.1, teams vary in the degree to which they use and employ the various structures and practices.

TABLE 4.1 Elements of Health Care Team Types

Type	Example Context	Advantages	Challenges	Communication Structures	Leadership
Ad hoc	Reduce central line infection	Single-minded focus on specific issue using correct mix of expertise and experience	Different perspectives, potential for conflict, motivation to do work, attendance issues	Face-to-face meetings important; keeping records online for distributed work	Keep team focused, on track, maintain morale and shared expectations
Nominal	Patients of Primary Care MD	Primary care physician involved in care provided by specialists; continuity of care	Responsibility for this rests with MD, if busy, then omissions, other problems can occur	Formal channels: lab and consult reports, medical records, dyadic interactions	MD is center of hub and spoke system of communication
Unidisciplinary	Physical therapy	Depth in specialty, consults, backup; sense of identification with team	Communication with other disciplines due to 'silo'-like focus	Formal and informal meetings, formal channels, handoffs	Vary from centralized to shared structure, based on discipline
Multidisciplinary	Cancer treatment of individual patients	Range of expertise from multiple disciplines Learning from others	Communication barriers due to discipline-based frames of reference Forging common team culture/ identity	Patient medical records, briefings, checklists, formal meetings, sites for informal interaction build awareness, trust	Goal is to harmonize disciplines, shared or single leadership, care coordinators may be common
Interdisciplinary	Hospice care	Increased linkages of expertise by disciplines Flexible, adaptive, collaborative	Managing heavy communication load Conflict Unbalanced input and representation by discipline	Formal and informal meetings, medical records, checklists, sites for informal interaction build awareness, trust, fewer status differences	Varies: some have designated, others are distributed. Point person needed for each case. Adaptive based on situation
Transdisciplinary	Long-term care	More cross-disciplinary skills, enabling flexible, adaptive caregiving and clear communication	Potential dilution and erosion of disciplinary skills; reputation of team, morale issues	Briefings, formal and informal meetings, checklists, medical records, sites for informal interaction to share information	Similar to interdisciplinary; situation is big factor as is leader capability. Instilling confidence and pride important

Each of the six team types has a particular set of advantages and strengths and also faces specific problems and challenges that must be met if the team is to function effectively. We believe that each type of team system will be most effective if its configuration of communication structures and practices is set up to enable it to capitalize on its strengths and address its challenges. In the next section, we expand on this translation of theory into practice with the concept of multiteam systems.

Translating Theory Into Practice: Multiteam Systems

As the previous section indicates, some types of teams—multidisciplinary, inter-disciplinary, and transdisciplinary—are "microcosms" of multiteam systems in that, if sufficiently large, they may embody disciplinary subteams that must coordinate with one another. Each team type, however, is potentially a distinctive team in a multiteam system in which its inputs, processes and outputs represent the overall work of the team but also, smaller sections of activity, which Marks, Mathieu and Zaccaro (2001) denote as "performance episodes." These episodes describe specific actions that a team would take, such as surgery of a patient in an operating room. For example, an interdisciplinary surgical team may handoff a patient to a multidisciplinary intensive care unit that then transfers the patient to a transdisciplinary long-term care facility that ultimately hands the recovering patient off to an interdisciplinary home health care team.

Each team in our typology represents a somewhat different type of MTS. The *ad hoc* team focused on reducing central line infections likely functions in a hospital environment where they would get input from other teams, such as surgical teams, rapid response teams (a team that takes action to prevent further deterioration of hospitalized patients in distress), and continuous quality improvement teams. These teams would benefit from decreased infections and the reduced level of complications would be an input to their work. A *nominal care* group organized around a primary care physician could hand patients off to *unidisciplinary* teams such as radiologists and pharmacists. In this case, the output of the nominal care group would be the input for the unidisciplinary team. Because the primary care physician continues to be involved in overseeing the treatment, information and often the patient would flow back to the doctor in charge.

When a *multidisciplinary* team provides care for an individual cancer patient, they may coordinate their care with members of other teams, such as patient transport team or chemo or radiation teams. They likely realize their work through process interdependence, such as sharing information, coordinating sequential actions, and managing an evolving treatment plan. Hospice care teams are typically *interdisciplinary* teams where social workers, nurses, pharmacists, physicians, pastoral care and more work together in the same setting. They may share input interdependencies in the form of shared facilities, space, supplies, etc. (Mathieu et al., 2001). These teams may accomplish their goals by working together or, in the case of pastoral care; they may come into play more toward the end of the care episodes. *Transdisciplinary* teams, as noted, have greater levels of collaboration and mutual trust. A team like this in a long-term care facility will experience input interdependency (shared facilities, etc.) and process interdependencies (communication, coordination, collaboration). As with all MTSs, the key challenges are effective coordination among teams and ensuring a proper balance between individual team goals and the goals of the entire system. Neither set of goals should be sacrificed at the expense of the other.

Other Factors to Consider

Health care professionals operate in complex environments characterized by time pressure, multiple decision-makers, rapidly changing, ambiguous situations, information overload, and serious consequences for error (Baker et al., 2005). These professionals working in health care teams do not operate in isolation but are shaped by a number of environmental factors that need to be considered in the process of applying theory. The value of a systems theory/IPO framework lies in understanding that health care teams are situated within multiple contexts: societal, organizational, clinical, and team, each of which are considered here below.

At the societal level, research from cross-national comparisons of health care systems suggest that the U.S. has more fragmented care delivery, less coordination of health care professionals, and more duplication of resources than most other major developed countries (Squires, 2011). To address these shortcomings in the U.S., Accountable Care Organizations (ACO) were created (as part of the Patient Protection and Affordable Care Act) in order to improve the coordination and delivery of care to greater numbers of patients. Teams and teamwork are an important element of ACOs and these structural changes have led to changes in care delivery processes. This is an example of how inputs from the broader societal environment (policies, investments) shape organizational structure and capabilities, which then influence team processes and patient outcomes.

Organizational contexts that need to be considered in the process of utilizing IPO/HCT theory in health care organizations (HCOs) include goals, structure, rewards, resources, training and technology (Lemieux-Charles & McGuire, 2006). The goals of the HCO are related to the type of organization, whether it is a hospital, long-term care facility or a small clinic, which would influence the type of teams present in that context. For example, surgical teams in hospitals are different than provider teams in long-term care facilities. HCO structure could include buildings (including their design), equipment, and finances, each of which would impact HCT delivery processes and patient outcomes (Donabedian, 1966). There is growing interest in health care design research that examines how design and the built environment impact hospital teamwork, communication, workflow, and patient care (see Aakhus & Harrison, this volume; Barbour et al., this volume; Guinther, Carll-White, & Real, 2014 and Zimring et al., 2008 for examples). Organizational rewards, resources, training and technology are also important factors that shape how teams work. When people are rewarded for teamwork, they tend to be good team members. Organizations that have sufficient resources, training, and technology inputs are likely to have satisfactory team processes and outcomes.

The clinical environment is significant, for example, teamwork may look different in an ICU than in a primary care clinic. Inputs, processes, outputs will differ across clinical environments. Surgical teams are more likely to have inputs that are formal, such as formal team briefings, structured communication checklists, and formal handoffs. In many social and organizational contexts, these formal structures are required. On the other hand, according to the *Wall Street Journal*, primary care team members may meet in more informal "huddles" during the day to review incoming patients and identify any concerns (Landro, 2014). Teams that work in geriatric care, primary care, and emergency departments (see Barbour et al., this volume) may tend to rely more on structures such as sites for informal interactions (such as hallways or break rooms) and informal communication networks (see Doerfel, this volume, on the importance of networks). The communication processes in these latter teams may be comprised of informal talk and backstage communication while in surgical teams they may be information exchange, requests for assistance, and other formal types of communication. Team outputs are likely to vary but different types of clinical teams will naturally have distinct outcomes. Surgical teams may be focused on how communication impacts quality of care, delays in care, wasted time, adverse events or procedural errors. Outputs of teams in nursing homes or hospice care, because they are in longer-term contexts, may be more oriented toward team cohesion, morale, and retention. We should note here that these patterns may differ across types of teams, depending on societal, organizational, clinical and team factors (such as composition). For instance, we could find a surgical team where members have worked together over a long period of time. As such, they may know each other so well that they could add informal communication to the required formal structures and processes already in place.

The team context is important and the type of team (e.g., ad hoc, multidisciplinary, etc.) can influence how the IPO framework can be understood. We have described above an example of what this would look in an *ad hoc* team that addressed central line infections. A *nominal care* group, directed by a physician who sends patients to other specialists but remains in contact with the patient and the specialist, will likely rely on communication structures such as channels for routine information exchange (electronic, paper, etc.) and channels for ongoing verbal interaction (face-to-face, electronic, etc.). Communication processes in nominal care groups may be fairly routine, requesting or providing information, acknowledging others' communication and requests for assistance. Outputs may include quality of care and efficiency.

Communication in *unidisciplinary* teams may depend on the clinical context and discipline. For example, inputs for hospital nurses could include formal handoffs, communication channels for routine information exchange and problem solving, and sites for informal interaction. A group of family practice MDs working in a clinic may be much less formal, as they cover for each other and interact about patients, so they may not rely on formal handoffs as much as hospital nurses. Processes and outputs would also be distinct. Nurses could engage in backstage, informal talk (processes) to address team tensions in order to boost team cohesion and morale (outputs). They also routinely ask for help to have outputs such as efficient and timely care. Family practice doctors may request or provide information, ask for or give feedback, and all members of the team could voice their ideas. The outputs of this team would likely be primarily oriented to quality of care.

It is likely that *multidisciplinary, interdisciplinary,* and *transdisciplinary* teams share many communication inputs, processes and outputs, but they may be distinct by gradations. Greater degrees of interdependence and team motivation are likely to lead to higher levels of interaction. A transdisciplinary team that has worked together closely over time may engage in both formal communication structures (briefings, checklists, handoffs) and informal communication sites (hallways, patient rooms) *to a greater extent* than multidisciplinary and interdisciplinary teams. It is likely that they also have more informal communication networks in place that extend up and down the organizational hierarchy than other types of teams. For example, if the team needed a supervisor's support for a decision, they may have informal ties to upper management that would allow them to quickly contact someone who could get things done. These informal ties are important for building social capital (see Chewning, this volume) and the ability to get tasks accomplished. And if nurses needed a room cleaned out quickly in order to get a patient in, they may have the kind of informal relationship with housekeeping staff that would make that happen too. These same kinds of things can happen in all teams, but they are more likely to happen in teams characterized by shared mental models, effective communication, mutual trust, and transactive memory structures (Hollingshead et al., 2011; Salas et al., 2005), all of which are more pronounced in transdisciplinary teams.

Challenges of Implanting Theory Into Practice

There are a number of challenges facing the successful application of a systemic IPO framework in practice. Health care organizations function within a complex environment and carry a competing array of challenges and demands carried out by highly distinct professional clinical staff. To be successful in employing teams in health care, a number of pitfalls must be recognized, addressed, and avoided. Organizational input factors such as leadership, culture, trust, and learning can support teamwork. If these are lacking, then team processes and outcomes will not be realized and patients can suffer.

Leadership and management support for teams in health care organizations is crucial for building effective health care teams (Taplin, Foster, & Shortell, 2013).

Teams flourish in organizations where they are authorized to make decisions and carry them out. Top management support for health care team autonomy leads to collaboration, communication, teamwork, and coordination (Dietz et al., 2014). One consequence of reduced leadership support for teams is diminished teamwork in the form of problem solving, conflict management, decision-making, and quality of care. Further, a lack of management support for teams is indicative of an individualistic mindset, a belief that individuals make better decisions than teams. However, a systems approach to understanding health care processes is what is needed. As the Institute of Medicine's *To Err is Human* report revealed, there is a persistent belief in health care that errors are personal failings. Yet it is systemic issues such as short-staffing, high workloads, poor communication and other issues that lead to patient care problems and many of these can be addressed through effective leadership (IOM, 2000; Ramanujam & Rousseau, 2006).

A second and very important challenge is culture, which is perhaps even more crucial than leadership. An organizational culture that supports teamwork will be characterized by behaviors, beliefs, values, and communication that encourage and promote teams, such as a HCO that rewards employees for team participation. On the other hand, a culture that does not support teamwork could be one characterized by silence, a major problem in health care (Gardezi, Lingard, Espin, Whyte, Orser & Baker, 2009; Maxfield, Grenny, Lavandero, & Groah, 2005). A culture that supports silence could look something like this: a nurse is hesitant to directly challenge a physician's medication order that they believe is incorrect, so they discuss it with their manager or a pharmacist (which takes more time) or they stay silent, which is even worse for patients (IOM, 2000; Ramanujam & Rousseau, 2006). Silence, unfortunately, is embedded in many health care organization cultures due to status differences and medical hierarchies, where direct communication is discouraged. A culture of silence is an unsafe system for patients and health care professionals alike (see Bisel and Zanin, this volume, for more on the moral mum effect).

A third important challenge is trust. When trust is broken or simply absent, then teamwork is missing. Instead of emphasizing collaboration and coordination, too often the focus is on defensiveness, blame, and other dysfunctional elements. The Institute of Medicine (2004) found that when hospitals view staff as costs (rather than assets), emphasize efficiency over patient safety, and have poor communication practices, there is a loss of trust. As you can imagine, this is a problem when it comes to quality of patient care. On the other hand, when staff and teams feel trust, they are more likely to have the interest of the organization (system) in mind when they act and are less likely to expect any short-term payoff to their behaviors. Open and honest communication can only thrive in an environment of trust. Open systems, where information flows between individuals, teams, departments, and organizations in health care, are successful when trust is present.

A fourth challenge that needs to be addressed is learning, a vital ingredient in HCTs, HCOs and individual professionals. A unique feature of HCOs is that the workforce is comprised of multiple professions, physicians, nurses, pharmacists, etc., who have been trained and socialized into their professions before they enter the organization (Clark, 1997). To improve teamwork, interprofessional education and training has been developed where students of various health care professions (medicine, nursing, pharmacy) learn with students of other professions (World Health Organization, 2010). The idea behind this training is for students to learn to collaborate with other professions in order to reduce future professional silos. This will lead to improved teamwork and likely a reduction in medical hierarchies. This will also enhance communication, which Weaver, Dy and Rosen (2014) have found to be among the most common teamwork competencies HCOs would like to improve. Weaver et al. suggest that learning appropriate assertiveness communication can counter cultures of silence and improve task-related feedback, conflict management and mutual trust (see Canary, this volume, on learning organizations).

It is important to understand that conflicting demands and ineffective communication are two primary pitfalls to be avoided in developing a collaborative, interdisciplinary context where teams can flourish. To address these challenges, successful health care delivery often requires multiteam systems where teams work together and communicate within the team and they also communicate and work with other teams in the system. However, there are times when tensions exist between the goals of an individual team and that of the MTS. For example, in a *nominal care* setting, a physician may gather information from a nurse about the patient then interact with other professionals, including pharmacy, radiology, occupational/physical therapy, labs, and perhaps even administrative staff (in case there was an insurance or finance-related question). But these other professionals may be in systems where there are staff shortages, heavy workloads, lack of resources, or have little ability or knowledge of communication. The physician wants additional information and possibly insight into diagnosis in a timely fashion, yet may experience frustration due to the conflicting demands of the other professionals.

Conclusions

In this chapter, we utilized systems theory and an input-process-output framework as a basis for understanding communication in health care teams. To illustrate this phenomenon in practice, we described how our generic typology of health care teams accounts for different communication processes in order to be effective. We applied these principles further with a look at multiteam systems in health care as well as a consideration of additional factors such as societal, organizational, clinical, and team contexts. We briefly deliberated on how challenges of leadership, culture, trust, and learning are important for team communication in health care organizations. We believe that patients who are cared for by teams and nurses such as Katie Burns at the University of Kentucky hospital will benefit from this enhanced awareness of how communication inputs and processes impact outcomes for patients, staff, teams, and health care organizations.

DISCUSSION QUESTIONS

1. In considering systems theory, are there ways to change inputs in order to impact processes? Are there ways to transform processes so as to improve outcomes?
2. How do health care teams improve the quality of communication in hospitals, clinics, and other health care contexts?
3. How does communication "make a difference" in patient outcomes? In staff/provider satisfaction?
4. What type of team would you like to be on if you worked in health care? Why?

Suggested Reading

Haynes, A. B., Weiser, T. G., Berry, W. R., Lipsitz, S. R., Breizat, A. S., & Dellinger, E. P., et al. (2009). A surgical safety checklist to reduce morbidity and mortality in a global population. *New England Journal of Medicine, 360*, 491–9.

Poole, M. S. & Real, K. (2003). Groups and teams in health care: Communication and effectiveness. In T. L. Thompson, A. M. Dorsey, K. I. Miller, & R. Parrott (Eds.) *Handbook of health communication* (pp. 369–402). Mahwah, NJ: Lawrence Erlbaum Publishers.

Real, K. & Poole, M. S. (2011). Health care teams: Communication and effectiveness. In T. L. Thompson, R. Parrott, & J. Nussbaum (Eds.) *The Routledge Handbook of Health Communication* (2nd ed., pp. 100–116). New York: Routledge.

References

Baker, D., Gustafson, S., Beaubien, J., Salas, E., & Barach, P. (2005). Medical teamwork and patient safety: The evidence-based relation. Agency for Healthcare Quality and Research, Rockville, MD.

Centers for Disease Control (CDC) (2012). Central Line-associated Bloodstream Infection. Retrieved from http://www.cdc.gov/hai/bsi/bsi.html.

Clark, P. G. (1997). Values in health care professional socialization: Implications for geriatric education in interdisciplinary teamwork. *The Gerontologist, 37*(4), 441–451.

Dietz, A. S., Pronovost, P. J., Benson, K. N., Mendez-Tellez, P. A., Dwyer, C., Wyskiel, R., & Rosen, M. A. (2014). A systematic review of behavioural marker systems in healthcare: What do we know about their attributes, validity and application? *BMJ Quality & Safety, 23*, 1031–1039.

Donabedian, A. (1966). Evaluating the quality of medical care. *The Milbank Memorial Fund Quarterly*, 166–206.

Ellingson, L. L. (2003). Interdisciplinary health care teamwork in the clinic backstage. *Journal of Applied Communication Research, 31*, 93–117.

Fernandez, R., Kozlowski, S. W. J., Shapiro, M. J., & Salas, E. (2008). Toward a definition of teamwork in emergency medicine. *Academic Emergency Medicine, 15,* 1104–1112.

Gardezi, F., Lingard, L., Espin, S., Whyte, S., Orser, B., & Baker, G. R. (2009). Silence, power and communication in the operating room. *Journal of Advanced Nursing, 65,* 1390–1399.

Guinther, L., Carll-White, A., & Real, K. (2014). One size does not fit all: A diagnostic post-occupancy evaluation model for an emergency department. *Health Environments Research & Design, 7*(3), 15–37.

Hackman, J. R. (1987). The design of work teams. In J. W. Lorsch (Ed.), *Handbook of organizational behavior* (pp. 315–342). Englewood Cliffs, NJ: Prentice-Hall.

Haynes, A. B., Weiser, T. G., Berry, W. R., Lipsitz, S. R., Breizat, A. S., & Dellinger, E. P., et al. (2009). A surgical safety checklist to reduce morbidity and mortality in a global population. *New England Journal of Medicine, 360,* 491–9.

Hollingshead, A. B., Gupta, N., Yoon, K., & Brandon, D. P. (2011). Transactive memory theory and teams: Past, present, and future. In E. Salas, S. M. Fiore, & M. P. Letsky (Eds.). *Theories of team cognition: Cross-disciplinary perspectives* (pp. 421–455). London: Routledge.

Institute of Medicine (2000). *To err is human: Building a safer health system.* National Academy Press: Washington, DC.

Institute of Medicine (2004). *Keeping patients safe: Transforming the work environment of nurses.* National Academies Press: Washington, DC.

Joint Commission (2005). *The Joint Commission guide to improving staff communication.* Oakbrook Terrace, IL: Joint Commission Resources.

Landro, L. (2014, Feb. 17). The doctor's team will see you now. *Wall Street Journal.* Retrieved from http: www.wsj.com.

Lemieux-Charles, L. & McGuire, W. L. (2006). What do we know about health care team effectiveness? A review of the literature. *Medical Care Research and Review, 63,* 263–300.

Lingard, L., Regehr, G., Orser, B., Reznick, R., Baker, G.R., Doran, D., et al. (2008). Evaluation of a preoperative checklist and team briefing among surgeons, nurses, and anesthesiologists to reduce failures in communication. *Archives of Surgery, 143,* 12–17.

Marks, M. A., Mathieu, J. E., & Zaccaro, S. J. (2001). A temporally based framework and taxonomy of team processes. *Academy of Management Review, 26*(3), 356–376.

Mathieu, J. E., Marks, M. A., & Zaccaro, S. J. (2001). Multiteam systems. *International handbook of work and organizational psychology, 2,* 289–313.

Maxfield, D., Grenny, J. Lavandero, R., & Groah, L. (2005). *The Silent Treatment.* Retrieved from http://www.silenttreatmentstudy.com/silencekills/.

McGrath, J. E. (1984). *Groups: Interaction and performance.* Englewood Cliffs, NJ: Prentice-Hall.

O'Daniel, M. & Rosenstein, A. H. (2008). Professional communication and team collaboration. In Hughes, R. G. (2008). Chapter 33: Professional Communication and Team Collaboration. *Patient safety and quality: An evidence-based handbook for nurses vol 1* (pp. 271–284). Agency for Healthcare Quality and Research, Rockville, MD.

Poole, M. S. (2014). Systems Theory. *The SAGE handbook of organizational communication* (pp. 49–74). Thousand Oaks, CA: Sage.

Poole, M. S. & Real, K. (2003). Groups and teams in health care: Communication and effectiveness. In T. L. Thompson, A. M. Dorsey, K. I. Miller, & R. Parrott (Eds.) *Handbook of health communication* (pp. 369–402). Mahwah, NJ: Lawrence Erlbaum Publishers.

Ramanujam, R. & Rousseau D. (2006). The challenges are organizational not just clinical. *Journal of Organizational Behavior, 27,* 811–827.

Real, K. & Poole, M. S. (2011). Health care teams: Communication and effectiveness. In T. L. Thompson, R. Parrott, & J. Nussbaum (Eds.) *The Routledge handbook of health communication* (2nd ed., pp. 100–116). New York: Routledge.

Salas, E., Sims, D. E., & Burke, C. S. (2005). Is there a "Big Five" in teamwork? *Small Group Research, 36*(5), 555–599.

Salas, E., Cooke, N. J., & Rosen, M. A. (2008). On teams, teamwork, and team performance: Discoveries and developments. *Human Factors: The Journal of the Human Factors and Ergonomics Society, 50*(3), 540–547.

Squires, D. A. (2011). The US health system in perspective: A comparison of twelve industrialized nations. *Issue Brief (Commonwealth Fund), 16*, 1.

Taplin, S. H., Foster, M. K., & Shortell, S. M. (2013). Organizational leadership for building effective health care teams. *The Annals of Family Medicine, 11*(3), 279–281.

University of Kentucky News (2014). *Gill Heart Institute Nurse's Skills Contribute to Patient Care.* Retrieved from http://uknow.uky.edu/content/gill-heart-institute-nurses-skills-contribute-patient-care.

Weaver, S. J., Dy, S. M., & Rosen, M. A. (2014). Team-training in healthcare: A narrative synthesis of the literature. *BMJ Quality & Safety, 23*(5), 359–372.

World Health Organization (2010). *Framework for action on interprofessional education and collaborative practice.* Geneva: WHO Press.

Zimring, C. M., Ulrich, R. S., Zhu, X., DuBose, J. R., Seo, H. B., Choi, Y. S., . . . & Joseph, A. (2008). A review of the research literature on evidence-based healthcare design. *Health Environments Research & Design, 1*(3), 15–37.

5

DECISION-MAKING IN MEDICAL TEAMS

Torsten Reimer, Tillman Russell, and
Christopher Roland

Dr. James Jaggers, transplant surgeon at Duke University Hospital, gasped in terror upon receiving the immunology lab technician's call: the new organs freshly implanted in young Jesica Santillan's body did not match her blood type. In February of 2003, a team of twelve doctors and nurses, responsible for successfully performing Jesica's heart and double-lung transplant, fatally neglected to check the match of her blood type with her donor. Instead of publically announcing the tragedy, the hospital decided to keep quiet and search for a donor internally. Jesica's body rapidly deteriorated. After roughly two weeks, she finally received a second transplant, but it was too late. Jesica had suffered irreversible brain damage and was in a vegetative state, prompting the excruciating decision of attending physician Dr. Eva Grayck to turn off the machine keeping Jesica alive (see Kopp, 2003).

In the aftermath of Jesica's death, Duke University Hospital performed a root cause analysis of the medical team's performance to pinpoint when and why the error occurred and to prevent future occurrences (Diflo, 2006). Analyses revealed a breakdown in communication amongst medical team members. Specifically, the procurement coordinator did not relay Jesica's blood type to the transplant surgeon nor did the transplant surgeon request this information from the procurement coordinator. Likewise, after procuring the organs from New England, the procurement surgeon returned to Duke where neither the blood type, nor the donor, was confirmed until the operation was nearly complete (Diflo, 2006). Official review of this tragedy resulted in the institution of changes in organ donation and transplant procedures on a global scale (Diflo, 2006).

Like police, fire-fighting, and military teams, medical teams routinely perform tasks in which faulty decision-making can have dire consequences, a fact gravely illustrated by Jesica's preventable demise (Cannon-Bowers, Salas, & Converse, 1993). In this chapter, we review research on medical teams demonstrating that communication and coordination amongst the members of those teams is critical for their performance (e.g., see Tschan, Semmer, Hunziker, & Marsch, 2011). The tragedy of Jesica Santillan's death illustrates how task-relevant information processing can be derailed by a team's failure to communicate, process, and integrate critical information. Ample research on professional teams including medical teams has been conducted within an input-process-output framework (Forsyth, 2010; Real & Poole, 2011) and has been described through an information-processing lens (e.g., see Reimer, Park, & Hinsz, 2006; Russell & Reimer, 2015). We follow this tradition by focusing on the effects of input variables and processing characteristics on a specific outcome, the decisions that are made by medical teams.

Many of the organizational and psychological variables that have been studied in research on decision-making in medical teams can be classified into one of three categories (see Figure 5.1 for an overview): (a) characteristics of the task environment (e.g., time pressure and coordination requirements); (b) the structure of the team (e.g., team size and composition); and (c) process variables that characterize team interaction (e.g., information sharing and transactive memory systems). In the following sections, we use these three categories to review and integrate research pertinent to information processing and decision-making in medical teams. Thereby, we repeatedly refer to two interrelated themes: first, we reflect on how the described theories and empirical studies can be translated into practice by health organizations to improve medical decision-making; and second, we explicitly describe boundaries and additional factors that have to be taken into account when applying the described models. We will conclude with a discussion of the ecological rationality of the described models and highlight some key lessons that can be learned from the reviewed literature on decision-making in medical teams.

Task Environment

As the events surrounding Jesica Santillan's death tragically underline, medical teams often operate under complex, stressful environments with high information load (Tschan et al., 2011). The highly precarious and perilous working conditions of these task environments can easily increase vulnerability to faulty team decision-making (Russell & Reimer, 2015; Salas, Burke, & Samman, 2001). In this section, we focus on two task characteristics that frequently pose immense challenges to medical teams: time pressure and the coordination requirements of their task environment.

Time Pressure

Medical teams often work under stress. This holds in particular for surgery teams, emergency teams, and intensive care unit (ICU) teams who often have to make

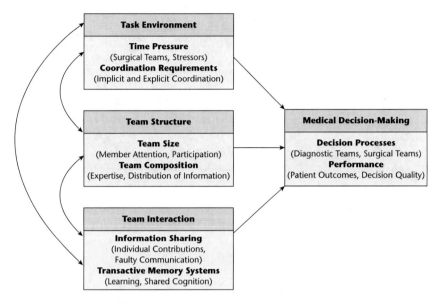

FIGURE 5.1 Overview of Medical Team Decision-Making.

decisions under high time pressure and information load. Research exploring the impact of acute and chronic environmental stressors on nurses and doctors in ICU teams found that recognition of potential patient fatality contributes to team member workload and stress (Piquette, Reeves, & LeBlanc, 2009). In addition to the intense and unpredictable environmental demands, team members' awareness that one wrong decision could cause patient fatality adds to their level of stress (Piquette et al., 2009).

Along with other stressors, time pressure is a key environmental parameter that can impair the quality of medical decisions. Medical team research that explored the effect of time pressure on nurses' decision-making performance in acute care found that time pressure reduced nurses' ability to detect the need of appropriate intervention and also the tendency to report this need (Thompson et al., 2008).

Time pressure can increase the quantity and severity of communication and decision errors. Research investigating teams in other high-stakes environments suggests that most teams under intense time pressure do not simply employ slow, analytic decision-making strategies, but rather look for cues which signal a situation is similar to one experienced in the past (Klein, 1997; Salas et al., 2001; Simon, 1987). If the cue(s) signal the presence of a similar environment, the team will make a similar decision based on this evidence (Klein, 1997; Simon, 1987). These team decision-making strategies decrease the experience of stress under time pressure and the need for excessive cognitive expenditure (Salas et al., 2001).

Another strategy to deal with high time pressure consists in the reliance on experts. With increased time pressure, nurses have been shown to rely more on colleagues with clinical experience for advice on making the best decision given the circumstances (McCaughan, Thompson, Cullum, Sheldon, & Thompson, 2002; Parahoo, 2000; Retsas, 2000). Use of such a frugal decision heuristic (i.e., "follow-the-expert") may be adaptive for medical teams under environmental constraints such as time pressure (Reimer & Hoffrage, 2006; Reimer, Mata, & Stoecklin, 2004). Critically, the follow-the-expert heuristic, as well as strategies that capitalize on the success of past behaviors and routines, hinge on the ability of medical team members to identify experts as well as the ability to be adaptive and to recognize changes in the environment (Tschan et al., 2011; Reimer, Bornstein, & Opwis, 2005).

Coordination Requirements

Medical teams have to coordinate their actions. This can typically be done in various ways. Importantly, the way medical teams coordinate their behaviors should match the demands of the task to be effective. For example, surgical teams typically do not only work under high time pressure but, at the same time, they also have to process large amounts of quantitative information. The information also has to be monitored, updated, and communicated often because surgical teams typically have different experts and personnel joining the team only for part of the procedure (Bogenstätter et al., 2009). The coordination requirements for these teams are very different from the coordination requirements of a diagnostic team that tries to come up with a diagnosis. Ideally, medical teams select different decision-making procedures and strategies for those two situations.

Tschan et al. (2011) conducted a study with medical professionals in which they tested if groups adapt their strategies to the task demands. They simulated two different situations. The first scenario was a cardiac arrest scenario that required resuscitation. In this situation, the diagnosis was clear and task requirements were prescribed by guidelines. Time pressure was high. Thus, the situation called for decisive action with minimal delays. A directive leadership style was most appropriate. The second scenario was a diagnostic task scenario in which the diagnosis was difficult and team members had conflicting cues. This second scenario called for explicit reasoning and a more democratic leadership style that explicitly invited contributions from team members. The authors reasoned that in the diagnostic task, members should share their information with the whole team and "talk to the room." A micro-analysis of the coordination behaviors in those two scenarios supported the authors' hypotheses and revealed that clear leadership was related to performance in the resuscitation but not the diagnostic task. Conversely, "talking to the room" was related to performance in the diagnostic but not the resuscitation scenario.

Implicit vs. Explicit Coordination

High time pressure in medical teams increases the need for accurate and efficient anticipation of team member action. To be effective and help coordinate actions instead of impair group performance, communication itself has to be coordinated (Reimer, Neuser, & Schmitt, 1997). Teams who face similar stressful situations repeatedly can improve their coordination efforts by coordinating their actions explicitly and discussing their strategies in a training session under low time pressure conditions to prepare for implicit coordination processes during times of high time pressure.

Implicit coordination is coordination accomplished without need for overt communication of individual plans, activities, or responses (Macmillan, Entin, & Serfaty, 2004). Team members know who has to do what. Implicit coordination of team member knowledge, skills, and abilities typically requires, initially, that group members explicitly discuss their expertise and specific roles. During an initial phase of *explicit* coordination, team members discuss and coordinate individual team member plans, actions, and responses (Macmillan et al., 2004).

Implicit coordination provides advantages for teams under intense task load by reducing time and cognitive resource expenditure (Macmillan et al., 2004). Instead of each member having to continuously communicate situation and task-relevant information, the team possesses shared cognition, permitting rapid action with low communication overhead (Macmillan et al., 2004). Given past experience with team member conduct, proficiency, and talent, team members can anticipate how other members will respond. The effectiveness of this implicit or tacit coordination depends on the extent to which team members learn and make adjustments when their anticipations are incorrect (Wittenbaum, Stasser, & Merry, 1996).

Team Structure

Coordination requirements do not only depend on task characteristics but are also strongly affected by the size and composition of a team. Typically, groups differ along a number of compositional dimensions, including members' expertise and personalities, basic values and beliefs, cognitive capacity, gender, and race (Adamowicz et al., 2005).

According to research on diversity in groups, homogeneity of team members with regard to their objectives, knowledge, task representation, individual preferences, and choices is crucial to understanding information processing. In this section, we focus on two structural dimensions of medical teams that have been shown to influence team interactions and decision-making (see Figure 5.1): the size and composition of medical teams.

Team Size

Team size refers to the number of members who are involved in a medical procedure. Since medical teams often operate in dynamic environments, the number of team members can greatly vary and change during a procedure such as a surgery. While some research suggests larger medical teams yield more positive patient outcomes than smaller teams (Bower, Campbell, Bojke, & Sibbald, 2003; Haward et al., 2003; Lemieux-Charles & McGuire, 2006), advantages associated with greater team size are often attenuated by the increased likelihood of member distraction and inefficiency (Adamowicz et al., 2005; Russell & Reimer, 2015).

Increase in medical team size often causes a decrease in member participation and team effectiveness. Empirical studies with medical teams found a negative relationship between medical team size and team participation such that, as medical team size increases, team members tend to show a decrease in team task engagement (Lemieux-Charles & McGuire, 2006; Poulton & West 1999; Shortell et al., 2004; Vinokur-Kaplan, 1995). Other research has reported similar results with respect to team effectiveness. In their study of primary care quality improvement (QI) teams, Shortell et al. (2004) proposed a curvilinear relationship between size and team effectiveness. In their study, increased team size was associated with increases in QI up to a certain threshold, but beyond this threshold, it was associated with decreases in QI.

The larger the size of a medical team, the more challenging are the communication and coordination processes and the development of shared mental models, consequently increasing the likelihood of communication and decision-making errors (Cassera, Zheng, Martinec, Dunst, & Swanström, 2009; Pendharkar, 2007). Palazzolo, Serb, She, Su, and Contractor (2006) found that team size was negatively associated with the average amount of communication amongst team members, expertise recognition accuracy, and knowledge differentiation.

It is also more challenging for large teams to be efficient than for small teams. Research shows, for example, that larger surgery teams need more time than smaller teams. Research investigating the impact of team size (operationalized as surgery team turnover rates) on surgery procedure time found that, independent of surgical complexity, as team size increased the surgical procedure time also increased (Cassera et al., 2009). Regression analyses showed that, accounting for variance contributed by all other variables, simply adding one individual to a surgical team increased procedure time by approximately 15 minutes. This increased time combined with high turnover rates decreases the likelihood that explicit communication will occur and shared team cognition will develop amongst team members. Teams that are too large easily lack effective and efficient implicit as well as explicit coordination which can greatly increase the likelihood of decision-making errors.

Team Composition

Team size is one important characteristic of the structure of medical teams that has been shown to influence group communication and a variety of outcome variables. The composition of medical teams is another important structural dimension that has effects on how teams process and discuss information, and ultimately, on their decisions. Typically, medical teams are highly diverse and consist of members that have different roles, education, tenure, and expertise. This diversity is necessary to perform complex tasks like a surgery but also poses various communication challenges to medical teams. The relationship between expertise diversity and task performance is often not linear but depends on other variables (Mannix & Neale, 2005).

Van der Vegt and Bunderson (2005), for example, found that team identification moderated the relationship between diversity and performance in multidisciplinary teams (also see Reale & Poole, this volume). The authors focused on multidisciplinary teams in the oil and gas industry that had similar characteristics like medical teams. They examined expertise diversity's relationship with team learning and team performance under varying levels of collective team identification. In teams with low collective identification, expertise diversity was negatively related to team learning and performance; where team identification was high, those relationships were positive.

Expertise diversity can only promote medical team performance if members are able to identify situations in which they should speak up because they have critical, task-relevant information that is not known to everybody. Larson, Christensen, Franz, and Abbott (1998) demonstrated that critical information is often not mentioned in diagnostic teams. Larson et al. (1998) asked physicians in teams of three to diagnose two hypothetical medical cases. Some of the information about each case was given to all team members prior to discussion (shared information), whereas the rest was divided among them (unshared information). The materials were constructed such that the teams had to consider some unshared information to be able to identify the most appropriate diagnosis. Team leaders were consistently more likely than other members to ask questions and to mention unshared information. Similar to many studies on hidden profiles in other domains, though, the authors observed that the medical teams had great difficulties identifying the most appropriate alternative (Christensen & Abbott, 2000; see Reimer, Reimer, & Hinsz 2010, for an exception).

This result was replicated in a follow-up study, in which the discussion of information among mixed-status clinical teams was examined while constructing differential diagnoses (Christensen et al., 2000). Twenty-four teams, each consisting of a resident, an intern, and a third-year medical student, were given two hypothetical patient cases to discuss and diagnose. The teams' overreliance on previously shared information and their inability to appropriately utilize unique information was detrimental when a correct diagnosis demanded the inclusion of such information. The authors concluded that clinical discussions that require the consideration of uniquely held information may be susceptible to error.

As the discussion of unshared information may affect group decisions, mechanisms that increase the likelihood that group members would discuss crucial unshared information items can be critical (Reimer, Reimer, & Czienskowski,

2010). Moreover, research suggests that the formation of strong and stable preferences prior to group discussion affects how groups deliberate about choice alternatives (Reimer & Hoffrage, 2012). Groups that are composed of members with strong preferences have a tendency to negotiate and integrate their individual preferences. Conversely, groups that enter discussions without individual preferences, focus more on information received at the meeting (Milch, Weber, Appelt, Handgraaf, & Krantz, 2009; Reimer et al., 2010). In situations in which it is crucial for a medical team to consider unshared information in order to be able to form good decisions, it may be wise to introduce a decision task as new business and to ask team members to deliberate without forming individual preferences and opinions. To increase decision quality, it may be necessary to compose teams based on the extent to which team members do have or do not have strongly formed preferences for a decision alternative prior to discussion. Omitting critical information can have tragic consequences as in Jesica's case in which the involved doctors did not discuss her blood type. In the following section, we look more closely at additional communication errors beyond the omission of critical information.

Team Interaction

Medical teams cannot achieve their goals and complete their tasks without effective and efficient communication. Similar to aircraft crews in the cockpit (Forsyth, 2010), tragedies in the operation room and other medical settings have been repeatedly attributed to communication failures and errors (Greenberg et al., 2007). In this section, we discuss characteristics of the interaction and discussion within medical teams by focusing on two research areas that have been studied extensively: research on information sharing and on transactive memory systems (see Figure 5.1).

Information Sharing

As the case of Jesica Santillan illustrates, communication errors can cause major damage. Greenberg et al. (2007) conducted an extensive surgical review of communication breakdowns resulting in injury to patients. Of the 444 surgical malpractice claims reviewed, 60 were identified as being a direct consequence of communication error which resulted in harm to patients. Within those cases, the authors identified a total of 81 communication errors with a range of 1 to 6 errors per case. Omitting key pieces of information was a frequent problem (49%) but not the only one and not the most frequent one. The most frequent error referred to inconsistencies in practitioner's descriptions of a patient's status (74% of 60 cases). Inaccurate information transmission was identified in 44% of the studied cases. Uncertainty as to the roles, responsibility, or leadership of team members occurred in 58% of cases.

In a similar vein, Lingard et al. (2004) documented 421 communication events in an extensive field study in operating rooms (OR), finding that 30% had some failure in communication. Communication failures commonly concerned communication that was inappropriate to the situation (45%), inaccurate information (35%), not achieving communicative objectives (21%), and communication episodes in which key team member were not represented (24%). While not all communication failures adversely affect team outcomes, it was found that 36% of communication failures resulted in an observable effect on the OR system processes. These effects included inefficiency, tensions between team members, delay, inconvenience to patients, and error in OR procedures.

Information which is inaccurate or incomplete has emerged as a major issue in medicine (Ford, Killebrew, Fugitt, Jacobsen, & Prystas, 2006). Despite its pervasiveness, little research has examined the causes of errors in transmitting information. Utilizing a high-fidelity patient simulator, Bogenstätter et al. (2009) studied the causes of information transmission error between first responding nurses and joining physicians in an emergency cardiac arrest incident. It was found that approximately 18% of the information that was transmitted to incoming responders was inaccurate—specifically information containing numerical values such as dosage frequency or defibrillation strength. Information that was older was less likely to be accurate as a consequence of the high memory load requirements of the cardiac arrest situation. Additionally, it was found that information which was explicitly communicated, such as transfer-appropriate encoded information (e.g., communicating the total rather than individual defibrillations), was strongly associated with greater information accuracy. This research suggests that communication which can alleviate constraints on working memory is integral for medical practitioners.

The described studies illustrate the profound importance of communication and the grave implications its misuse can have in professional medical settings. Team communication is particularly important when complex task demands necessitate increased team information processing effort. Several research programs—including research on shared mental models (SMM) and transactive memory systems (TMS)—pointed out that the key to high team performance in such situations is the development of a shared understanding of the task, the individual members' goals, expertise and roles, and of teamwork, which facilitate implicit coordination.

Transactive Memory Systems

Several studies demonstrate the relevance of transactive memory systems for medical teams. In a transactive memory system, team members rely on each other as sources of task-relevant information. Transcending the confines of any individual team member memory store, a transactive memory system involves members interdependently utilizing each other's knowledge and expertise to complete organizational tasks.

To develop an effective TMS, teams should be trained together or have at least opportunities to work together repeatedly. Using a cardiopulmonary resuscitation (CPR) simulation, Hunziker et al. (2009) compared the performance of pre-formed first responder teams with prior team-building experience against emergent, ad hoc first responder teams. The authors found that ad hoc team performance and decision-making were less effective compared to pre-formed teams, providing less hands-on care and delayed shock treatments. The results mimic findings of studies that have been conducted in the manufacturing industry (Liang, Moreland, & Argote, 1995). Liang et al. (1995) found that teams that learned together how to assemble radios developed better-structured and more accurate transactive memory systems and had higher performance scores later on compared to teams in which members learned the same procedure individually.

Research on transactive memory systems underlines that accurate, shared meta-knowledge about "who knows what" may assist professional teams in mastering complex tasks. In line with this assumption, studies have shown that groups which can accurately detect the expertise of other group members tend to make better decisions (Littlepage, Schmidt, Whistler, & Frost, 1995).

Transactive memory systems are effective to the extent they are accurate. Tschan et al. (2009) found evidence of an illusory transactive memory system in newly formed medical teams. Using an emergency diagnostic simulation based on a patient simulator, the study assessed the diagnosis and decision-making of 20 groups composed of physicians. Analysis uncovered that many diagnoses were inaccurate as a consequence of a false assumption; namely, that the physician who possessed important, decision-relevant information would share it. Group members developed an illusory transactive memory system by forming the false assumption that when another group member has important and relevant information they will communicate it.

The study by Tschan et al. (2009) demonstrates that inaccurate meta-cognitive assumptions can impair group performance. Likewise, Burtscher, Kolbe, Wacker, and Manser (2011) found evidence suggesting that the similarity and accuracy of team mental models affected team performance in anesthesia. Thirty-one two-person teams consisting of anesthesia residents and anesthesia nurses were video-taped during a simulated anesthesia induction. Team mental models were assessed with a concept-mapping technique. As expected, the study revealed that team mental model similarity and accuracy affected team performance.

Ecological Rationality: The Match Between Decision Strategies and Characteristics of the Environment

Many decisions in the health care system are made by teams and groups. Medical decision-making involves gathering, sharing, and processing information with the goal of collective response. Compared to individuals, groups provide increased memory capacity, augmented information exchange, and enhanced information-processing capabilities (Hollingshead, 2001; Hautz, Kämmer, Schauber, Spies, & Gaissmaier, 2015). We reviewed research that indicates that medical teams do have much in common with other professional groups and outlined how some common observations in professional groups apply to medical teams. From an organizational perspective, it is important to see which tasks medical teams typically face to be able to identify and develop decision strategies that match the requirements of the task.

Unfortunately, there is not one simple strategy or recipe that guarantees the best medical decisions in all situations and under all circumstances. Rather, the challenge for medical teams (as for individual health care professionals) consists in selecting decision strategies that are adaptive (see Kämmer, Gaissmaier, Reimer, & Schermuly, 2014). The goal should be to adapt decision strategies to the requirements of the task and the medical setting and to form decisions that are ecologically rational (Rieskamp & Reimer, 2007; Todd & Gigerenzer, 2012). Whenever possible, organizations should shape the information environment and decision context such that they are as decision-maker friendly as possible. An important outcome of the research tradition on ecological rationality consists in the insight that decision-making can be greatly facilitated by developing decision models and tools that do not only provide good decisions but are also highly transparent and easy to use and communicate. For example, researchers and practitioners have developed fast and frugal decision trees that help form a diagnosis in areas in which decisions routinely have to be made under time pressure. Specifically, Fischer et al. (2002) developed a simple heuristic to form a decision on whether children with community-acquired pneumonia should be prescribed macrolides. The heuristic only looks at a child's age and for how long a child had fever to make this decision. Likewise, Green and Meehl (1997) suggested a fast and frugal decision tree for deciding whether or not a patient has a high risk of ischemic heart disease and should thus be sent to the coronary care unit. Both models have replaced more complex decision procedures that had been used before. The new decision tools are much more frugal and, thus, they can be learned and applied as well as communicated much more easily than more complex models.

Decision strategies that are as elegant and user-friendly as those developed by Fischer and colleagues (2002) and by Green and Meehl (1997) do not exist for many decision-making situations. Hopefully, more frugal models will be developed and tested in the future, including fast and frugal heuristics for groups and teams (see Reimer & Hoffrage, 2012). The study of ecological rationality prompts us to focus our attention not only on the decider but also on the environment. In this context, the following classification of frequent environments and tasks for medical teams is very helpful.

Manthous and Hollingshead (2011) described scenarios for three critical care situations: resuscitations, daily rounds, and quality control teams. The authors demonstrate that these medical scenarios have certain task characteristics which necessitate specific organizational responses and leadership styles.

The *resuscitation* scenario is extremely critical and time-sensitive and decisions have immediate, life-or-death implications on patients being treated. As a consequence, an autocratic leadership style is most appropriate. This style reinforces the accountability and accuracy of team members which this high-stakes situation demands. At times, this situation requires team members to advance beyond their typical roles, so the development of a shared understanding of the team's task and composition of expertise should be facilitated.

Daily rounds are characterized by short- but not immediate-term responses which have critical implications on the life of patients. As this situation encompasses much of the time that team members spend together, it represents an excellent team-building opportunity. As a result, this situation asks for a democratic rather than an autocratic leadership style. With a highly distributed knowledge base which develops on daily rounds, psychological safety is required to promote team members to contribute while team members should simultaneously be accountable to share their best ideas with the team.

Finally, *quality control* teams are composed of multi-disciplinary members tasked with innovating new medical practices and addressing systemic problems. This situation is defined by low time constraints, and the team processes are non-emergent. As a result, team leaders should benefit from employing democratic approaches. According to the authors, ideally, all approaches should promote psychological safety to ensure that members are comfortable contributing to team initiatives and share critical information. Classifications like the one by Manthous and Hollingshead (2011) help us understand the specific requirements for team functioning and to enable medical teams to adapt their strategies.

Recommendation for Organizations and Practitioners

Medical teams often operate in health care environments with high time pressure and high information processing demands. How can health organizations and practitioners assist their medical teams in performing at their peak under such workplace demands? Teams must learn to adapt their decision-making strategies to match environmental constraints. Team training sessions can provide an important way for teams to increase the effectiveness of decision strategy adaptation. Conducted for new medical team members, team training sessions may focus on learning the most important cues relevant to decision-making under different medical situations. Training which emphasizes cue learning can facilitate improvement of medical team decision-making in actual workplace scenarios. Training should also facilitate the development of differentiated and accurate transactive memory systems and provide opportunities for teams to explicitly discuss coordination strategies for high-stress situations and develop routines where appropriate.

As the reviewed literature demonstrates, the effectiveness of medical teams in terms of patient outcomes as well as team efficiency and coordination are greatly influenced by the effectiveness of team member communication. Practitioners can benefit from noting that effective communication is measured by the quality rather than the mere amount of communication. Practitioners should work to develop a shared understanding of the information and expertise that each team member provides in order to ensure that all relevant information is considered.

Typically, what is shared among group members will more strongly affect a group's decision than that which is not shared (Kerr and Tindale, 2004). This impact of sharing includes team members' factual knowledge and also pertains to the sharing of concepts, preferences, and individual choices. The strategic use of team members' expertise and diversity provides an important tool for organizations. The literature on decision-making in medical teams demonstrates that the size and composition of teams can greatly affect team functioning and decision-making. These characteristics should be taken into consideration when forming teams and assigning decision tasks to teams.

These research findings on medical teams can be easily applied. The wise application of the reviewed literature may help reduce the risk of medical catastrophes like the heartrending death of Jesica Santillan. In Jesica's case, a faulty transactive memory system, coordination problems, and a failure of communication were at the heart of the decision-making catastrophe. The transplant surgeon, procurement coordinator, and the procurement surgeon all failed to request or check the match of Jesica's blood type with her donor based on faulty assumptions about the intentions and actions of other team members (Diflo, 2006).

The grim price Jesica paid for the medical team decision-making error illustrates the importance of communication and task-relevant information processing in medical teams. Effective communication and decision-making in medical teams can be extremely perilous given the unique contextual constraints intrinsic to typical medical team situations. A more accurate and comprehensive understanding of how task characteristics, team structure, and team process variables affect medical team performance can contribute to preventing tragedies like Jesica's. An adequate understanding of how each of these classes of variables affects team performance can assist in the important team duty of learning to select and develop decision strategies that match the complex task requirements of medical teams.

DISCUSSION QUESTIONS

1. What are typical decisions that are made by medical teams?
2. What are common challenges that medical teams face when they form decisions?
3. How does communication affect the quality of decisions in medical teams, and how can communication processes be improved?
4. How can the concept of ecological rationality help organizations facilitate decision-making in medical teams?

Suggested Reading

Manthous, C. A. & Hollingshead, A. B. (2011). Team science and critical care. *American Journal of Respiratory and Critical Care Medicine, 184*(1), 17–25.

Tschan, F., Semmer, N. K. Hunziker, S., & Marsch, S. U. (2011). Decisive action vs. joint deliberation: Different medical tasks imply different coordination requirements. In V. G. Duffy. (Ed.). *Advances in human factors and ergonomics in healthcare* (pp. 191–200). Boca Raton: Taylor & Francis.

References

Adamowicz, W. A., Hanemann, M., Swait, J., Johnson, R., Layton, D., Regenwetter, M., Reimer, T., & Sorkin, R. (2005). Decision strategy and structure in households: A "groups" perspective. *Marketing Letters, 16,* 387–399.

Bogenstätter, Y., Tschan, F., Semmer, N., Spychiger, M., Breuer, M., & Marsch, S. (2009). How accurate is information transmitted to medical professionals joining a medical emergency? A simulator study. *Human Factors, 51,* 115–125.

Bower, P., Campbell, S., Bojke, C., & Sibbald, B. (2003). Team structure, team climate and the quality of care in primary care: An observational study. *Quality and Safety in Health Care, 12,* 273–279.

Burtscher, M. J., Kolbe, M., Wacker, J., & Manser, T. (2011). Interactions of team mental models and monitoring behaviors predict team performance in simulated anesthesia inductions. *Journal of Experimental Psychology: Applied, 17,* 257–269.

Cannon-Bowers, J. A., Salas, E., & Converse, S. A. (1993). Shared mental models in expert team decision making. In N. J. Castellan, Jr. (Ed.), *Individual and group decision making: Current issues* (pp. 221–246). Hillsdale, NJ: Lawrence Erlbaum Associates.

Cassera, M. A., Zheng, B., Martinec, D. V., Dunst, C. M., & Swanström, L. L. (2009). Surgical time independently affected by surgical team size. *The American Journal of Surgery, 198,* 216–222.

Christensen, C. & Abbott, A. S. (2000). Team medical decision making. In G. B. Chapman, & F. A. Sonnenberg (Eds.), *Decision making in health care: Theory, psychology, and applications* (pp. 183–210). Cambridge, UK: Cambridge University Press.

Christensen, C., Larson, J. R., Abbott, A., Ardolino, A., Franz, T., & Pfeiffer, C. (2000). Decision making of clinical teams: Communication patterns and diagnostic error. *Medical Decision Making, 20,* 45–50.

Diflo, T. (2006). The transplant surgeon's perspective on the bungled transplant. In K. Wailoo, J. Livingston, & P. Guarnaccia (Eds.), *A death retold: Jesica Santillan, the bungled transplant, and paradoxes of medical citizenship* (pp. 70–81). Chapel Hill, NC: University of North Carolina Press.

Fischer, J. E., Steiner, F., Zucol, F., Berger, C., Martignon, L., Bossart, W., Altwegg, M., & Nadal, D. (2002). Use of simple heuristics to target macrolide prescription in children with community-acquired pneumonia. *Archives of Pediatrics & Adolescent Medicine, 156,* 1005–1008.

Ford, C. D., Killebrew, J., Fugitt, P., Jacobsen, J., & Prystas, E. M. (2006). Study of medication errors on a community hospital oncology ward. *Journal of Oncology Practice, 2,* 149–154.

Forsyth, D. R. (2010). *Group dynamics* (5th edition). Belmont, CA: Cengage.

Green, L. A. & Meehl, D. R. (1997). What alters physicians' decisions to admit to the coronary care unit? *Journal of Family Practice, 45,* 219–226.

Greenberg, C. C., Regenbogen, S. E., Studdert, D. M., Lipsitz, S. R., Rogers, S. O., Zinner, M. J., & Gawande, A. A. (2007). Patterns of communication breakdowns resulting in injury to surgical patients. *Journal of the American College of Surgeons, 204*, 533–540.

Hautz, W. E., Kämmer, J. E., Schauber, S. K., Spies, C. D., & Gaissmaier, W. (2015). Diagnostic performance by medical students working individually or in teams. *JAMA, The Journal of the American Medical Association, 313*, 303–304.

Haward, R., Amir, Z., Borrill, C., Dawson, J., Scully, J., West, M., & Sainsbury, R. (2003). Breast cancer teams: The impact of constitution, new cancer workload, and methods of operation on their effectiveness. *British Journal of Cancer, 89*, 15–22.

Hollingshead, A. B. (2001). Cognitive interdependence and convergent expectations in transactive memory. *Journal of Personality and Social Psychology, 81*, 1080–1089.

Hunziker, S., Tschan, F., Semmer, N. K., Zobrist, R., Spychiger, M., Breuer, M., Hunziker, P. R., & Marsch, S. C. (2009). Hands-on time during cardiopulmonary resuscitation is affected by the process of teambuilding: A prospective randomised simulator-based trial. *BMC Emergency Medicine, 9*, 3.

Kämmer, J., Gaissmaier, W., Reimer, T., & Schermuly, C. C. (2014). The adaptive use of recognition in group decision making, *Cognitive Science, 38*, 911–942.

Kerr, N. L. & Tindale, R. S. (2004). Group performance and decision making. *Annual Review of Psychology, 55*, 623–655.

Klein, G. (1997). The recognition-primed decision (RPD) model: Looking back, looking forward. In C. E. Zsambok & G. Klein (Eds.). *Naturalistic decision making* (pp. 285–292). Hillsdale, NJ: Lawrence Erlbaum Associates, Inc.

Kopp, C. (2003, March 16). The anatomy of a mistake. *CBS News*. Retrieved from http://www.cbsnews.com/news/anatomy-of-a-mistake-16-03-2003/.

Larson Jr., J. R., Christensen, C., Franz, T. M., & Abbott, A. S. (1998). Diagnosing groups: The pooling, management, and impact of shared and unshared case information in team-based medical decision making. *Journal of Personality and Social Psychology, 75*, 93–108.

Lemieux-Charles, L. & McGuire, W. L. (2006). What do we know about health care team effectiveness? A review of the literature. *Medical Care Research and Review, 63*, 263–300.

Liang, D. W., Moreland, R., & Argote, L. (1995). Group versus individual training and group performance: The mediating role of transactive memory. *Personality and Social Psychology Bulletin, 21*, 384–393.

Lingard, L., Espin, S., Whyte, S., Regehr, G., Baker, G. R., Reznick, R., Bohnen, J., Orser, B., Doran, D., & Grober, E. (2004). Communication failures in the operating room: An observational classification of recurrent types and effects. *Quality and Safety in Health Care, 13*, 330–334.

Littlepage, G. E., Schmidt, G. W., Whistler, E. W., & Frost, A. G. (1995). An input-process-output analysis of influence and performance in problem-solving groups. *Journal of Personality and Social Psychology, 69*, 877–889.

MacMillan, J., Entin, E. E., & Serfaty, D. (2004). Communication overhead: The hidden cost of team cognition. In E. Salas & S. M. Fiore (Eds.), *Team cognition: Understanding the factors that drive process and performance* (pp. 61–82). Washington, DC: American Psychological Association.

Manthous, C. A. & Hollingshead, A. B. (2011). Team science and critical care. *American Journal of Respiratory and Critical Care Medicine, 184*, 17–25.

Mannix, E. A. & Neale, M. A. (2005). What differences make a difference? The promise and reality of diverse teams in organizations. *Psychological Science in the Public Interest, 6*, 31–55.

McCaughan, D., Thompson, C., Cullum, N., Sheldon, T. A., & Thompson, D. R. (2002). Acute care nurses' perceptions of barriers to using research information in clinical decision-making. *Journal of Advanced Nursing, 39*, 46–60.

Milch, K. F., Weber, E. U., Appelt, K. C., Handgraaf, M. J., & Krantz, D. H. (2009). From individual preference construction to group decisions: Framing effects and group processes. *Organizational Behavior and Human Decision Processes, 108*, 242–255.

Palazzolo, E. T., Serb, D. A., She, Y., Su, C., & Contractor, N. S. (2006). Coevolution of communication and knowledge networks in transactive memory systems: Using computational models for theoretical development. *Communication Theory, 16*, 223–250.

Parahoo, K. (2000). Barriers to, and facilitators of, research utilization among nurses in Northern Ireland. *Journal of Advanced Nursing, 31*, 89–98.

Pendharkar, P. C. (2007). A comparison of gradient ascent, gradient descent and genetic-algorithm-based artificial neural networks for the binary classification problem. *Expert Systems, 24*, 65–86.

Piquette, D., Reeves, S., & LeBlanc, V. R. (2009). Stressful intensive care unit medical crises: How individual responses impact on team performance. *Critical Care Medicine, 37*, 1251–1255.

Poulton, B. C. & West, M. A. (1999). The determinants of effectiveness in primary health care teams. *Journal of Interprofessional Care, 13*, 7–18.

Real, K. & Poole, M. S. (2011). Communication and effectiveness. In T. L. Thompson, R. Parrott, & J. F. Nussbaum (Eds.), *The Routledge handbook of health communication* (pp. 100–116). New York, NY: Routledge.

Reimer, T. (2001). Attributions for poor group performance as a predictor of perspective-taking and subsequent group achievement: A process model. *Group Processes and Intergroup Relations, 4*, 31–47.

Reimer, T., Bornstein, A. L., & Opwis, K. (2005). Positive and negative transfer effects in groups. In T. Betsch & S. Haberstroh (Eds.), *The routine of decision making* (pp. 175–192). Mahwah, NJ: Lawrence Erlbaum Associates.

Reimer, T. Park, E. S., & Hinsz, V. B. (2006). Shared and coordinated cognition in competitive and dynamic task environments: An information-processing perspective for team sports. *International Journal of Sport and Exercise Psychology, 4*, 376–400.

Reimer, T. & Hoffrage, U. (2006). The ecological rationality of simple group heuristics: Effects of group member strategies on decision accuracy. *Theory and Decision, 60*, 403–438.

Reimer, T. & Hoffrage, U. (2012). Simple heuristics and information sharing in groups. In R. Hertwig, U. Hoffrage, & the ABC Research Group (Eds.), *Simple heuristics in a social world* (pp. 266–286). New York: Oxford University Press.

Reimer, T., Mata, R., & Stoecklin, M. (2004). The use of heuristics in persuasion: Deriving cues on source expertise from argument quality. *Current Research in Social Psychology, 10*, 69–83.

Reimer, T., Neuser, A., & Schmitt, C. (1997). Unter welchen bedingungen erhöht die kommunikation zwischen den gruppenmitgliedern die koordinationsleitstung in einer kleingruppe? *Zeitschrift für Experimentelle Psychologie, 44*, 495–518.

Reimer, T., Reimer, A., & Czienskowski, U. (2010). Decision-making groups attenuate the discussion bias in favor of shared information: A meta-analysis. *Communication Monographs, 77*, 121–142.

Reimer, T., Reimer, A., & Hinsz, V. B. (2010). Naïve groups can solve the hidden-profile problem. *Human Communication Research, 36,* 443–467.

Retsas, A. (2000). Barriers to using research evidence in nursing practice. *Journal of Advanced Nursing, 31,* 599–606.

Rieskamp, J. & Reimer, T. (2007). Ecological rationality. In R. F. Baumeister & K. D. Vohs (Eds.), *Encyclopedia of social psychology* (pp. 273–275). Thousand Oaks, CA: Sage.

Russell, T. & Reimer, T. (2015). Risk communication in groups. In H. Cho, T. Reimer, & K. A. McComas (Eds.), *The SAGE handbook of risk communication* (pp. 272–287). Los Angeles, CA: SAGE.

Salas, E., Burke, C. S., & Samman, S. N. (2001). Understanding command and control teams operating in complex environments. *Information, Knowledge, Systems Management, 2,* 311–323.

Shortell, S. M., Marsteller, J. A., Lin, M., Pearson, M. L., Wu, S. Y., Mendel, P., Cretin, S., & Rosen, M. (2004). The role of perceived team effectiveness in improving chronic illness care. *Medical Care, 42,* 1040–1048.

Simon, H. A. (1987). Making management decisions: The role of intuition and emotion. *The Academy of Management Executive (1987–1989), 1,* 57–64.

Thompson, C., Dalgleish, L., Bucknall, T., Estabrooks, C., Hutchinson, A. M., Fraser, K., de Vos, R., Binnekade, J., Barrett, G., & Saunders, J. (2008). The effects of time pressure and experience on nurses' risk assessment decisions: A signal detection analysis. *Nursing Research, 57,* 302–311.

Todd, P. M. & Gigerenzer, G. (2012). *Ecological rationality: Intelligence in the world.* New York, NY: Oxford University Press.

Tschan, F., Semmer, N. K., Gurtner, A., Bizzari, L., Spychiger, M., Breuer, M., & Marsch, S. U. (2009). Explicit reasoning, confirmation bias, and illusory transactive memory: A simulation study of group medical decision making. *Small Group Research, 40,* 271–300.

Tschan, F., Semmer, N. K. Hunziker, S., & Marsch, S. U. (2011). Decisive action vs. joint deliberation: Different medical tasks imply different coordination requirements. In V. G. Duffy. (Ed.), *Advances in human factors and ergonomics in healthcare* (pp. 191–200). Boca Raton: Taylor & Francis.

Van der Vegt, G. S. & Bunderson, J. S. (2005). Learning and performance in multidisciplinary teams: The importance of collective team identification. *Academy of Management Journal, 48,* 532–547.

Vinokur-Kaplan, D. (1995). Treatment teams that work (and those that don't): An application of Hackman's group effectiveness model to interdisciplinary teams in psychiatric hospitals. *The Journal of Applied Behavioral Science, 31,* 303–327.

Wittenbaum, G. M., Stasser, G., & Merry, C. J. (1996). Tacit coordination in anticipation of small group task completion. *Journal of Experimental Social Psychology, 32,* 129–152.

6

IMPROVING PATIENT ACCRUAL TO RESEARCH STUDIES AND CLINICAL TRIALS THROUGH COMMUNICATION DESIGN INTERVENTIONS

Susan E. Morgan and Ashton Mouton

The effective treatment and cure of many diseases, including cancer, is largely dependent on the enrollment of adequate numbers of patients to clinical trials and other research studies. However, the rate of accrual to many important clinical trials is woefully inadequate, and a large number of otherwise promising trials are discontinued due to lack of patient participation (Kolata, 2009). While a number of studies point to patient-based barriers such as age, race/ethnicity, distrust of the medical system, altruistic ideals, mood at the time of recruitment, and socioeconomic-driven variables such as the availability of transportation to study sites and education/literacy levels (Schmotzer, 2012), other factors significantly impact the recruitment process as well. For example, there are also a number of physician-based impediments including financial disincentives for recruitment to clinical trials (such as loss of revenue stream due to referral out of practice), lack of commitment to a research mission, and negative physician attitudes toward a particular trial (IOM, 2012). Even in major hospitals, "encouraging participation is not part of their routine practice or . . . their priorities, quality plan, or metrics" (IOM, 2012, p. 67). Researchers have also pointed out that many physicians simply lack the ability to communicate well about research with their patients, and lack the knowledge to answer patient questions that might arise about a specific study (Ford et al., 2011; Paramasivan et al., 2011). In one study, cancer patients described a clinical trial communication process with physicians and staff that was characterized both by tremendous information overload and by gross over-simplification (Stevens & Ahmedzai, 2004).

Organizational Barriers to Patient Recruitment

In addition to provider- and patient-based issues, there are critical system-based organizational barriers to patient recruitment. These are quite varied in nature. First, most health care organizations where poor and underserved populations seek care do not have the infrastructure to support patient recruitment processes (Castel, Negrier, & Boissel, 2006; Green, White, Barry, Nease, & Hudson, 2005; Probstfield & Frye, 2011). Physicians working in academic medical settings are more likely to refer patients to clinical trials because of the availability of supportive infrastructure (Siminoff, Ravdin, Colabianchi, & Sturm, 2000). In contrast, most clinics do not have trained staff or the time needed to discuss studies with patients or to obtain informed consent. Signing patients up for studies is only the first step; once enrolled, staff must continue to invest the time needed to prevent patients from dropping out. "Substantial costs are necessary to enroll and retain diverse populations . . . For [minority and underserved populations] extra time is needed to gain individual and community acceptance. Balancing the need to enroll . . . understudied populations and developing outreach strategies to support their participation is an ongoing challenge" (Probstfield & Frye, 2011, p. 1798). Thus, simple organizational staffing issues—which nonetheless represent significant costs to the system—are to blame for a lack of accrual.

Second, it is very difficult and time-consuming to identify patients who might qualify for participating in particular research studies or trials (Cuggia, Besana, & Glasspool, 2011; IOM, 2012). Generally, there are a number of specific criteria that patients must meet in order to be considered for participation. For example, patients must often be of a particular age, have a certain medical condition (and either have or lack other co-morbidities), and so on. In order to assess whether patients meet these criteria, a staff member must go through individual patient files to scan all pertinent information and then flag the files of patients who are likely to be eligible for the study. Technology can potentially facilitate this process; automatic alert systems, which use electronic health records to flag patients who qualify for study participation, have already been developed (Cuggia et al., 2011; Embi et al., 2005; Kho, Zafar, & Tierney, 2007). Unfortunately, such systems are not only expensive, but there is little to no interoperability across different electronic health record (EHR) systems. This means that these alert systems have to be developed for each EHR system separately and, correspondingly, the details of each study or trial would have to be entered into every individual alert system (Cuggia et al., 2011).

Third, in addition to knowing the studies for which a patient qualifies, knowledge that a patient would be interested in participating in a clinical trial or research study is also very helpful to the clinical trial recruitment process. Previous participation in a research study or clinical trial is a strong predictor of subsequent interest in participation in future studies (Trauth, Jernigan, Siminoff, Musa, Neal-Ferguson, & Weissfeld, 2005; Schutt, Schapira, Maniates, Santiccioli, Henlon, & Bigby, 2010). This can easily be summed up with the old expression, "The best predictor of future behavior is past behavior." This necessitates, of course, a system that keeps track of past participation in research studies and perhaps aggregates participants into a pool from which they can be more easily contacted to enroll in future studies.

Fourth, physicians and clinic staff may be unconvinced of the benefits to patients that would be associated with study participation, or have strong feelings about the desirability of one treatment arm relative to another (IOM, 2012; Paramasivan et al., 2011; Probstfield & Frye, 2011; Ulrich et al., 2012). While this may appear to be a provider-based issue, some scholars have indicated that organizational culture may be to blame (Embi & Tsevat, 2012). Ironically, while physicians want to provide the "best" treatment for their patients, many are unwilling to participate in the (research) process of determining precisely which treatment is indeed the most effective. The organizational culture of many medical practices, even large hospitals, undervalues the importance of research and provides few rewards or recognitions to physicians who advance knowledge through research. Part of the blame may be due to the fact that medical training includes little on the process or importance of research, and few physicians are socialized to value the research process. What may be helpful is fostering more contact between enthusiastic investigators and the physicians from whose practices patients must be recruited. Currently, most of the principal investigators who create and lead studies generally have little or no contact with the physicians, nurses, and recruiters who discuss these studies with patients (Castel et al., 2006). However, when physicians have a sense of involvement with the research being conducted in their clinic or practice, they are far more supportive (Reed, Barton, Isherwood, Baxter, & Roeger, 2013).

At an even more basic level, the ways in which research studies and clinical trials are developed are problematic to the goal of physician support and involvement (IOM, 2012). A rheumatoid arthritis research network in Nebraska (the Rheumatoid Arthritis Investigational Network, or RAIN) was developed to remedy the problems associated with the usual top-down approach by bringing together practicing rheumatologists from across the region to discuss the most pressing questions that physicians have about the best ways to treat patients. These led to the development of research studies and trials to answer these questions, as well as protocols that met the approval of physicians' own patient populations. The results of these physician- and patient-centered studies were subsequently published in leading medical journals, demonstrating that researcher/scientist-initiated investigations are not the only means by which to create valuable medical insights.

Finally, the ways in which clinics are physically structured and the ways in which workflows are organized significantly impact the recruitment process (Reed et al., 2013). For example, recruitment in waiting rooms can be a way to minimize disruptions to the workflow (Bodurtha et al., 2007; see also Barbour, Gill, and Dean, this volume, and Harrison, this volume, for a discussion of space and design related to health and message processes). However, discussing a patient's qualifications for trial participation in this setting can present problems with maintaining patient privacy and confidentiality. This represents a fundamental tension that requires special attention. Nonetheless, the design of recruitment processes that minimize the impact of research on day-to-day operations is key to maintaining a positive relationship between (non-physician) recruiters and the staff of a medical practice (McSweeney, Pettey, Fischer, & Spellman, 2009).

While these issues exist regardless of the socioeconomic status of potential research participants, these barriers are particularly acute in the recruitment process of minority and underserved populations. For example, poverty compounds issues of access to clinical settings where recruitment for clinical trials and research studies generally takes place. Additionally, lower education and literacy levels inhibit the process of obtaining informed consent, requiring additional time from already-overburdened staff members, compounding staffing issues. At the same time, it is critical to have participation from all patients across racial, ethnic, and socioeconomic backgrounds in order to conduct valid tests of the efficacy of treatment protocols and other approaches to alleviating suffering from disease (see Aakhus and Harrison, this volume, for a discussion of how these barriers lead to structural violence). Thus, it is important to identify ways to facilitate the enrollment of underrepresented groups to research studies and clinical trials. Figure 6.1 illustrates the interplay of variables impacting successful recruitment of patients to clinical trials, including those experienced by physicians and patients, and those that are imposed by the system itself. The variables within the model that are potential sites of invention and intervention through Communication Design include:

- Infrastructure to support study enrollment and execution
- Barriers to (physician) participation, including the time needed to recruit patients and the disruption of clinic workflow caused by recruitment processes
- Knowledge that a patient is suitable for a study
- Complexity of trial/demand on physician
- Communication skills to describe the study
- Communication behaviors (physician recommendation of study, amount of information offered)
- Study offered to patient.

In this chapter, we pay particular attention to several systems-based barriers, including infrastructure support, identification of eligible patients, and key barriers to physician participation in the research study recruitment process. It should be said that while models help to identify the variables that require attention in order to improve outcomes, they cannot tell us how to accomplish

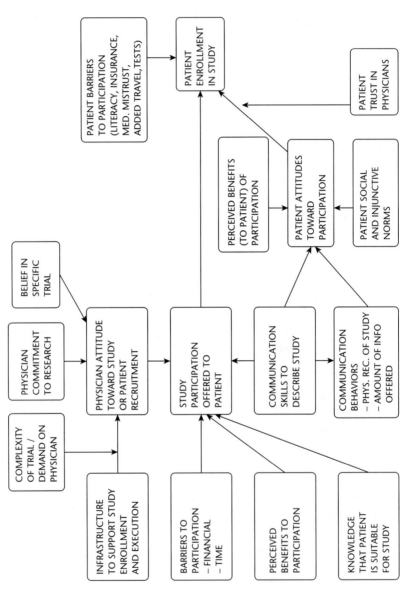

FIGURE 6.1 Model of Clinical Trial Accrual.

this change. However, Communication Design identifies a process by which to create new systems of interaction, using the variables specified in other theories or models (Harrison, 2014). Thus, it serves as a lens through which we can more clearly see current states and envision better ways of structuring systems of interaction.

Communication Design

Communication Design is an approach to organizing and communicating that has been underutilized in terms of its potential applications to organizational and health contexts. Because the Communication Design process is centered on transforming current practices (which are assumed as a "given" or "the way things are") into something that more closely matches "ideal" practices (Aakhus, 2007), this approach holds great promise for creating deliberate change in health care organizations, particularly those that serve underprivileged and underserved populations. Designing communication processes and interaction protocols with patients who have limited basic or health literacy and who may be intensely distrustful of the intentions of researchers seems to typify the kind of quandary that Aakhus (2007) has in mind when he describes the purpose of Communication Design:

> A central puzzle that people face, from a design perspective, is how to make communication possible that was once difficult, impossible or unimagined. Communication Design happens when there is an intervention into some ongoing activity through the invention of techniques, devices, and procedures that aim to redesign interactivity and thus shape the possibilities for communication. The relationship between interaction and communication, which is a central problem for communication theory, is a central problem for design.
>
> *(p. 112)*

Communication Design practices consider not only the negative consequences of poor communication protocols, but also the ideals to which they aspire. This is termed "design wisdom," which "shifts thoughts from focusing only on avoiding undesirable states to focusing on intentional actions that lead to states of reality which are desirable and appropriate" (Nelson & Stolterman, 2003, p. 17). Thus, Communication Design is the manifestation of larger (but often unrecognized) abstract principles and values, such as justice and equality. However, our Communication Design choices can serve to either match or contradict a core set of values. An exploration of existing communication protocols in health care organizations can reveal where better choices can be made in order to more faithfully represent social values and ideals.

Surprisingly, Communication Design has rarely been applied to health issues (for a couple of exceptions in the area of health communication campaign design, see Harrison et al., 2010; Harrison et al., 2011; Harrison, 2014), although there is considerable breadth of contexts to which it has been applied. These contexts include alternative dispute resolution processes (Harrison, 2003, 2004, 2007, 2013; Harrison & Doerfel, 2006; Harrison, Hopeck, Desrayaud, & Imboden, 2013), public deliberation processes (Aakhus, 2007), work processes (Ballard & McVey, 2014), and the operationalization of safety procedures (Barbour & Gill, 2014). Additionally, Jackson and Aakhus (2014) identify one drug abuse prevention intervention ("Keepin' it REAL") developed by Hecht and Miller-Day (see Hecht & Miller-Day, 2007) as closely adherent to Communication Design principles. In all areas of application, though, a Communication Design approach helps to highlight helpful and harmful practices, relative to the values held by society or the organizational system in which these processes are situated.

The efforts required to redesign communication practices and protocols can be well worth the trouble because such interventions can dramatically affect observed outcomes. For example, alternative dispute resolution systems such as mediation have carefully attended to issues like clearly defining conflict resolution processes, turn-taking in face-to-face discussions between disputants, and avoidance of interruptions, all of which serve to create a balance in the power held by each disputant (e.g., Aakhus, 2003; Harrison, 2014; Harrison and Morrill, 2004). This balance of power not only leads to greater engagement by all parties in a dispute, it creates greater trust in the organizations which use these systems, improves chances for repairing and restoring previously damaged relationships between organizational actors, and avoids the reification of existing power relationships (whereby the more powerful disputant imposes his or her will on the less powerful disputant).

Specifically related to our work on clinical trial recruitment, a Communication Design approach can be translated into specific communication protocols in the recruitment process for underprivileged/underserved populations. While the literature in the area of clinical trial and research study recruitment is fragmented, with widely divergent views of the source of problems with accrual, we have collected data from clinical trial recruiters themselves. This study represents one of the very few attempts to talk to people who are closest to the process of recruitment to obtain their views about the impact of organizations themselves on recruitment success. Using thematic analytic processes with NVivo, we analyzed transcripts from a pilot study of three focus groups of full-time professional clinical trial recruiters (N = 13). The recruiters in our study recruited primarily from underprivileged and underserved patient populations in diverse settings, including hospitals, clinics, patient homes, community-based settings (such as fairs and festivals), and over the phone.

The Impact of Health Systems on Clinical Trial Recruitment

Some of the above-mentioned system variables and communication issues have already been attended to through the creation of a system of professional recruiting by specialized employees often termed "research assistants" (RAs). These professional recruiters tend to be employed by a central agency or organization and are trained on the details of each study prior to the recruitment process (Kho, Zafar, & Tierney, 2007). In addition, the recruiters in our study receive de facto communication training through a shadowing process during the early months of their employment, and some receive additional training through seminars and conferences; however, they still experience organizational barriers in their recruitment work. In the passages that follow, barriers mentioned above are highlighted from the points of view of our participants, and then points of intervention from the perspective of Communication Design are highlighted.

First, recruiters experience a variety of system-based barriers to recruitment because of a lack of infrastructure to recruit, which is demonstrated in the following vignettes:

> Example 1, Genne: Where I'm at though, my office is in the basement. The patients are upstairs, so I can't ask someone who's 85 to come down to the basement, you know, to my office. So I have to find a spot within the clinic somewhere, a free spot, if I can find one, to recruit the patients. A lot of times, the clinic has, especially with the new system that they installed— it's supposed to be faster, more efficient for the patient, but it's not—we are waiting, the patients are waiting three and four hours to be seen sometimes. So now you're waiting for that patient because you don't have any place to recruit them, so you have to wait until they get into their room to recruit these patients.

> Example 2, Peter: The problem we have a lot is where it says contact, there is a section specifically for it, they put contact the doctor at, and the doctor's not at that number. It's the nursing staff or it's a front desk somewhere. Give a specific contact. Say contact this person, and give someone who is going to answer that, because when there are questions, we all know how hard it is to get ahold of the doctor let alone tie them down for 20–30 minutes asking questions.

> Example 3, Larissa: You guys are lucky, you guys have Spanish speakers. Like when I need a Spanish speaker, I have to pay someone hourly to work on my studies, you know, to make sure that it's cost-effective.

These comments illustrate some of the challenges that recruiters must overcome that are simply inherent to the physical set-up or geographic isolation of the clinic environment. Genne explains the struggles recruiters have with attaining a suitable space in the clinic to recruit or carry out recruitment procedures. In fact, many of our participants detailed struggles with recruiting in waiting rooms, time constraints in clinic rooms, and finding different places to recruit depending on the layout of the clinic. Peter highlights the challenges associated with time investment to make sure patients complete enrollment or stay enrolled in the study. When patients need more information from their doctor or the PI, the recruiters provide the contact information, but patients drop out or fail to sign up for a trial because they are unable to reach the person from the contact numbers. Finally, Larissa details the challenges with recruiting non-English speakers to trials because of the lack of staff to translate.

Second, recruiters experience system-based challenges in identifying eligible and interested patients, which the following passages highlight:

> Example 1, Janine: I think it's also important that [doctors] don't make assumptions about their patients and what they will or won't consent to. We just had that today at [Clinic]; the doctors don't think they have a Type II population there [. . .] It is the main population!
>
> Ronja: Tuesday when I was over there, there was four patients in there being seen for diabetes. There was four kids over there; they were there for diabetes.
>
> Janine: They assume that [the patients] are not going to want to do that.
>
> Example 2, Elizabeth: We get a page when there's an eligible patient in one of the five clinics, so five of the six of us have a pager at any time, and originally the proposal that one did is that that was the only way we could interview the patients is if we were in the clinic, got the page, or if we're out of clinic, got the page, but got to the clinic before the doctor went in the room after the patient was already in a private space, usually the exam room. So the farthest clinic is seven miles that way, the closest clinic is over there, but you have to park who knows where and run in. [. . .] So we sat down with the expectation of amending and suggested [. . .] the option of us being able to catch them on the phone if we miss them in the clinic, and in fact we've at this point recruited more people over the phone than we have in clinic.

Janine and Ronja recount how recruiters struggle with doctors who assume their patients are uninterested. On the other hand, some of the recruiters discussed the lack of barriers encountered when physicians provide a list of eligible patients for the recruiters to approach. Other innovative approaches have been implemented in addition to having doctors identify patients. However, Elizabeth explains that even when they have a programmed computerized system that identifies eligible patients when they check in at the clinic, organizational and system-based barriers prevent recruitment during the visit.

Third, physicians, nurses, and other clinic staff create barriers to successful clinical trial recruitment in the clinic setting. The following vignettes illustrate the complexities created for recruitment through relationships with physicians and other clinic staff.

> Example 1, Janine: There is often a big disconnect between the doctors who are in charge of the study and the staff. [. . .] And so getting into the facility to get around and recruit people, because just because the doctor has said we're gonna do the study does not mean that the staff is all aware, and you are in their clinic space and territory and all that. So you really need a lot of support from the person who's sending you there.

> Example 2, Veronica: The relationship with the physician, mostly if the physician is on board, everyone else kind of falls in place because we have gone to them and said this is the study, this is how long it will take and that we are not going to impede on your flow, [. . .] but once that doctor is on board, normally the staff will fall into place and they will say "she's here to do that study" and they kind of dictate the environment a lot, and it doesn't hurt to take them stuff too.

> Example 3, Veronica: I would say something that I get comments from physicians is they want to know your final paper, they would like to know what the results are, you know, I'd like you to follow up. Sometimes we don't always do that with the studies that we do. They constantly ask me, well how did it come out or we'd like to see it. So that's a big, I think that if they do that it would make things go so much better because they could see the end of the project. [. . .] We're in there all the time constantly with new projects and so just telling them the end result would be nice.

Janine identifies challenges in communication with physicians. She explains that while doctors give permission for recruiters to approach their patients, they do not often inform the rest of the clinic staff about the agreement. Other participants in our study described barriers associated with doctors forgetting about the recruiters or the study altogether. Another challenge stems from the doctor's relationships with their patients. Veronica, on the other hand, explains that a good relationship with the physician can aid recruitment practices because the doctor can impact the entire clinic. When the clinic as a whole is unaware of recruitment, organizational challenges are paramount.

Furthermore, some physicians would like incentives for their participation or would like to know the results of the study, and recruiters do not have the ability to grant incentives or share the PI's results. Similarly, nurses and other clinic staff also impact recruitment.

> Example 1, Lynette: A good introduction from the nurse to the patient can mean everything, like "oh this lady is going to come in and talk to you, she's really nice." Bang. In. No problem.

> Example 2, Larissa: You need to befriend the nurses. The nurses are your first line of defense and typically they have to go back in there after the doctor is done. [. . .] So if you talk to those nurses ahead of time. When you get there, just remind them, like I'm here today and kind of point them out, they'll keep them.

Lynette and Larissa explain the benefits of including nurses in the recruitment process, but all of the participants commented on the challenges to recruitment if nurses were not aware of the research process, did not know the recruiter, or felt as if the recruiters were in the way or invading their territory. Our participants also mentioned other clinic staff, such as medical assistants, who impacted recruitment, both positively and negatively.

Finally, clinic structure and workflow in the clinic also hinder recruitment in clinical trials, as illustrated in the following testimonies:

> Example 1, Larissa: So a lot of times I have just a brief window between the time the nurses finish vitals and sit them in the room until the resident or the physician comes in and so I just have to give it to them all in a nutshell, like this is what it is; this is what it truly is. If we have a pre-screener, they take the pre-screener, and if they're eligible, setting them up with the consent form, give them time to read through it, write down questions, but if you're interested when I come back, we'll talk about it.

> Example 2, Veronica: When they step into that room, no matter who it is, we have to leave, and I don't care what we're doing, so we have to; now sometimes, they have gotten comfortable with me and they say "you can stay" or they'll go into the next room and say "Veronica I'll let you stay" but that's over a long, long time. Years of communicating and everything.

> Example 3, Elizabeth: I will definitely not interrupt clinic flow. You can let me know anytime if I should go in and talk to somebody and I have another space set aside so if the person decides to participate, they can go in the dietician's room with me, we won't be taking up an exam room. But I think personalities aside, you can't control for that, it does take some time

for people and the staff in a busy clinic trying to, every week they have some new thing they have to do, some new regulation or whatever, to just earn their trust so that they see that you're not going to be one more thing that they have to worry about.

Evident in these testimonies is the barrier of space and time to recruit. Many of the recruiters talked at length about the amount of time they have to enter a room, recruit a patient, and then leave before the physician came in the room. Some recruiters, as evidenced in Larissa's description above, will go back into the room with the patient after the physician is done, but none of the recruiters will interrupt or delay a physician or nurse entering the patient's room. These problems are exacerbated when patients are late for appointments or when the clinic is behind schedule because there is even less time for recruitment in those situations.

Transformation/Redesign of the Recruitment System

Findings from this study constitute formative research which, when viewed through the lens of Communication Design, suggests a number of points of possible intervention. As stated above, a Communication Design approach, with the aim of redesigning interactivity, would find the points where transformation is possible to improve practices (Aakhus, 2007). We propose that a health care organization can be set up in such a way that communication about clinical trials and other research studies can be facilitated (or at least not impeded by barriers). The time required to make the offer of a clinical trial is already built into the design of the communication process of many clinics because professional recruiters approach patients to explain the details of the study and to obtain their written consent, as evidenced above. This addresses the understaffing issue with which many clinics (and trials seeking to enroll patients) struggle. However, the recruiters also experience barriers to successful recruitment.

Many of the communication issues they face (mentioned above) can be addressed within a Communication Design framework. First, addressing infrastructure concerns, a Communication Design intervention would facilitate identification of how clinical trial recruitment processes can be structured in ways that meet higher-order goals, such as the concern for patient safety and confidentiality in suitable spaces as well as the elimination of distractions that detract from comprehension of study information, which in turn enhances the likelihood of obtaining informed consent. In addition, a Communication Design intervention would identify contact information as well as translation services as potential sites for improvement and would structure future studies to eliminate these barriers through communication protocols. Second, when assessing how to find eligible and interested patients, a Communication Design intervention would target tools that both trigger and facilitate communication processes as important. Finding ways to improve current systems such as the computerized pager notifications or a registry that identifies eligible patients would be sites for communicative improvement. In addition, Communication Design approaches would also consider communication between PIs, physicians, nurses, and recruiters in the clinic. All of these actors influence recruitment for better or worse, and a Communication Design approach would identify which communicative behaviors create unnecessary barriers to recruitment. For example, if physicians and nurses need to know about recruitment procedures, a Communication Design intervention would suggest a specific protocol for introductions between recruiters and clinic staff at the initiation of each study. Finally, a Communication Design approach could identify moments in clinic flow which facilitate or impede recruitment of underserved populations and make suggestions for the improvement of patient flow.

Other Factors Impacting the Utilization of Communication Design in Health Care Organizations

The entirety of the Communication Design approach revolves around taking into account all of these considerations when creating improvements to communication processes. For example, the workflow of clinics is designed to maximize efficiency for physicians and creates certain difficulties for recruiters who want to talk to patients about research study participation. While recruiters have a fairly wide range of levels of educational attainment (high school degree to Master's degree), their lower status relative to physicians, nurses, and even other clinic staff members provides them with the least amount of power to assert themselves in this context, regardless of the legitimacy of their need for space and time with both patients and physicians (see Lammers & Proulx, this volume, Myers & Gaillard, this volume, and Barbour, Gill, & Dean, this volume, for further discussion of the role of status and professions in health care). The health care environment itself also poses restrictions on what recruiters can say to patients and where they can say it. For example, recruiters are constrained by the semi-public nature of waiting rooms and the need to maintain patient confidentiality about information about their illness (i.e., the very condition that would qualify them for study participation). Suitable space and support to speak with patients is crucial to recruitment. A Communication Design approach would highlight issues of space and confidentiality as points of transformation in the recruitment process.

Potential Pitfalls to Avoid

There are a number of potential pitfalls that may be avoided with careful attention to formative research as part of the Communication Design process.

One of the most important of these potential pitfalls is the unwitting incorpora-
tion of unintended consequences into the new system. "A new design brings
a shadow with it. There are always unintended consequences associated with
design, many of which are negative. This is related to another . . . [outcome]—
the loss of opportunities. When a design is brought into the world and made real,
its very presence excludes other opportunities" (Nelson & Stolterman, 2003,
p. 262). While insights from professional study recruiters help to illustrate key
Communication Design principles and help to advance theorizing in this context, we have to be cautious about simply adopting the recommendations that
are inherent in their perspectives. The following questions should be considered:
if we open up the clinic system more fully to recruitment, is there potential for
researchers to abuse/exploit the patient population? Would the extra time it takes
to recruit cut into the number of patients who can be seen by providers and/or
increase patient wait time more than in the status quo? These and other questions
should be seriously considered before interventions are implemented. Ultimately,
it is hoped that readers will deepen their understanding that simply "improving
communication" between patients and providers (or in this case, recruiters) is not
enough. Rather, it is critical to attend to communication processes and to delib-
erately intervene through Communication Design in order to improve desired
outcomes. At the same time, no amount of excellence in the design of communication protocols can substitute for the development of community partnerships
and outreach in minority and underserved communities (Michaels et al., 2011).

Future Theorizing of Communication Design and Clinical Trials

A Communication Design approach is closely related to a systems theory approach
in that it acknowledges that changing one set of practices may require addressing other interrelated issues (Nelson & Stolterman, 2003). Indeed, clinical trial
recruitment would likely be placed into the category of "wicked" problems rather
than "tame" ones, as it is the type of problem where each issue is symptomatic of
yet another complicated issue (Nelson & Stolterman, 2003). For example, limited
basic and health literacy prevents many people who belong to underprivileged
populations from understanding important information about specific research
and clinical trials from which they might benefit from participation. Addressing
the root of this problem would necessarily entail addressing issues of gross inequities in the quality of the U.S. educational system. Similarly, clinical trials that
require insurance coverage for participation inherently exclude those who do not
have adequate coverage (i.e., the poor and underserved); resolving this problem
requires universal access to health care. Future theorizing in the area of clinical
trial recruitment should attend to these systemic problems and identify potential areas for intervention. Multidisciplinary research in communication, policy,

health care, education, nursing, etc. is needed to address "wicked" problems associated with clinical trial recruitment of underserved populations.

Particularly instructive for the issue of research study recruitment is Ballard and McVey's (2014) study on the impact of temporality on work and interaction processes. Research recruiters in our study are primarily embedded in three time frames: the immediate recruitment process, which takes only minutes; the day-long rhythm of the work-life of the clinic; and a long-term relationship time frame, in which recruiters foster a sense of trust and friendly acquaintanceship with patients in order to ease the recruitment process for future studies with these same patients. The patients with whom recruiters interact, however, are embedded in somewhat different time frames which govern their research participation. In addition to the immediate recruitment process and a (possible) relationship time frame, patients are embedded in a time frame that governs their illness or medical condition, or at least their perception of it. Those with chronic diseases that last for years or a lifetime, such as diabetes, may respond differently to the offer of trial participation than those with temporally brief illnesses. Ballard and McVey (2014) demonstrate that it is possible to incorporate temporality into the design of communication processes within organizations, though theorizing has not identified what happens to communication processes when actors' temporal frames are mismatched.

Conclusion

One obvious route to increasing accrual rates to studies is to reduce barriers that are created by the organizational system itself. Recruiters often struggle to simply find the physical space they need to discuss research studies and clinical trials with patients. Participating in the research process simply is not a priority for most physicians and other medical staff, which may be why recruiters are not designated a space to work, even when recruiters work in one clinic for the majority of their hours during the working week, sometimes for years on end. Instead, recruiters must nimbly negotiate for a small amount of patient time wherever and whenever they can be fit into "the clinic workflow." Failing to do so means running the risk of being denied access to patients, which leads to a failure to recruit, which in turn leads to lower accrual for research studies. The relative success of this group of professionals, then, is a testament to their ability to carefully negotiate physical space and time concerns, as well as their ability to build positive relationships with staff and physicians.

Another system that recruiters must navigate is the information system that identifies some patients as being potentially qualified to participate in a study. A reasonably functional information system that can search electronic health records for a study's eligibility criteria has yet to be developed, so identifying patients qualified for a study is a time-consuming process. Recruiters sometimes simply do this in person at a clinic where the most likely patients are seen. Ironically, they sometimes appear to be more aware of the medical conditions of patients than the patients' own physicians. Worse, physicians can be dismissive of potential interest by patients, creating unnecessary frustrations for recruiters. However, in the case of relatively rare diseases and conditions, the system of professional study recruitment can lead to additional system-based difficulties. Recruiters often have to drive significant distances to meet with a single patient, and of course, discussing a study is no guarantee that a patient will be interested in participating. These are all problems that could be addressed with a significant culture shift in the medical system where study recruitment is seen as an inherently valuable activity that directly and positively impacts patient care, albeit over the long term.

Finally, we would be remiss if we did not mention the larger social system within which recruiters must operate. Many patients struggle with language and basic literacy issues, and worse, with a medical system that has often been guilty of perpetuating significant abuses. While poverty, illiteracy, and medical distrust are extremely difficult to address through the design of interventions, we believe that it is possible to make other changes that can transform communication within a health care context that will increase the successful accrual of patients to research studies and clinical trials. Redesigning communication protocols around recruitment should, in turn, lead to improved treatments for a wide variety of diseases and medical conditions, creating a ripple effect that will improve the quality of life for patients and their families.

DISCUSSION QUESTIONS

1. Think about an organization with which you are familiar or have frequent involvement. How might a Communication Design intervention help move that organization from "the way things are" to a more "ideal" state?
2. Clinical trial recruitment is only one application of a Communication Design approach. What other communicative goals related to health care might benefit from a Communication Design intervention? Explain.
3. Other than those listed in the chapter, what are some potential pitfalls to avoid when planning a Communication Design intervention?
4. Which other variables depicted in the model of clinical trial recruitment might be well-suited to interventions developed using a Communication Design approach?

Suggested Reading

Aakhus, M. (2007). Communication as design. *Communication Monographs, 74*, 112–117.
Institutes of Medicine (2012). *Envisioning a Transformed Clinical Trials Enterprise in the United States: Establishing an Agenda for 2020: Workshop Summary.* Washington, DC: The National Academies Press.

References

Aakhus, M. (2003). Neither naïve nor normative reconstruction: Dispute mediators, impasse, and the design of argumentation. *Argumentation: An International Journal on Reasoning, 17*, 265–290.

Aakhus, M. (2007). Communication as design. *Communication Monographs, 74*, 112–117.

Ballard, D. I. & McVey, T. (2014). Measure twice, cut once: The temporality of communication design. *Journal of Applied Communication Research, 42*, 190–207.

Barbour, J. B. & Gill, R. (2014). Designing communication for the day-to-day safety oversight of nuclear power plants. *Journal of Applied Communication Research, 42*, 168–189.

Bodurtha, J. N., Quillin, J. M., Tracy, K. A., & Borzelleca, J. (2007). Recruiting diverse patients to a breast cancer risk communication trial: Waiting rooms can improve access. *Journal of the National Medical Association, 99*, 917–922.

Castel, P., Negrier, S., Boissel, J.-P. (2006). Why don't cancer patients enter clinical trials? A review. *European Journal of Cancer, 42*, 1744–1748.

Cuggia, M., Besana, P., & Glasspool, D. (2011). Comparing semi-automatic systems for recruitment of patients to clinical trials. *International Journal of Medical Informatics, 80*, 371–388.

Embi, P. J., Jain, A., Clark, J., & Harris, C. M. (2005). Development of an electronic health record-based clinical trial alert system to enhance recruitment at the point of care. *AMIA Annual Symposium Proceedings Archive*, 231–235.

Embi, P. J. & . Tsevay, J. (2012). The relative research unit providing incentives for clinician participation in research activities. *Academic Medicine, 87*(1), 11–14.

Ford, E., Jenkins, V., Fallowfield, L., Stuart, N., Farewell, D., & Farewell, V. (2011). Clinicians' attitudes towards clinical trials of cancer therapy. *British Journal of Cancer, 104*, 1535–1543.

Green, L. A., White, L. L., Barry, H. C., Nease, D. E., & Hudson, B. L. (2005). Infrastructure Requirements for Practice-Based Research Networks. *Annals of Family Medicine 3 Supplement, 1*(1), S5–S11.

Harrison, T. R. (2003). Victims, targets, protectors and destroyers: Using disputant accounts to develop a grounded taxonomy of disputant orientations. *Conflict Resolution Quarterly, 20*, 307–329.

Harrison, T. R. (2004). What is success in ombuds processes? Evaluation of a university ombudsman. *Conflict Resolution Quarterly, 21*, 313–335.

Harrison, T. R. (2007). My professor is so unfair: Student attitudes and experiences of conflict with faculty. *Conflict Resolution Quarterly, 24*, 349–368.

Harrison, T. R. (2014). Enhancing communication interventions and evaluations through communication design. *Journal of Applied Communication Research, 42*, 135–149.

Harrison, T. R. & Doerfel, M. L. (2006). Competitive and cooperative conflict communication climates: The influence of ombuds processes on trust and commitment to the organization. *International Journal of Conflict Management, 17*, 129–153.

Harrison, T. R., Hopeck, P., Desrayaud, N., & Imboden, K. (2013). The relationship between conflict, anticipatory procedural justice, and design with intentions to use ombudsman processes. *International Journal of Conflict Management, 24*(1), 56–72.

Harrison, T. R., Morgan, S. E., Chewning, L. V., Williams, E. A., Barbour, J. B., DiCorcia, M. J., & Davis, L. (2011). Revisiting the worksite in worksite health campaigns: Evidence from a multi-site organ donation campaign. *Journal of Communication, 61*, 535–555.

Harrison, T. R., Morgan, S. E., King, A. J., DiCorcia, M. J., Williams, E. A., Ivic, R. K., & Hopeck, P. (2010). Promoting the Michigan organ donor registry: Evaluating the impact of a multi-faceted intervention utilizing media priming and communication design. *Health Communication, 25,* 700–708.

Harrison, T. R. & Morrill, C. (2004). Ombuds processes and disputant reconciliation. *Journal of Applied Communication Research, 32,* 318–342.

Hecht, M. L. & Miller-Day, M. (2007). The drug resistance strategies project as translational research. *Journal of Applied Communication Research, 35,* 343–349.

IOM (Institute of Medicine) (2012). *Envisioning a Transformed Clinical Trials Enterprise in the United States: Establishing an Agenda for 2020: Workshop Summary.* Washington, DC: The National Academies Press.

Jackson, S. & Aakhus, M. (2014). Becoming more reflective about the role of design in communication. *Journal of Applied Communication Research, 42,* 125–134.

Kho, A., Zafar, A., & Tierney, W. (2007). Information Technology in PBRNs: The Indiana University Medical Group Research Network (IUMG ResNet) Experience. *Journal of the American Board of Family Medicine, 20,* 196–203.

Kolata, G. (2009). Lack of study volunteers is said to hobble fight against cancer. *New York Times.* New York, NY.

McSweeny, J. C., Pettey, C. M., Fischer, E. P., & Spellman, A. (2009). Going the distance: Overcoming challenges in recruitment and retention of Black and White women in multisite, longitudinal study of predictors of coronary heart disease. *Research in Gerontological Nursing, 2,* 256–264.

Michaels, M., Weiss, E. S., Guidry, J. A., et. al. (2011). The promise of community-based advocacy and education efforts for increasing cancer clinical trials accrual. *Cancer Education, 27,* 67–74.

Nelson, H. G. and Stolterman, E. (2003). *The design way: Intentional change in an unpredictable world.* Englewood Cliffs, NJ: Educational Technology Productions.

Paramasivan, S., Huddart, R., Hall, E., Lewis, R., Birtle, A., & Donovan, J. L. (2011). Key issues in recruitment to randomised controlled trials with very different interventions: A qualitative investigation of recruitment to the SPARE trial (CRUK/07/011). *Trials, 12,* 78.

Probstfield, J. L. & Frye, R. L. (2011). Strategies for recruitment and retention of participants in clinical trials. *JAMA, 306,* 1798–1799.

Reed, R. L., Barton, C. A., Isherwood, L. M. Baxter, J. M., & Roeger, L. (2013) Recruitment for a clinical trial of chronic disease self-management for older adults with multimorbidity: A successful approach within general practice. *BMC Family Practice, 14,* 125–131.

Schmotzer, G. L. (2012). Barriers and facilitators to participation of minorities in clinical trials. *Ethnicity & Disease, 22,* 226–230.

Schutt, R. K., Schapira, L., Maniates, J., Santiccioli, J. Henlon, S., & Bigby, J. A. (2010). Community health workers' support for cancer clinical trials: Description and explanation. *Community Health, 35,* 417–422.

Siminoff, L. A., Ravdin, P., Colabianchi, N., & Sturm, C. M. S. (2000). Doctor-patient communication patterns in breast cancer adjuvant therapy discussions. *Health Expectations, 3,* 26–36.

Stevens, T. & Ahmedzai, S.H. (2004). Why do breast cancer patients decline entry into randomised trials and how do they feel about their decision later: A prospective, longitudinal, in-depth interview study. *Patient Education and Counseling, 52,* 341–348.

Trauth, J. M., Jernigan, J. C., Siminoff, L. A., Musa, D., Neal-Ferguson, D., & Weissfeld, J. (2005). Factors affecting older African American women's decisions to join the PLCO cancer screening trial. *Journal of Clinical Oncology, 23*(34), 8730–8738.

Ulrich, C. M., Zhou, Q., Ratcliffe, S. J., Ye, L., Grady, C., & Watkins-Bruner, D. (2012). Nurse practitioners' attitudes about cancer clinical trials and willingness to recommend research participation. *Contemporary Clinical Trials, 33*, 76–84.

7

WORK SPACE, GENDERED OCCUPATIONS, AND THE ORGANIZATION OF HEALTH

Redesigning Emergency Department Communication

Joshua B. Barbour, Rebecca Gill, and Marleah Dean

Communication in health care organizations involves complex problems of uncertainty and information management, multiple competing and collaborating professions, pressing resource constraints, and high-stakes outcomes (Barbour, 2010; Dean & Oetzel, 2014), paralleling, for example, communication in settings such as nuclear power plants (Barbour & Gill, 2014), fire departments (Myers & McPhee, 2006), and other risky workplaces (Barbour & James, forthcoming; Real, 2008). The presence of such issues in health care contexts, such as in hospital emergency departments (EDs), makes them particularly important settings for study (Eisenberg, Baglia, & Pynes 2006; Eisenberg et al., 2005).

Taking care with communication in such settings means acknowledging and accounting for the material conditions in and through which communication unfolds (Aakhus & Laureij, 2012; Ashcraft, Kuhn, & Cooren, 2009), including the spatial and temporal (Ballard, 2014; Harrison, 2014; Harrison et al., 2011). We contend that intervening in professionalized, knowledge-intensive organizing such as the provision of health care means coming to terms with more than the challenges of sending and receiving messages or installing the right equipment.

That is, theorizing the gendered, power-laden character of organizing and how it becomes expressed in and through, for example, the arrangement of an organization's physical environment can elucidate what have otherwise been intractable problems of interprofessional communication (e.g., the persistence of medical error despite the widespread recognition of it as a problem, Ulrich et al., 2008). The health, safety, and well-being of individuals and organizations are intertwined with the physical spaces in which organizing occurs, and physical space enables and constrains role performances and interactions (Elsbach & Pratt,

2007). However, whereas research has tended to focus on the design of spaces for physiological health and well-being, in particular in health care settings, we know much less about the design of workspaces to support healthier and safer organizational communication (Ulrich et al., 2008).

As such, our chapter focuses on the intersection of (a) discursive patterns, (b) work space, and (c) health and (d) organizational communication. We contend that broader Discourses in medical work are (re)produced in everyday communication and reflected in the arrangement of physical space, and that one tool for useful intervention in the organizing of health care is in understanding communication as designed (Aakhus, 2007; Aakhus & Jackson, 2005; Jackson & Aakhus, 2014). To make this case, we draw on examples from research on health care organizations and health in organizations (Harrison, 2014; Real, 2010) and one ED in particular—EmergiCare.

Throughout our chapter, we offer examples from EmergiCare to illustrate our claims. This exemplar demonstrates that it is *in the rethinking of communication that seemingly disconnected concerns for the gendered discourse of organizations, physical space, and communication dynamics may be integrated.* The design choices made about the organization of physical working space at EmergiCare "reveal how important aspects of organizational and professional life are organized around the possibilities for orchestrating interactivity to facilitate some forms of communication while inhibiting other forms" (Aakhus & Laureij, 2012, p. 42). Communication redesign offers a space for the consideration of what might be instead. In this, insights about health care organizing may provide resources for improving the health of organizations and the organization of health.

Communication at EmergiCare

EmergiCare is a Level 1 Trauma and Academic Medical Center ranked among the top 100 US hospitals. It is located in a densely populated Southwestern US city and sees approximately 70,000 patients per year. The adult emergency department (versus the pediatric one) has two sides, Manzia and Sundano, which are divided by a solid wall. Each has a nurse's and physician's station with patient rooms around the perimeter (see Figure 7.1).

Communication in EDs is distinctive compared to other health care organizations as EDs provide 24-hour care and are fraught with time constraints, dialectic tensions, limited resources, and high patient influx, as well as being marked by uncertainty and unpredictability (Dean & Oetzel, 2014; Eisenberg et al., 2006). Health care professionals in EDs have several roles and responsibilities, must make quick decisions, and deal with multiple hierarchies and expertise (Eisenberg et al., 2005). EDs are intense physical spaces susceptible to accidents, medical errors, and staff injury (Ulrich et al., 2008).

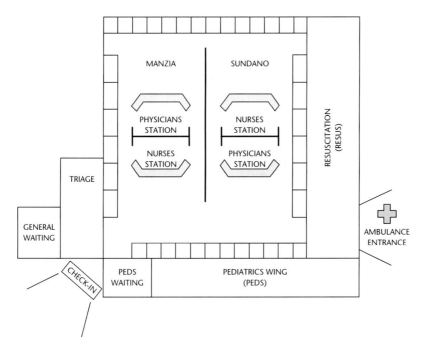

FIGURE 7.1 Graphic Representation of EmergiCare.[1]

Organizing for Health Through a Lens of Macromorphic Discourse

As demonstrated throughout this volume, productive possibilities emerge at the nexus of health and organizational communication scholarship. Our contribution is to present and consider how Discourse—a concept drawn from the work of Michel Foucault and others—influences and shapes communication in medical contexts, and specifically in EDs, while accounting for the physical environment of organizations in particular (an aspect of materiality overlooked in strictly discursive approaches, Vásquez & Cooren, 2013). Although there are a number of levels of analysis at which we could define discourse (see Alvesson & Karreman, 2000; Fairhurst & Putnam, 2004), our approach here is to understand it as a "macromorphic" phenomenon, meaning that we are interested in the social-level patterns of communication that extend across and beyond particular situations and contexts but which nonetheless affect them. We use the term macromorphic to retain the idea that these Discourses are not fixed but are becoming. In this, Discourse is analytically distinct from, though entwined with, institutional and meso-level explorations of health care organizing (e.g., Barbour & Lammers, 2007; Eisenberg et al., 2005; Lammers & Barbour, 2006), which tend to be tethered more to specific organizations, professions, and institutions.

Macromorphic Discourse has been described as "an assemblage of knowledge that creates 'truth effects'" (Tracy & Trethewey, 2005, p. 169), thereby (re)producing and regulating beliefs, attitudes, and behaviors. Such truth effects "fix" particular assumptions and normalize "the way things are" so that to resist Discourse would risk being perceived as eccentric or inappropriate, as not "following the 'rules'", or as an outsider (Alvesson & Willmott, 2002). Such beliefs and behaviors are (re)produced in medicine in the perceived status of the physician and the concomitant roles that nurses, patients, and others are expected to play. Physicians are given leave to analyze patients' bodies through a seemingly expert "medical gaze," thus enacting a kind of regulatory power over patients' bodies and choices (Foucault, 1963, 1973). For patients to "flip the script" and self-diagnose (or even offer medical advice to physicians!) would appear bizarre. And yet, although patients' involvement in their own medical care has initially been perceived as unorthodox, the increasing participation of patients in medicine (Street et al., 2009) demonstrates that Discourse can indeed change, given time and space (Alvesson & Willmott, 2002; Scott, Ruef, Mendel, & Caronna, 2000; Trethewey, 1997).

The Character of Occupations

Recognizing that the field of medicine is "[not] immune from the values, mores, and prejudices of the wider society" (Gamble, 2000, p. 168–169), we turn our attention to the work undertaken within this field. Specifically, our interest is in recent attention to occupations as themselves possessing characteristics that shape the performance of work (Ashforth, Rogers, & Corley, 2011; Barbour & Lammers, 2015; Cheney & Ashcraft, 2007). Arguments around this suggest, "much like organizations, occupations are distinguished by collective identities, in that we treat lines of work as typified by central, abiding, and unique features" (Ashcraft, 2013, p. 8). Ashcraft's (2013) "glass slipper" metaphor illuminates how occupations are perceived as a singular, fixed "thing" (e.g., that declaring oneself as a "physician" speaks for itself), and yet are constructed in and through the ongoing patterning of communication:

> Much like Cinderella's shoe, occupational identity is an artifact manufactured through artifice [where] the "magic" behind the making of occupational identity quickly fades into presumption of authenticity. The invention becomes forgotten as such, taken instead as an accurate description of what an occupation entails.
>
> *(p. 16)*

Occupational discourses are thus "transcendent" and collective, informing our thinking about how to do a job or what it "should" be like (Scott, 2008). Scholarly inquiry along these lines has also examined the occupations of pilot (Ashcraft, 2007), veterinarian (Lammers & Garcia, 2009), fundraiser (Meisenbach, 2008), lawyer (Kuhn, 2009), entrepreneur (Gill & Larson, 2014), and scientist (Wells, 2013), among others. Accordingly, this perspective helps us theorize how medical professionals develop an identity that informs, and is informed by, their occupation (Apker & Eggly, 2004; Barbour & Lammers, 2007; Lammers & Barbour, 2009) to enable interventions in interprofessional communication (Barbour, 2010).

One important facet of the glass slipper metaphor is that it highlights that occupations are not necessarily "one size fits all." Rather, occupational Discourses are formed through and alongside the social identities perceived to be the "right fit" for the occupation, including the idealized gender, ethnicity/race, sexuality, age, and so forth, of the worker in that role (Acker, 1990; Allen, 2004; Ashcraft, 2007; Trethewey, 1997; Wells, 2013). Occupational Discourse is therefore "ordered" by assumptions regarding the appropriate behaviors, bodily appearances, and performance of tasks that inform who is perceived as being fit for the job, and also influences judgments and evaluations of those working in the position. Thus, we understand and examine work and organizing through the communication of difference (Ashcraft, 2011).

The importance of occupational Discourse for our focus here is that it helps us recognize not only the bias of occupations, but also that, accordingly, people are influenced to shape or comport themselves, their communication, and even the arrangement of work space to "fit" that occupation (Alvesson & Willmott, 2002; Ashcraft, 2013). That is, in seeking to look and act the part of the occupation, people navigate the occupational "image" when they enact their "role," meaning that "the latter (i.e., occupational identity *communication*) negotiates the former (i.e., occupational identity *discourse*) in the context of everyday work life" (Ashcraft, 2007, p. 12, emphasis in original).

Understanding Discourse as organizing occupations underscores a central claim of our chapter: *that we cannot positively or meaningfully intercede in the organization of health care without also understanding the significant and enduring influences of Discourse on medical workers' understanding of what they do and why they do it.* The "transmission" of communication is not just improved by enhancing communication competencies but also by recognizing the Discursive patterns in medical work that shape practice. As such, we now turn to a focused discussion of how medical professions possess their own socio-occupational identity, and how this identity influences the "doing" of these occupations.

The Importance of Occupational Discourse for Medical Work

Following from claims regarding occupations as characterized and ordered through assumptions of difference, we now consider the gendering of medical occupations and how this shapes communication. Overall, occupational segregation literature has illuminated how assumptions of femininity and masculinity are "patterned in and through" occupations, often presuming a "masculine" or "feminine" body as being more suited to a particular job (see Acker, 1990). Particularly in the case of "professional" work, women have historically been segregated into passive, unskilled, and "assistance-based" positions such as secretarial or service work, and men into active, skilled, and often prestigious and leadership positions such as managers and experts (see Ashcraft, 2013, for an extensive review).

In medical Discourse, assumptions of masculinity inform the historical associations of medicine as requiring a strong stomach, quick decision-making, emotional detachment, and long hours—qualities and characteristics seen as inappropriate for women or those with "feminine" dispositions (Pringle, 1998). These associations continue to be prevalent today, where physicians are constructed (and construct themselves) as masculine, hands-on, technical, and possessing particular body parts needed for their work (e.g., "balls," Hinze, 1999). Indeed, Apker and Eggly (2004) found that medical residents learned to adopt ways of thinking and acting that reinforced historically masculine ideologies. During morning report conferences, for instance, residents who offered opinions and explanations culled from their own life experiences were corrected and guided by faculty toward "preferred," biomedical and technologically informed explanations.

Contrasting this is the association of feminine qualities with nurses. The occupation of "nurse" has historically involved being a helpmate to a physician (Davies, 2003) and requiring a soft touch, the expression of care and concern, and an unassuming nature. While managerial tasks have more recently been added to nursing duties (Halford & Leonard, 2006), and some organizations have developed higher-status nursing roles (Apker, Propp, & Zabava Ford, 2005), the perception that the primary responsibility of nurses is to provide soothing and sympathetic touch and talk remains dominant. For instance, McMurray (2011) found that although general practitioners supported nurses' efforts to become Advanced Nurse Practitioners, the general practitioners did not accept the nurses' abilities to diagnose patients once certified.

Such gendered Discourses are brought into relief by, for example, the specific labeling of men in nursing as "male nurses," which has the effect of distinguishing them from the *presumed* sex of people in this occupation (i.e., female). Moreover, when men *are* present in the nursing field, they are often disassociated from emotional work and (re)associated with technical and managerial work (Hallam, 2000). As such, gender segregation occurs even within nursing, further compounding care as feminine and technical knowledge as masculine.

Entwined with the gendered character of these occupations is that they are also underpinned by ethnic/racial, class, and heteronormative assumptions where the "standard" medical professional is white, middle-upper or middle class, and heterosexual (indeed, such assumptions are inherent in the notion of a "professional" more generally, Cheney & Ashcraft, 2007). The patriarchal and rational physician and the gentle and caring nurse are images that contrast with other powerful stereotypes of, for instance, the angry black man or woman and evoke assumptions of genteel whiteness (for this discussion in the context of entrepreneur discourse, see Knight, 2005). Illuminating this, Gamble (2000) noted that racial and ethnic minority medical students had been "mistaken (even by medical professionals) for janitors, maids, and dietary workers" (p. 165) and recalled "being asked to leave the doctors' eating area because we did not fit the picture of the typical physician" (p. 165). In addition to drawing attention to the discrimination and tokenism that medical professionals of color may experience, Gamble's account highlighted the racial and ethnic characteristics *that make up the physician and nurse occupations* themselves. The intersecting of these social identities is noted in her realization: "I would not just be a physician, but a black woman physician. I recall thinking that if I had been a white woman, the patient would have mistaken me for a nurse rather than a maid" (pp. 167–168).

The historical character of macromorphic Discourse matters here, because it frames and undergirds how we think about medical work, our judgments about the quality and importance of different sorts of medical work, and how we attempt to intervene in it. In short, the associated expectations for everyday communication and role performance are informed by the gendered, raced, and classed Discourses of medical work. Because physicians are expected to gather and give information to make a diagnosis as well as be efficient (Apker & Eggly, 2004; Dean & Oetzel, 2014), and nurses are expected to be caring, demonstrate compassion and build relationships (e.g., Davies, 2003), individuals in these positions seek to enact these roles, thereby reinforcing the Discourse.

Occupational Communication at EmergiCare

At EmergiCare, communication patterns reflected the social identities of medical occupations as gendered, specifically, but also as subtly incorporating assumptions of class and race/ethnicity. Physicians, most often but not always males, used *case talk*. Case talk meant communication should be direct and assertive (Mulac, 2006). Case talk displayed knowledge and control. Case talk served to confirm and challenge medical judgments among those in the know. Case talk involved forceful opinions and authoritative directions. Case talk evidenced a control of emotion (Guerrero, Jones, & Boburka, 2006), without common articulations of sympathy or understanding (Eisenberg, 2002).

Comfort talk, on the other hand, was typically used by nurses, who were most often but not always female. Comfort talk meant providing support for patients (Guerrero et al., 2006; Mulac, 2006) through informative but encouraging messages (Ellingson & Buzzanell, 1999). Comfort talk demonstrated responsiveness to patients, helping them feel valued and important (Chatham-Carpenter & DeFrancisco, 1998). Comfort talk created space for patients to express their emotions and opinions without disrupting the overall nursing work.

Gendered Discourse at EmergiCare

Case and comfort talk reflect macromorphic Discursive occupational norms, revealing distinct communication purposes and goals. Case talk exhibits what is typically coded as masculine. Physician case talkers diagnosed and interpreted patient symptoms, sought the confirmation of other physicians, gave directions, and informed patients of problems. Case talk emphasized thorough, rational thought as a means for solving medical problems.

In contrast, comfort talk exemplifies what is typically coded as feminine. Nurse comfort talkers (all female except the nurse in charge of the ED nurses) engaged in positive talk, asked about feelings, and provided context for the patient. Comfort talk was a vehicle for helping patients understand their circumstances, share their story, and cope with the medical process. It stressed listening and empathy. These communication styles are gendered in that they are (re) produced in and of the historical occupational identity of being a physician or a nurse and the associated communication expectations for those roles.

Thus far, we have constructed a picture of occupational Discourse that suggests that it is fixed and inescapable. However, although we believe that Discourse is highly pervasive and regulatory, we recognize that the social, created nature of it means that it can be resisted, altered, and reformed. That is, "occupational identities are contrived, and this means they could be otherwise" (Ashcraft, 2013, p. 17; see also Trethewey, 1997). Therefore, our next objective is to explore how we might effectively "interrupt" the Discourse that seems to influence physician and nurse communication patterns—focusing, in our case, on the use of space at EmergiCare. Specifically, we highlight here our normative assumption that because ED professionals engage in complex, knowledge-intensive conversations important to patient care and safety, we should strive to assist them in capitalizing on the diversity of expertise held by physicians *and* nurses, enhancing their collaboration and communication.

"Interrupting" Occupational Discourse in Practice

We want to accompany our recognition of occupational Discourse as present in medical work with consideration of how we can best interrupt Discourse to better understand and improve medical practice. To this end, we take a communication design approach (see also Aakhus & Harrison, this volume and Morgan & Mouton, this volume), which offers a useful theoretical framework for intervening in the communicative and material conditions in which organizations emerge (Aakhus & Laureij, 2012; Barbour & Gill, 2014). Design is about the formation of "ideal things out of a cloud of possibilities" (Nelson & Stolterman, 2012, 2012, p. 7), and "transforming something given into something preferred" (Aakhus, 2007, p. 112). In this, communication design attends to what might be learned in the creation or reformation of messages, conversations, systems of interaction, and communication technologies.

The mix of occupational Discourse here characterized by technical complexity, medical uncertainty, and gender, ethnicity/race, and other social identities, must be considered in making design decisions (even if it is to overlook facets of it). We see this, for instance, in Harrison et al.'s (2011) analysis of the effectiveness of organ donation campaigns in driver licensing bureaus, where they described the encounter as encompassing a dizzying combination of material and discursive factors: ". . . the physical layout of [licensing] offices, and includ[ing] activities and interactions such as entering the [licensing] offices, standing in line, reading materials, being greeted, moving from one line to another, and ending with the final interaction with the clerk who completes the desired transactions" (pp. 807–808). Their intervention sought to re-craft the interactivity and messaging of the encounter, where, although not every step could be optimized, the design of the interaction was nonetheless informed by theory, practice, and the exigencies of the moment. Harrison and colleagues exemplify how design requires moving from the universal to the particular by making choices about how communication *could possibly* occur (Nelson & Stolterman, 2012).

Thinking of communication as designed reflects the understanding that people attempt to "do" things with language and interactivity (Aakhus & Laureij, 2012), and in doing so addresses the communication situation as they understand it (Lammers, 2011; O'Keefe & Lambert, 1995). Communicators must grapple with gendered Discourses in particular spaces even if they only seek to ignore it, or endeavor to resist or acquiesce to it. The patterns of communication that are constructed within Discourse over time reflect exigent power differences and material constraints and resources. That is, not all voices involved in the arrangement and performance of work—including regarding participation, identity presentation, turn-taking, communicative topics, and so forth—have equal power. In this sense, being powerful means being able to shape communication and thus influence what knowledge and practices are created in what format (Aakhus, 2007; Aakhus & Laureij, 2012; Barbour & Gill, 2014). Arguably, occupational Discourse informs the limits of this.

Bringing Material Conditions of Work Into the Merging of Discourse and Design

Communication as design invites us to think about the physical space of health organizations like EDs in terms of how the arrangement of space reflects *choices* influenced by relevant and encumbering occupational Discourse (Lammers, 2011). Organizing is corporeal at the same time as it is communicative (Ashcraft, 2007; Ashcraft et al., 2009). Our chapter joins efforts to contend with space in communication scholarship (e.g., Vásquez & Cooren, 2013), though we construe our focus more narrowly than the more general project because we are concerned with the physical environments of organizations, defined by Elsbach and Pratt (2007) as including:

. . . all of the material objects and stimuli (e.g., buildings, furnishings, equipment, and ambient conditions such as lighting and air quality) as well as the arrangement of those objects and stimuli (e.g., open-space office plans and flexible team work spaces) that people encounter and interact with in organizational life.

(pp. 181–182)

More specifically, Elsbach and Pratt summarized research on the use of space into four streams: (1) enclosures and barriers, (2) adjustable work arrangements, equipment, and furnishing, (3) personalization of work spaces, and (4) nature-like ambience. These dimensions shape possibilities for role performance, for instance, where the positioning and use of rooms, offices, and hallways convey particular sensibilities or identities, "organiz[ing] an ensemble of possibilities (e.g., by a place in which one can move) and interdictions (e.g., by a wall that prevents one from going further)" (De Certeau, 1984, p. 98).

The disposition of occupations is therefore (re)produced and navigated alongside the above dimensions. Space and place can enable and constrain role performances and interactions linked to status and gender (Elsbach & Pratt, 2007; Gill & Larson, 2014), for instance, by locating those with less status in more visible and immoveable spaces but supporting flexibility of movement for those with higher status. In the case of medical professionals, physicians typically have freedom of distance and nurses tend to be situated in and around the same space. Busy and continuously moving, nurses "[buzz] around repetitive spatial patterns," whereas physicians are more likely to be "still—the thinker—or walking purposefully toward a goal—the doer" (Halford & Leonard, 2006, p. 93).

In fact, it may be hard to overstate the importance of the physical spaces in which communication unfolds. In their study of worksite health campaigns, Harrison et al. (2011) argued:

. . . when looking at the 'doing of work' within organizational 'communities,' individuals engage in action within a physical space that both limits and facilitates certain types of activities and communication. They do so not in isolation, but through developing working relationships of various degrees of influence with their colleagues, and they communicate and share information through the use of available channels within an organization. These constitute the basic interaction environment of the workplace.

(p. 536)

Interest in aesthetics, layout, and arrangement of work spaces has a long history (Becker, 1981; Davis, Leach, & Clegg, 2011), in particular as it relates to human health (Ulrich, 1984), which is not surprising because physical spaces have direct effects on health, safety, and well-being (General Services Administration, 2009; National Institute of Building Sciences, 2015). Recently, office space has received renewed attention as organizations experiment with open space offices and temporary work space assignments (Konnikova, 2014) and attempt to figure out the best way to create work environments conducive to knowledge work (cf., Demarco & Lister, 2013). The physical environment at work is particularly important because of the effects it has and because of the longevity and cost of design choices (Elsbach & Pratt, 2007). This is especially true in health care design. Ulrich et al. (2008) argued, "Many hospital settings have not been redesigned, although jobs have been changed, and as a result, hospital environments often increase staff stress and reduce effective care delivery;" however, there is "a growing and convincing body of evidence suggesting that improved hospital design can make the jobs of staff easier" (p. 145).

Features of Physical Environments

The evidence on *particular work space features* is mixed, limiting the recommendations that may be reasonably made in the design of work spaces such as hospitals and other health care settings. Ulrich et al.'s (2008) review of over 600 health care design studies found some empirical evidence for the relationships between staff outcomes (e.g., injuries, stress, effectiveness, and satisfaction) and specific aspects of the physical environment (e.g., single-bed rooms, access to daylight and appropriate lighting, views of nature, family zones, carpeting and noise-reducing finishes, ceiling lifts, nursing floor layout, decentralized supplies, and acuity-adaptable rooms); however, strong evidence was only available for the relationship between the presence of ceiling lifts and staff injury reductions. It is likely that, rather than there being "one best arrangement," the effects of physical space are mediated in and through individuals' perceptions and communicative action. For example, looking at the effects of office location on intentions to make use of ombudsmen, Harrison (2013) found that the location itself had little influence but that *perceptions* of the location's ability to protect confidentiality were meaningful. Particular individuals and interactions also have distinctive needs and goals for particular spaces. Ulrich et al., for instance, found that, whereas dim lighting improved patient–provider communication, bright lighting was associated with reductions in medical error.

Underlying Mechanisms

In light of this complexity, scholars have tried to transcend the mix of findings by conceptualizing the *mechanisms* underlying the effects of particular aspects of the physical environment such as proximity, privacy, or social interference (albeit with mixed results, Elsbach & Pratt, 2007). In Harrison et al.'s (2011) theorization of the effects of physical structure on interaction, they posited that physical space may be related to the density of relationships among organizational members, where organizations are like pinball machines: "The tighter the bumpers, the more the pinball bounces around, comes into contact with other bumpers, and moves into all areas of the board" (p. 537) and proximity increases interaction (see Monge, Rothman, Eisenberg, Miller, & Kirste, 1985). Although Harrison et al. found that density had no effect on knowledge or attitudes about the campaign intervention, or had unanticipated effects, they nonetheless called for additional study of physical space in organizing, highlighting the difficulty of operationalizing aspects of space design. There are infinite factors to measure and infinite ways to measure them (e.g., numbers of floors, cubicles, break rooms, exercise areas, childcare facilities, nature of workspace [office type], and vending machine areas), and particular office space choices interact in complex ways with other aspects of environment and communication.

Work Space and Interaction as Designed Objects at Emergicare

At EmergiCare, *case and comfort talk* mapped onto the physical layout in unsurprising ways. Case talk occurred most often at the physician's station, their "home base." The interaction that occurred here tended to only involve the physicians and in this way, the station "contained" medical expertise. Here, physicians ordered medicines and tests and engaged in consultations with other physicians, exchanging information and confirming and challenging interpretations, gathered around charts or computers. The presence of nurses here was specific and bounded, and here there was no need for comfort talk. Nurses dropped off forms, and when they did talk with physicians it was to provide or obtain information.

The *nurse's station* was "home base" for the nurses, though nurses were often moving between their station and patients' rooms (Halford & Leonard, 2006). This station was thus largely a site of interaction between nurses to coordinate and confirm care. The nurse's station evidenced more permeable boundaries than the physician's station, as nurses entertained technicians as well as patients and their families here, providing information and comfort talking. Physicians rarely entered this area, and when they did it was to obtain information.

The communicative activity in EmergiCare was highly formatted (e.g., scheduled handoffs, formalized patient intake procedures) but also in flux. Nurse and physician communication intertwined against and in the layout, where these occupational groups were linked to spaces that (re)produced the macromorphic occupational images traced in and onto the distinct spaces.

A Discourse-Design Approach in Practice

Overall, our contention is that communication design can be useful for bridging concerns involving occupational Discourse, the material conditions of work, and day-to-day interaction. These approaches focus attention to the *context* in which design choices are made and offer resources for understanding those choices.

In practice, the key pitfall to avoid is assuming that it is possible or advisable to optimize space to serve one ideal or interest. Rather, communication design choices involve ongoing trade-offs and balances (Aakhus, 2001; Aakhus & Rumsey, 2010). It is in the analysis of the spatial/communicative arrangements as designed objects reflecting relevant occupational Discourses that the integration becomes visible.

Re(Design) at EmergiCare

At EmergiCare we imagined three intentional changes (Nelson & Stolterman, 2012). First, the work of organizing the ED could include physicians as well as nurses. A whiteboard accessible to the entire ED that displays key patient and care information could support de-segregated collaboration. Nurses suggested this intervention (e.g., "a central communication board"). Second, responsibility for the day-to-day organizing of the ED could rotate among nurses and physicians. An ED organizer could track patient status, facilitate visitors, and reflect on communication among patients, nurses, and physicians, helping the ED "see" its own interaction. Third, EmergiCare could consider re-situating the work stations or remove the wall separating them to encourage more impromptu collaboration integrating case and comfort talk. Implementing these recommendations would provide nurses and physicians alike with a more holistic understanding of the work performed by others in and across the ED. Such efforts reflect a communication design intervention. This intervention may challenge long-standing medical images of the male, all-knowing physician and the female, helpmate nurse, and any such effort should begin by recognizing the entrenched and enduring character of such Discourses.

In other words, the physical environment should be organized to accomplish the functional requirements of work and space in ways that acknowledge, mitigate, and remake the character of occupational Discourse. Not only is design specific to sites of engagement (Nelson & Stolterman, 2012; Stolterman, Mcatee, Royer, & Thandapani, 2008), but space and place are linked to identity formation, negotiation, and regulation (Gill & Larson, 2014; Vásquez & Cooren, 2013) that reflect status dynamics (Elsbach & Pratt, 2007). Future directions of research should explore the ways in which space influences communication between patients and providers and examine how the gendered occupations of health care roles influence communication.

The physical layout of work environments (e.g., location of patient rooms, hallways, nurse and physician stations) can impede and enhance communication amongst providers. Ulrich et al. (2008) underscored the importance of communication among and between patients, providers and families, but lamented, "it is unfortunate that there is not much research on how the built environment enhances or hinders communication" (p. 137). For EmergiCare, then, we posed suggestions for (re)designing physician–nurse communication. Yet, we also acknowledge the difficulty in changing Discourse for practical ends and, in this sense, suggest that a Discourse-Design approach be conceived as a long game. Moreover, we recognize that suggestions for change can have the effect of creating more work and require additional effort and commitment, as well as developing novel problems. Executing communication design changes in organizing, as with organizational change in general, is neither simple nor straightforward.

DISCUSSION QUESTIONS

1. Imagine that you are trying to improve a communication process in your organization. Who are the key players, and what assumptions do they have about how communication works? How are those assumptions consistent and contradictory? What are the implications of those assumptions for practice?

2. How would you redesign the physical work space at EmergiCare (or in your own organization)? Would simply changing the physical layout change the communication dynamics at play? Why or why not?

3. Reflecting on your own place of work, how do you resist and acquiesce to assumptions of difference, such as gender assumptions, relevant to how and why you work? Put another way, are you expected to enact practices that reflect feminine or masculine ideals? How so? What does this mean for your day-to-day interactions?

4. The next time you visit a health care provider, how might you communicate to encourage case or comfort talk? What might be reasons for doing so?

Note

1 The authors wish to thank Heather Pitts for her assistance in creating Figure 7.1.

Suggested Reading

Apker, J. & Eggly, S. (2004). Communicating professional identity in medical socialization: Considering the ideological discourse of morning report. *Qualitative Health Research, 14*, 411–429.

Barbour, J. B. & Gill, R. (2014). Designing communication for the day-to-day safety oversight of nuclear power plants. *Journal of Applied Communication Research, 42*, 168–189.

Dean, M. & Oetzel, J. G. (2014). Physicians' perspectives of managing tensions around dimensions of effective communication in the emergency department. *Health Communication, 29*, 257–266.

References

Aakhus, M. (2001). Technocratic and design stances toward communication expertise: How GDSS facilitators understand their work. *Journal of Applied Communication Research, 29*, 341–371.

Aakhus, M. (2007). Communication as design. *Communication Monographs, 74*, 112–117.

Aakhus, M. & Jackson, S. (2005). Technology, interaction, and design. In K. Fitch & R. Sanders (Eds.), *Handbook of language and social interaction* (pp. 411–436). Mahwah, NJ: Lawrence Erlbaum Associates, Inc.

Aakhus, M. & Laureij, L. V. (2012). Activity materiality, and creative struggle in the communicative constitution of organizing: Two cases of communication design practice. *Language and Dialogue, 2*, 41–59.

Aakhus, M. & Rumsey, E. (2010). Crafting supportive communication online: A communication design analysis of conflict in an online support group. *Journal of Applied Communication Research, 38*, 65–84.

Acker, J. (1990). Hierarchies, jobs, bodies: A theory of gendered organizations. *Gender and Society, 4*(2), 139–158.

Allen, B. J. (2004). *Difference matters: Communicating social identity*. Prospect Heights, IL: Waveland Press.

Alvesson, M. & Karreman, D. (2000). Varieties of discourse: On the study of organizations through discourse analysis. *Human Relations, 53*, 1125–1149.

Alvesson, M. & Willmott, H. (2002). Identity regulation as organizational control: Reproducing the appropriate individual. *Journal of Management Studies, 39*, 619–644.

Apker, J. & Eggly, S. (2004). Communicating professional identity in medical socialization: Considering the ideological discourse of morning report. *Qualitative Health Research, 14*, 411–429.

Apker, J., Propp, K. M., & Zabava Ford, W. (2005). Negotiating status and identity tensions in healthcare team interactions: An exploration of nurse role dialectics. *Journal of Applied Communication Research, 33*, 93–115.

Ashcraft, K. L. (2007). Appreciating the 'work' of discourse: Occupational identity and difference as organizing mechanisms in the case of commercial airline pilots. *Discourse & Communication, 1*, 9–36.

Ashcraft, K. L. (2011). Knowing work through the communication of difference: A revised agenda for difference studies. In D. K. Mumby (Ed.), *Reframing difference in organizational communication studies: Research, pedagogy, practice* (pp. 3–29). Thousand Oaks, CA: Sage.

Ashcraft, K. L. (2013). The glass slipper: "Incorporating" occupational identity in management studies. *Academy of Management Review, 38*, 6–31.

Ashcraft, K. L., Kuhn, T. R., & Cooren, F. (2009). Constitutional ammendments: "Materializing" organizational communication. *The Academy of Management Annals, 3*, 1–64.

Ashforth, B. E., Rogers, K. M., & Corley, K. G. (2011). Identity in oganizations: Exploring cross-level dynamics. *Organization Science, 22*, 1144–1156.

Ballard, D. I. (2014). Measure twice, cut once: The temporality of communication design. *Journal of Applied Communication Research, 42*, 190–207.

Barbour, J. B. (2010). On the institutional moorings of talk in health care. *Management Communication Quarterly, 24*, 449–456.

Barbour, J. B. & Gill, R. (2014). Designing communication for the day-to-day safety oversight of nuclear power plants. *Journal of Applied Communication Research, 42*, 168–189.

Barbour, J. B. & James, E. P. (forthcoming). Collaboration for compliance: Identity tensions in the interorganizational regulation of a toxic waste facility. *Journal of Applied Communication Research.*

Barbour, J. B. & Lammers, J. C. (2007). Health care institutions, communication, and physicians' experience of managed care: A multilevel analysis. *Management Communication Quarterly, 21,* 201–231.

Barbour, J. B. & Lammers, J. C. (2015). Measuring professional identity: A review of the literature and a multilevel confirmatory factor analysis of professional identity constructs. *Journal of Professions and Organization, 2,* 38–60.

Becker, F. D. (1981). *Workspace: Creating environments in organizations.* Westport, CT: Praeger Publishers.

Chatham-Carpenter, A. & DeFrancisco, V. (1998). Women construct self-esteem in their own terms: A feminist qualitative study. *Feminism and Psychology, 8,* 467–489.

Cheney, G. & Ashcraft, K. L. (2007). Considering "The Professional" in communication studies: Implications for theory and research within and beyond the boundaries of organizational communication. *Communication Theory, 17,* 146–175.

Davies, K. (2003). The body and doing gender: The relations between doctors and nurses in hospital work. *Sociology of Health & Illness, 25,* 720–742.

Davis, M. C., Leach, D. J., & Clegg, C. W. (2011). The physical environment of the office: Contemporary and emerging issues. In G. P. Hodgkinson & J. K. Ford (Eds.), *International Review of Industrial and Organizational Psychology* (Vol. 26, pp. 193–235). Chichester, UK: Wiley.

De Certeau, M. (1984). *The practice of everyday life.* Berkeley, CA: University of California.

Dean, M. & Oetzel, J. G. (2014). Physicians' perspectives of managing tensions around dimensions of effective communication in the emergency department. *Health Communication, 29,* 257–266.

Demarco, T. & Lister, T. (2013). *Peopleware* (3rd ed.). Indianapolis, IN: Addison-Wesley Professional.

Eisenberg, E. M., Baglia, J., & Pynes, J. E. . (2006). Transforming emergency medicine through narrative: Qualitative action research at a community hospital. *Health Communication, 19,* 197–208.

Eisenberg, E. M., Murphy, A. G., Sutcliffe, K. M., Wears, R., Schenkel, S., Perry, S., & Vanderhoef, M. (2005). Communication in emergency medicine: Implications for patient safety. *Communication Monographs, 72,* 390–413.

Eisenberg, N. (2002). Empathy-related emotional responses, altruism, and their socialization. In R. J. Davidson & A. Harrington (Eds.), *Visions of compassion: Western scientists and Tibetan Buddhists examine human nature* (pp. 131–164). Oxford: Oxford University Press.

Ellingson, L. L. & Buzzanell, P. M. (1999). Listening to women's narratives of breast cancer treatment: A feminist approach to patient satisfaction with physician-patient communication. *Health Communication, 11,* 153–181.

Elsbach, K. D. & Pratt, M. G. (2007). The physical environment in organizations. *Academy of Management Annals, 1,* 181–224.

Fairhurst, G. T. & Putnam, Linda L. (2004). Organizations as discursive constructions. *Communication Theory, 14,* 5–26.

Foucault, M. (1963, 1973). *The birth of the clinic: An archeology of medical perception.* New York, NY: Vintage Books Random House.

Gamble, V. N. (2000). Subcutaneous scars. *Health Affairs, 19,* 164–169.

General Services Administration. (2009). *The new federal workplace: A report on the performance of six workplace 20–20 projects.* Retrieved from http://www.gsa.gov/graphics/pbs/GSA_NEWWORKPLACE.pdf.

Gill, R. & Larson, G. S. (2014). Making the ideal (local) entrepreneur: Place and the regional development of high-tech entrepreneurial identity. *Human Relations, 67*(5), 519–542.

Guerrero, L., Jones, S. M., & Boburka, R. R. (2006). Sex differences in emotional communication. In K. Dindia & D. J. Canary (Eds.), *Sex differences and similarities in communication* (2nd ed., pp. 241–261). Mahwah, NJ: Lawrence Erlbaum Associates.

Halford, S. & Leonard, P. (2006). *Negotiating gendered identities at work: Place, space and time.* New York, NY: Palgrave Macmillan.

Hallam, J. (2000). Nursing the image: Media, image, and professional identity. New York, NY: Routledge.

Harrison, T. R. (2013). The relationship between conflict, anticipatory procedural justice, and design with intentions to use ombudsman processes. *International Journal of Conflict Management, 24*, 56–72.

Harrison, T. R. (2014). Enhancing communication interventions and evaluations through communication design. *Journal of Applied Communication Research, 42*, 135–149.

Harrison, T. R., Morgan, S. E., Chewning, L. V., Williams, E. A., Barbour, J. B., DiCorcia, M. J., & Davis, L. A. (2011). Revisiting the worksite in worksite health campaigns: Evidence from a multi-site organ donation campaign. *Journal of Communication, 61*, 535–555.

Harrison, T. R., Morgan, S. E., King, A. J., & Williams, E. A. (2011). Saving lives branch by branch: The effectiveness of driver licensing bureau campaigns to promote organ donor registry sign-ups to African Americans in Michigan. *Journal of Health Communication, 16*, 805–819.

Hinze, S. W. (1999). Gender and the body of medicine or at least some body parts: (Re)constructing the prestige hierarchy of medical specialties. *The Sociological Quarterly, 40*, 217–239.

Jackson, S. & Aakhus, M. (2014). Becoming more reflective about the role of design in communication. *Journal of Applied Communication Research, 42*, 125–134.

Knight, M. (2005). The production of the female entrepreneurial subject: A space of exclusion for women of color? *Journal of Women, Politics and Policy, 27*, 151–159.

Konnikova, M. (2014, January 7). The open-office trap. *The New Yorker*.

Kuhn, T. (2009). Positioning lawyers: Discursive resources, professional ethics and identification. *Organization, 16*, 681–704.

Lammers, J. C. (2011). How institutions communicate: Institutional messages, institutional logics, and organizational communication. *Management Communication Quarterly, 25*, 154–182.

Lammers, J. C. & Barbour, J. B. (2006). An institutional theory of organizational communication. *Communication Theory, 16*, 356–377.

Lammers, J. C. & Barbour, J. B. (2009). Exploring the institutional context of physicians' work: Professional and organizational differences in physician satisfaction. In D. E. Brashers & D. J. Goldsmith (Eds.), *Communicating to manage health and illness* (pp. 319–345). Mahwah, NJ: Lawrence Erlbaum Associates.

Lammers, J. C. & Garcia, M. A. (2009). Exploring the concept of "profession" for organizational communication research: Institutional influences in a veterinary organization. *Management Communication Quarterly, 22*, 357–384.

McMurray, R. (2011). The struggle to professionalize: An ethnographic account of the occupational position of Advanced Nurse Practitioners. *Human Relations, 64*, 801–822.

Meisenbach, R. J. (2008). Materiality, discourse, and (dis)empowerment in occupational identity negotiation among higher education fund-raisers. *Management Communication Quarterly, 22*, 258–287.

Monge, P., Rothman, L., Eisenberg, E. M., Miller, K., & Kirste, K. (1985). The dynamics of organizational proximity. *Management Science, 31*, 1129–1141.

Mulac, A. (2006). The gender-linked language effect: Do language differences really make a difference? In K. Dindia & D. J. Canary (Eds.), *Sex differences and similarities in communication* (2nd ed., pp. 219–239). Mahwah, NJ: Lawrence Erlbaum Publishers.

Myers, K. K. & McPhee, R. D. (2006). Influences on member assimilation in workgroups in high-reliability organizations: A multilevel analysis. *Human Communication Research, 32*, 440–468.

National Institute of Building Sciences (2015). Whole building design guide Retrieved January 6, 2015, from http://www.wbdg.org/.

Nelson, H. G. & Stolterman, E. (2012). *The design way: Intentional change in an unpredictable world* (2nd ed.). Cambridge, MA: MIT Press.

O'Keefe, B. J. & Lambert, B. L. (1995). Managing the flow of ideas: A local management approach to message design. In B. Burleson (Ed.), *Communication Yearbook 18*, (pp. 54–82). Newbury Park, CA: Sage Publications.

Pringle, R. (1998). Sex and medicine: Gender, power and authority in the medical profession. Cambridge, UK: Cambridge University Press.

Real, K. (2008). Information seeking and workplace safety: A field application of the risk perception attitude framework. *Journal of Applied Communication Research, 36*, 339–359.

Real, K. (2010). Health-related organizational communication. *Management Communication Quarterly, 24*, 457–464.

Scott, W. R. (2008). Lords of the dance: Professionals as institutional agents. *Organization Studies, 29*, 219–238.

Scott, W. R., Ruef, M., Mendel, P. J., & Caronna, C. A. (2000). *Institutional change and healthcare organizations: From professional dominance to managed care.* Chicago, IL: The University of Chicago Press.

Stolterman, E., Mcatee, J., Royer, D., & Thandapani, S. (2008). *Designerly tools.* Paper presented at the Undisciplined! Design Research Society Conference, Sheffield, UK.

Street, R. L., Makoul, G., Arora, N. K., & Epstein, R. M. (2009). How does communication heal? Pathways linking clinician-patient communication to health outcomes. *Patient Education and Counseling, 74*, 295–301.

Tracy, S. J. & Trethewey, A. (2005). Fracturing the real-self-fake-self dictotomy: Moving toward crystallized organizational identities. *Communication Theory, 15*, 168–195.

Trethewey, A. (1997). Resistance, identity, and empowerment: A postmodern feminist analysis of clients in a human service organization. *Communication Monographs, 64*(4), 281–301.

Ulrich, R. S. (1984). View through a window may influence recovery from surgery. *Science, 224*, 420–421.

Ulrich, R. S., Zimring, C., Zhu, X., DuBose, J., Seo, H.-B., Choi, Y.-S., . . . Joseph, A. (2008). A review of the research literature on evidence-based healthcare design. *Health Environments Research and Design Journal, 1*, 101–165.

Vásquez, C. & Cooren, F. (2013). Spacing practices: The communicative configuration of organizing through space-times. *Communication Theory, 23*, 25–47.

Wells, C. (2013). Controlling "good science": Language, national identity, and occupational control in scientific work. *Management Communication Quarterly, 27*, 319–345.

8

MORAL DISSENT IN HEALTH CARE ORGANIZATIONS

Ryan S. Bisel and Alaina C. Zanin

Discussions of workplace ethics are often sterile, distant, obtuse, hypothetical, removed, and dry. Organizational ethics training and textbooks often fail to take seriously the context in which ethics are actually lived and experienced in the workplace in an ongoing manner. In actual practice, ethical and moral concerns tug at the heart and create anxiety and trepidation among health care professionals in everyday life, but such concerns are rarely discussed in the open, especially at work. Health care organizations present their own unique set of contextual factors in relation to ethical dilemmas and how ethical dilemmas get discussed.

Explaining the Workplace Moral Mum Effect

The *moral mum effect* refers to individuals' reluctance to label unethical behavior as unethical and has been documented to be typical among working adults (Bisel, Kelley, Ploeger, & Messersmith, 2011). Imagine a workplace situation in which you are asked by your boss to write a check from company funds to reimburse (what you know to be) his personal vodka-lunch with friends. Without question, you believe the reimbursement is unethical. What do you do? More to the point, what do you *say*? A program of research in organizational communication suggests (e.g., Bisel & Kramer, 2014) only a small minority (about 10%; Bisel et al., 2011) of working adults would deny the boss's request by labeling it as unethical publicly. In other words, very few of us would turn to our boss in this situation and *say*, "I can't because what you're asking me to do is unethical." The politically and communicatively skillful among us might instead opt for strategies that deny the request without the risk of accusing our boss of being unethical. We may respond by denying the request, but with reasons that do not require us to reveal our private objections based on ethics. In this situation, we could emphasize to the boss how a reimbursement will be difficult because of policy issues or financial constraints; we could feign confusion and ask for clarification, or even attempt to make a friendly joke.

When workers show a reluctance to label unethical workplace behavior, they are participating in a common language game of the workplace. This typical feature of human-language production can be explained by rules of politeness and patterns of sensemaking in work settings. Specifically, individuals understand implicitly that labeling their own or another's behavior as unethical represents a profound face threat to be avoided through silence (Morrison & Milliken, 2000), equivocation (Lucas & Fyke, 2013), politeness (Ploeger, Kelley, & Bisel, 2011), or issue crafting (Sonenshein, 2007). To say to a supervisor or a coworker, "I think what you are doing here is unethical," is a face threat of the highest order, even though it might actually be true. Labeling another's action, or request for action, as unethical holds the strong potential to wreak havoc on the maintenance of positive relationships. If labeling action or requests for action as unethical is so potentially damaging to images and relationships, and, at the same time, is such a rare occurrence in the workplace anyway, why discuss it further?

If organizational members cannot discuss the ethics of actions and requests for action, there is little chance that a group within an organization can give collective thought to its ethical mistakes and learn from those mistakes. Certainly, *individuals* may well be updating their thinking about how ethics should shape action in the workplace, but an *organization* will be unable to do so until members feel they can discuss the ethical implication of actual workplace practices with each other. In other words, group talk *is* group thought (Hirokawa & Rost, 1992). Groups cannot think or learn without communicating. When issues like ethics and morality are undiscussable within a group, the group is necessarily hindered from thinking about and learning from such issues together. Indeed, a group may be able to discuss ethics as the far-off distant ideals of esoteric philosophy, but making those ethics discussable in terms of the here-and-now is difficult because of the face-threatening implications such conversations often create. When it comes to speaking about moral or ethical concerns, the rules of politeness create a barrier to collective moral sensemaking because specific ethical assessments of particular situations are silenced. Given the potential for ethical catastrophe in health care organizations (e.g., the Veterans Administration's chronic fabrication of patient waiting lists; see Jaffe & O'Keefe, 2014), health care organizational leadership should seek to encourage the creation of social systems which detect, report, and remedy moral issues while they remain small and resolvable.

Increasingly, organizational scholars conceive of organizations—including health care organizations—as being similar to biological systems. In biology, the systems that adapt best to environmental hostility survive and thrive. For example, cacti are fit to survive the hostility of drought-prone environments because of adaptive mechanisms (e.g., spines, enlarged stems, special metabolism). Like plants, the human organizations that survive and thrive adapt to ever-changing environmental challenges; unlike plants, human organizations do so through the mechanisms of system-wide learning. The presence—or more likely the absence—of moral dissent in health care organizations is a matter of organizational learning, or, more accurately, a matter of organizational ignorance (i.e., not knowing; Bisel, Messersmith, & Kelley, 2012). Organizations learn when organizational members create, innovate, problem-solve, critique, and make sense of environmental challenges as well as how to meet those challenges and then change work practices accordingly (see Canary, this volume, for discussion of the complementary notion of organizational knowledge). But members of health care organizations will likely be unable to learn from ethical lapses within their systems if they are unable to discuss them publicly with one another. Moral dissent is a kind of critique and an attempt to make sense of how the organization is meeting environmental challenges: in this case, as *not* meeting the deeply-felt standards of right and wrong. To claim a work action or request for action is unethical is to offer a crucial resource or input for organizational moral learning and, ultimately, for maintaining organizational fitness. The perpetuation of unethical behaviors within health care organizations runs the risk of jeopardizing institutions' reputations, but also, could risk the health and well-being of health care providers and patients. When unethical behaviors become rampant within an organization, the organization's fitness wanes, making it increasingly susceptible to systemic catastrophe and failure.

The Moral Mum Effect as It Relates to Health Care Organizations

Thus far, studies of the moral mum effect have been conducted with samples of working adults (including those working in the health care industry), but these studies have not yet grappled with the specific dynamics of organizations within the health care industry. Bisel and Kramer (2014) argued the moral mum effect occurs, in part, when discrepancies exist between workers' private feelings that others' behavior is unethical, but they choose to invoke public justifications in line with financial or operational logics (e.g., it is not good for the bottom line; compare with Sonenshein, 2007). Thus, unethical actions are at times denied, but are rarely denied on ethical grounds, thereby creating a missed opportunity for growing the organization's moral learning capacity. It stands to reason, employees in the health care industry will show similar reluctance to label unethical behavior as unethical and may invoke public justifications which are in line with financial, operational, or bio-medical (Real & Street, 2009) logics typical of discourses of practice in modern medicine (Harter & Kirby, 2004). *Discourse of practice* refers to persistent ways of talking (and therefore ways of thinking) about the provision of health care common among health care practitioners. For example, a practitioner may verbally justify to colleagues obtaining informed consent from a patient through less-than-transparent means by arguing the treatment is needed for recovery without ever referencing ethical concerns (Olufowote, 2011). Here, the logic of "recovery" trumps other ways of seeing patients, such as individuals in need of dignity, and the legitimacy of their dignity-related concerns.

Discourses of Practice and the Moral Mum Effect

There are two major discourses of practice within modern medicine: the *biomedical* and the *biopsychosocial*. While the biopsychosocial model, discussed later in the chapter, has been proposed as an alternative to the biomedical model, the biomedical model remains as the dominant discourse within modern medicine. Specifically, the biomedical model underlies a discourse that promotes neutrality (e.g., decision-making without acknowledging the role of bias or emotion) and espouses scientific objectivity (e.g., diagnosing patients without regard to patients' own characterization of their health and illness). Harter and Kirby (2004) explain that the major tenants of the biomedical model emphasize (a) treating patient symptoms "rationally" rather than treating patients holistically and (b) managing uncertainty through scientific information seeking. This discourse disregards so-called "subjective," humanistic, and contextually-bound perspectives of how patients experience illness. Often, the biomedical perspective privileges the reality of the physician and marginalizes the reality of the patient. Imagine a doctor's visit in which you felt frustrated, unheard, rushed, or uncertain because of an interaction with a health care professional. Likewise, many of us would not express our discontent or disagreement with a supervising physician's diagnosis, given the face-threatening nature of the situation, our deeply-entrenched deference to power, and the structural constraints of time and money present in the modern medical system.

Consequently, the biomedical model of health care reinforces deeply embedded social identities, or roles, in which patients are viewed as uneducated, emotional, and irrational (Apker & Eggly, 2004), while doctors are cast as all-knowing omnipotent figures (Lupton, 1997). This casting reinforces the moral mum effect given the heightened power differential not only between physicians and patients, but among other organizational members as well (e.g., see Barbour, Gill, & Dean, this volume, for further discussion of power differentials in health care). Moreover, a biomedical discourse reinforces power structures where physicians gain compliance through technical expertise and authority.

Understanding how subtly private matters of morality and ethical concern get repackaged and repositioned in ordinary health care organizational discourse can be difficult. In order to illustrate theses social processes we draw from interview data that provides first-person insight into the public-private discrepancies about ethics that can arise in an ordinary health care organizational situation. We present the retrospective account as a first-person narrative, in order to invite readers to participate emotionally with our participant, Laura, as she struggles to find the words to confront her supervisor with her own moral objections about his conduct without risking his ego and her career. Then, we leverage the narrative to explain important concepts as well as offer recommendations for leaders who wish to cultivate authentic moral dialogue within health care organizations.

Focal Narrative: Being a Proxy for Patient Voice

Laura clasped Mrs. Garcia's frail hand as she evaluated swelling in her upper left arm. Laura stood on Mrs. Garcia's right side intentionally in order to give eye contact. Months earlier Mrs. Garcia suffered a stroke that paralyzed the left half of her face and arm. Laura pressed down Mrs. Garcia's arm asking, "Does this hurt?" "Does this hurt?" Each time, Mrs. Garcia winced. Clearly, she was in pain. Laura noted that Mrs. Garcia understood what she was asking, even though she was unable to speak.

Laura frowned. As a third-year medical student, even she knew that swelling was symptomatic of an edema, likely caused by an infection from previous surgery. If untreated, it could result in serious, even life-threatening complications. She felt a sense of frustration and unease. Laura knew why Dr. Howe, the attending physician, overlooked the complication—he had not taken the time to do a physical exam, or ask Mrs. Garcia how she was feeling. Even after Laura reminded Dr. Howe of Mrs. Garcia's partial paralysis, he stood on her left side. Consequently, Mrs. Garcia was unable to give him any nonverbal feedback.

Three days prior, Mrs. Garcia, an 80-year-old nursing home patient, was admitted to the hospital for a urinary tract infection. Dr. Howe ordered antibiotics but had not returned to check on Mrs. Garcia. To Laura, Dr. Howe seemed solely concerned with treating the infection and returning Mrs. Garcia to her nursing home. Laura knew she had to be an advocate for Mrs. Garcia, but she could not point out to Dr. Howe that he overlooked this symptom because of his carelessness, apathy, and bias against Mrs. Garcia. Earlier that day, he reminded Laura to "not spend too much time with any one patient" because they needed to "get through the patient list." Plus, Laura was not even a resident; she was just a lowly medical student. She felt she was in no position to tell her attending physician he was wrong, but remaining silent would be wrong as well. During rounds, Laura saw Dr. Howe in the hallway. She grabbed Mrs. Garcia's chart and approached him timidly. Laura coughed.

"Uh, Dr. Howe? Sorry, could I talk to you about something?"

"Yes Laura, briefly. What is it?" Dr. Howe said as he glanced in her direction.

"I was looking over Mrs. Garcia's chart this afternoon and I noticed she had surgery recently. Her upper arm is showing swelling. I know that often in geriatric patients that can be a sign of an edema. Do you think that could be something?" Laura said meekly.

Dr. Howe turned to face Laura, "Why were you looking through Mrs. Garcia's chart? Didn't I tell you to spend your time getting through the rest of the patients on the floor?"

Laura stammered, "I'm sorry, I took a little more time because I wasn't sure where the swelling was coming from. I wanted to collect more evidence to support my diagnosis. Also, I didn't want her to get discharged back to the nursing home, they find the swelling, and she gets sent right back to us."

Dr. Howe commented, "Oh, well, yes that would be a waste of time. We should probably take a look at that. Can I see her chart?"

Laura felt relieved. She did not have to tell Dr. Howe that he had made a serious error because of his carelessness and unethical treatment of Mrs. Garcia. She knew Mrs. Garcia was going to get the care she needed and she was able to tell Dr. Howe about the issue without overstepping her role as a medical student. *Win-win*, she thought.

As ordinary as this real-life medical dialogue might seem, it raises important questions: Was the way Laura handled this situation really a "win" for the organization? Was the outcome a "win" for Dr. Howe and his future patients?

Theorizing the Role of Biomedical Discourse in the Moral Mum Effect

A biomedical discourse reinforces that physicians are powerful because of their technical expertise. This underlying assumption is exemplified in Laura's reluctance to confront her attending physician about an incomplete diagnosis. If we consider all employees' private moral concerns to be important resources for organizational moral learning, Laura's contribution in this manner is important and should not be conflated with her inferior technical expertise to Dr. Howe. In other words, there *is* disparity between Laura and Dr. Howe's technical know-how, but that disparity does not necessarily imply that Dr. Howe is any more capable of sensing when and where current work efforts are falling short of moral excellence. In fact, Dr. Howe's professional and organizational socialization may be keeping him from sensing where current work efforts are falling short of moral excellence—socialization forces which Laura has not yet been influenced by as heavily (see Myers & Gaillard, this volume, for further discussion of socialization forces in the health care industry).

The biopsychosocial orientation is a counterview to the biomedical model and is characterized by a philosophy of *treating and valuing patients as whole persons* (Harter & Kirby, 2004). The biopsychosocial model of health care recognizes emotional, social, and contextual factors are relevant to the diagnosis and treatment of patients (Apker & Eggly, 2004). This orientation is in response to the biomedical model, which has been criticized for failing to recognize how patients experience illness and wellness in the broader context of their lives. A biopsychosocial orientation allows health care professionals to delve more deeply into a host of issues (e.g., socioeconomic level, relational abuse, culture and religious beliefs, mental illness) that may be contributing to—or manifest in—physiological symptoms. However, realistically, this approach to health care takes time, resources, and compassion that may be mentally and emotionally taxing on health care professionals (e.g., emotional labor and burnout, see Way & Tracy, 2012). With growing resource and staffing constraints, paired with greater demands placed on health care providers than ever before, providers and health care organizations are often influenced strongly by outside entities (e.g., insurance companies, Medicare), which can come to shape the way health care is provided. These structuring rules and resources influence medical discourse and consequently what behaviors get claimed as "ethical" in a health care organization.

Managed Care Versus Patient-Centered Care

A managed care model of health care has changed modern medical discourse. Managed care is an arrangement where insurance providers accept the risk for providing a set of health services—using a defined network of providers often for a specific population of patients—in return for fixed payments (Lammers & Duggan, 2002). Given governmental and public pressures on health care organizations to provide accessible, cost-effective health care, a managed care system emerged out of a movement to commodify and "ration" health care access and resources (Miller, Joseph, & Apker, 2000). In a managed care model, efficiency is rewarded over quality and has largely led to the disempowerment of physicians' decision-making (e.g., diagnostic testing must be cleared through insurance agencies before being ordered, see Lammers & Geist, 1997). Minogue (2000) explains:

> Physicians who view themselves as having ethical duties only to the patients are at odds with the new world of medicine. . . . Managed care logically requires that physicians become dual stewards . . . physicians have dual duties that require the development of new skills aimed at balancing the interests and wishes of patients with the financial integrity of the system.
>
> *(p. 442)*

A physician's obligation of "dual-stewardship" in managed care models creates financial, legal, and ethical tensions that must be negotiated regularly. For example, Real, Bramson, and Poole (2009) demonstrated that physicians are keenly aware of the "business of medicine" in terms of their own identity and role within health care organizations. However, Real et al. (2009) also found that physicians viewed medicine as a noble profession in which they are held to high moral and ethical standards. One participant explained, "I still think it's a very honorable profession and that you have more freedom to do the right or the wrong thing. There's more personal integrity involved in this than in any other occupation" (p. 580). Thus, health care providers have some autonomy to make ethical decisions, but at the same time are bound by structural constraints. The concurrent discourses of medicine as "noble" and as a "business" may not always be complementary and can be in competition.

In contrast with the managed care model of health care, there has been a call for a "patient-centered" approach to health care. Epstein et al. (2005) explain that patient-centered care is characterized by health care providers: (a) eliciting and understanding the patient's perspective (e.g., desires, experiences, needs), (b) enhancing shared understanding of the patient within his or her unique psychosocial context, and (c) including patients in their health care and treatment based on individual preference. Patient-centered care is an ideal, which many health care organizations strive to provide for their patients. However, there are several barriers to providing patient-centered care (e.g., economic and resource limitations) similar to the biopsychosocial perspective. While many health care organizations promote patient-centered care, the way in which care is actually provided in the minutiae of daily life may be quite different (see Berwick, 2009). As a result, the biomedical and managed care models dominate ways of talking (and therefore ways of thinking) present within modern medicine.

Future Directions for the Moral Mum Effect in Health Care Organizations

Given the ideological context of the biomedical and managed care models, paired with Bisel and Kramer's (2014) finding that workers are more likely to invoke justifications in line with financial or operational logics (i.e., logics that are closely in line with biomedical discourse), it is unlikely workers in the health care industry would label their colleagues and supervisors' behaviors as unethical overtly. We can easily imagine future research studies that document biomedical discourses in health care worker's public justifications for their private ethical objections. Take for example, medical student Laura's reluctance to confront her attending physician about his rushed and insensitive assessment of Mrs. Garcia in order to "get through the patient list." Laura believes privately that standardizing the amount of time spent with a patient and being pressured to do so is unethical. Moreover, she believes in a patient-centered approach to health care, where patients are active participants rather than lists of symptoms. Disregarding her private feelings, she justifies her actions publicly through financial and operational logics (e.g., "If I hadn't caught this other symptom she may have been sent back to the hospital from the nursing home, wasting time and money," or, "I need more time to collect more evidence to justify my diagnosis objectively") rather than ethical logics (e.g., "It's unethical to treat patients as lists of symptoms, we should be treating patients as whole persons").

Within this example we can see the logics of the biomedical model and managed health care take precedence over the voicing of ethics-based justification alternatives. The focal narrative illustrates how authentic ethical justifications can be absent in health care organizational discourse and how private ethical concerns are subtly replaced with other concerns in the content of organizational communication. Avoiding face threats, power differentials, and fear of retribution serve to mute voices of moral and ethical dissent. Ethnography paired with private retrospective interviews could be a useful combination for identifying public-private discrepancies about ethics in health care organizational talk. Likewise we could imagine language-production experiments like those created by Bisel and colleagues, which identify the regularity of biomedical justifications in the denial of unethical health care organizational requests.

Another promising avenue for extending the moral mum effect in health care organizations is to test whether the explicit *inclusion* of ethics talk in public organizational health care discourse by health care supervisors suppresses workers tendency to avoid labeling unethical requests as unethical. Here, moral talk contagion might be identified as the countervailing positive social process to workers' moral mum effect. Again, we can easily imagine a language production experiment in which health care workers are induced to believe their supervisors regularly describe health care tasks in terms of "ethics" and "morals." Then, workers could be asked to respond to an unethical request. Responses could be coded for the presence of moral talk as compared with a control group or workers who are induced to believe supervisors regularly describe situations in terms of biomedical logics. In the following, we discuss how leaders in health care organizations might overcome hegemonic discourses and the moral mum effect to foster organizational moral learning and adaptation.

Sensitivity to the Ethics of Health Care Organizations' Operations

Weick and Sutcliffe (2007) explained that organizations characterized by high reliability in accomplishing tasks that could threaten human life and well-being (e.g., health care organizations) tend to enact ongoing and vigilant sensitivity to operations. Health care organizations need to be reliable; to fail in the reliability of their performance means danger, injury, or death is close at hand. Sensitivity to operations allows high reliability organizations (HROs) to anticipate future failure by being "attentive to the front line where the real work gets done" (p. 12). While the phrase may sound a bit mysterious, pragmatically, *sensitivity to operations* tends to be accomplished through the cultivation of trusting human relationships in HROs. A common misconception about management is that nothing bad ever happens under the watchful eyes of truly great managers. A different view proposes that trouble is always inevitable and so great managers are the ones who identify trouble quickly while trouble is small and manageable. Poor managers are oblivious to how troubles are piling up and are being linked and amplified in intensity until catastrophe strikes (Weick & Sutcliffe, 2007). But, how do great managers actually identify trouble while it is minor and resolvable? The answer is both simple and complex: great managers identify trouble while it is small and resolvable *through others who trust them* enough to alert them to problems or potential problems. Achieving sensitivity to operations requires interpersonal trust.

The moral mum effect implies that remaining sensitive to the ethics of a health care organization's operation will be difficult. Of course, getting workers to speak up with their concerns about operations to management is always difficult (Kassing, 2011). When their private dissent includes concerns about ethics and morality, such ethical dissent is even less likely to be expressed to management (Kassing & Armstrong, 2002) in plain language without euphemisms (Lucas & Fyke, 2013) or be expressed directly without equivocation and polite circum-locutions (Bisel et al., 2012; Ploeger et al., 2011). Here, the need for trust and a sense of psychological safety (i.e., group members' sense they can take inter-personal risks; Bradley, Postlethwaite, Klotz, Hamdani, & Brown, 2012) among coworkers, supervisors, and subordinates is paramount because ethical discussions in the workplace are so rare and potentially damaging to public images and relationships. Coworkers need to know they will not be alienated for raising an ethical concern as an ethical concern and they need to know their coworkers and bosses can be trusted not to dismiss ethical concerns as irrelevant or naive. In addition to creating trusting relationships, Kassing (2011) recommends the development of organizational cultures where supervisors invite disagreement and scrutinize positive feedback. Over time, inviting disagreement and scrutiniz-ing positive feedback—in the context of trusting relationships—speaks into being a culture that values learning and the need to reflect constantly and update basic assumptions about how work should be accomplished (Argyris, 1990). Adding to Kassing's recommendation, we recommend inviting *moral* disagreement and scrutinizing the assumptions that workplace practices are always given the benefit of the doubt that they are morally excellent. In light of these recommendations, the capturing of moral dissent in health care organizations is obviously difficult and requires a multi-pronged approached. Yet, the building of trusting relation-ships remains central in these efforts (Bartolomé, 1993).

Supervisors who want to remain sensitive to the ethics of ongoing operations in health care organizations have to build such trusting relationships that they can "listen *through* indirectness" (Ploeger et al., 2011, p. 477, emphasis origi-nal). Since it is well documented that workers employ a variety of language forms to soften or even hide their private belief that an action or request for action is unethical, vigilant managers will have to accumulate enough experience with coworkers and subordinates that unusual nonverbal or verbal nuances can be detected. For example, weak signals like when a subordinate apologizes for no reason, appears to be confused, stutters, frowns, averts gaze, fails to comply, delays compliance, or is less available for conversations could each indicate the subordinate has private moral concerns that are not being shared forthrightly and publicly with the work team or supervisors. Take, for example, Laura's apologiz-ing, hedging, and stammering. Dr. Howe could have used these signals to iden-tify a subordinate who may be struggling with an ethical issue. Listening through indirectness involves identifying such weak signals and seeking gentle means of investigation. This would enable a leader to recognize when moral trouble may be afoot and whether that trouble can be identified while it remains small, resolvable, and learnable.

Managing the Silencing Effect of Power Differentials in Health Care Teams

Power differentials and hierarchies of prestige are common in health care teams. Team-based efforts are one of the most typical means through which health care is now delivered in the United States (see Real & Poole, this volume, for more on health care teams). Long-standing traditions, educational and pay differences, among many other factors, can contribute to team members' sense that they are not equals. That sense can cause workers with low status to make sense of their own private dissent as unwanted, mistaken, or even potentially damaging to themselves, if voiced. For instance, Bisel and Arterburn's (2012) study of the reasons why employees are reluctant to speak up to their bosses included participants' predictions that harm would come to them, or supervisors would not listen, if they spoke up freely. Likewise, participants also made sense of their withholding of dissent by questioning their own expertise and by constructing supervisors as ultimately responsible, thereby absolving themselves of their duty to voice dissent. It seems likely that health care team members, who have less status than other team members, would make sense of their silence in similar ways and avoid speaking up freely. Pronovost (2010) illustrates this point: "Perhaps most concerning is the response from nurses in participating hospitals when asked: 'if a new nurse in your hospital saw a senior physician placing a catheter but not complying with the checklist, would the nurse speak up.' The answer is almost always, 'there is no way the nurse would speak up'" (p. 204).

Nembhard and Edmondson (2006) found that leaders' inclusiveness in health care teams enhanced team members' sense of psychological safety, bolstering team members' willingness to speak up freely, and the team's ability to learn. *Leader inclusiveness* refers to leadership communication behavior that solicits input from team members and that demonstrates a deep appreciation for others' contributions without regard for status. These findings support the notion that leadership communication is a key to getting dissent, perhaps even moral dissent, from organizational members in health care settings. In light of Nembhard and Edmondson's (2006) findings, we recommend that leaders of organizational health care teams model communicative inclusiveness that also involves seeking and appreciating team member input regarding ethical concerns, without regard for team member status. All organizational members can serve as "moral barometers" or "ethics experts" for the organization; however, unfortunately, individuals may forget that, even though a team member has little technical expertise, tenure, or organizational authority, all individuals have ethical sensitivities. Leaders should be sensitive to their assumptions in order to cultivate moral organizational learning by listening through indirectness from *all* team members.

After Action Reviews as Sites of Authentic Ethical Dialogue

Recurring after action reviews (AARs) in health care organizations, like surgical morbidity and mortality conferences (M&Ms), are important sites of organizational learning in health care contexts and could be an important site for suppressing the moral mum effect's influence throughout a social system. Morbidity and mortality conferences are a common and recurring work practice in which surgeons meet in closed sessions to critique one another's technical performance and decision-making in the surgical theater. These conversations are preplanned and belong to a professional culture in which critique is common. In essence, M&Ms are planned conversational times designated for reflection and learning. Of course, not only surgeons need to reflect and learn from their own and others' mistakes; all kinds of workers can benefit from time to reflect. We recommend institutionalizing such after action reviews throughout health care organizations. AARs are likely to be keen opportunities to raise ethical concerns and invite others to discuss how current work practices could aspire to—not only avoid ethical failings—but achieve moral excellence in everyday work functions. However, while AARs are widely known to be important sites of organizational learning (Weick & Sutcliffe, 2007), after action review conversations themselves can unfold as struggles for power and impression management (e.g., Minei & Bisel, 2013) if they are not facilitated earnestly with the goal of sincere learning.

As difficult as it may be at first, we recommend leaders encourage dialogue that includes *specific* ethical assessments of *particular* medical decisions and actions—in all their ambiguity. Jovanovic and Wood's (2006) study of Denver City workers revealed ethics training was effective only when workers were encouraged to discuss particular and ambiguous ethical cases in which they themselves were *personally* involved. The researchers note the common tendency among people who discuss ethics do so in neutral and unemotional terms and in such a way as to distance oneself from the force of ethics in everyday life. The so-called "moral superiority of the uninvolved" threatens to make conversations about ethics in the workplace just another policy-driven, check-the-box, bureaucratic opportunity for cynicism. To avoid the othering that takes place in the dry, sometime absurd, hypothetical dilemmas so typical of business ethics courses, we recommend courageous leaders initiate such discussions by telling personal narratives of their own work life in which they had to struggle with the difficulty of making sense of an ethical situation. Indeed, such conversations are inherently face-threatening. However, these self-disclosures are the foundation of relational development, which might initiate reciprocity and allow leaders to gain insight into the often private moral judgments of employees and coworkers (Baack, Fogliasso, & Harris, 2000). Modeling how to discuss ethics as they pertain to particular decisions as well as praising others when ethics and ethical assessments are voiced publicly should suppress the moral mum effect.

Building trusting relationships is crucial to obtaining upward dissent, especially ethical dissent (Bartolomé, 1993), and is critical to accomplishing authentic team-based ethical dialogue.

Conclusion

Overall, this chapter provides a theoretical and applied link among the moral mum effect, discourses of practice, and organizational moral learning. We hope this chapter not only highlights how the absence of upward moral dissent can manifest in consequential ways in health care organizations, but also how communication theory can be applied to remedy this organizational communication phenomenon. Moral dissent is essential to building strong health care organizations. Together, leaders and frontline workers in the health care industry have the ability to cultivate an open climate of vigilance and trust in hopes of fostering morally adaptive organizations.

DISCUSSION QUESTIONS

1. Tell the story of a time you were reluctant to label another's actions or requests as unethical publicly, even though you privately had moral concerns.
2. How might the moral mum effect harm health care organizations, health care workers, and patients?
3. What are some strategies for suppressing the moral mum effect?
4. Imagine you are supervisor within a health care organization: Identify some message strategies for suppressing the moral mum effect.

Suggested Reading

Bisel, R. S. & Kramer, M. W. (2014). Denying what workers believe are unethical workplace requests: Do workers use moral, operational, or policy justifications publicly? *Management Communication Quarterly, 28*, 111–129.

Sonenshein, S. (2007). The role of construction, intuition, and justification in responding to ethical issues at work: The sensemaking-intuition model. *Academy of Management Review, 32*, 1022–1040.

References

Apker, J. & Eggly, S. (2004). Communicating professional in medical socialization: Considering the ideological discourse of morning report. *Qualitative Health Research, 14*, 411–429.

Argyris, C. (1990). *Overcoming organizational defenses: Facilitating organizational learning.* Englewood Cliffs, NJ: Prentice Hall.

Baack, D., Fogliasso, C., & Harris, J. (2000). The personal impact of ethical decisions: A social penetration theory. *Journal of Business Ethics, 24,* 39–49.

Bartolomé, F. (1993). Nobody trusts the boss completely: Now what? In Harvard Business Review Book Series. *The articulate executive: Orchestrating effective communication* (pp. 3–16). Boston, MA: Harvard Business School Publishing.

Berwick, D. M. (2009). What "patient-centered" should mean: Confessions of an extremist. *Health Affairs, 28,* W555–W565.

Bisel, R. S. & Arterburn, E. N. (2012). Making sense of organizational members' silence: A sensemaking-resource model. *Communication Research Reports, 29,* 217–226.

Bisel, R. S., Messersmith, A. S., & Kelley, K. M. (2012). Supervisor-subordinate communication: Hierarchical mum effect meetings organizational learning. *Journal of Business Communication, 49,* 128–147.

Bisel, R. S., Kelley, K. M., Ploeger, N. A., & Messersmith, J. (2011). Workers' moral mum effect: On facework and unethical behavior in the workplace. *Communication Studies, 62,* 153–170.

Bisel, R. S. & Kramer, M. W. (2014). Denying what workers believe are unethical workplace requests: Do workers use moral, operational, or policy justifications publicly? *Management Communication Quarterly, 28,* 111–129.

Bradley, B. H., Postlethwaite, B. E., Klotz, A. C., Hamdani, M. R., & Brown, K. G. (2012). Reaping the benefits of task conflict in teams: The critical role of team psychological safety climate. *Journal of Applied Psychology, 97,* 151–158.

Epstein, R. M., Franks, P., Fiscella, K., Shields, C. G., Meldrum, S. C., Kravitz, R. L., & Duberstein, P. R. (2005). Measuring patient-centered communication in Patient–Physician consultations: Theoretical and practical issues. *Social Science & Medicine, 61,* 1516–1528.

Harter, L. M. & Kirby, E. (2004). Socializing medical students in an era of managed care: The ideological significance of standardized and virtual patients. *Communication Studies, 55,* 48–67.

Hirokawa, R. Y. & Rost, K. M. (1992). Effective group decision making in organizations: Field test of the vigilant interaction theory. *Management Communication Quarterly, 5,* 267–288.

Jaffe, G. & O'Keefe, E. (2014, May 29). Calls for VA Secretary Eric Shinseki to resign intensify following watchdog report. *The Washington Post.* Retrieved from http://www.washingtonpost.com.

Jovanovic, S. & Wood, R. V. (2006). Communication ethics and ethical culture: A study of the ethics initiative in Denver city government. *Journal of Applied Communication Research, 34,* 386–405.

Kassing, J. W. (2011). *Dissent in organizations.* Malden, MA: Polity Press.

Kassing, J. W. & Armstrong, T. A. (2002). Someone's going to hear about this: Examining the association between dissent-triggering events and employees' dissent expression. *Management Communication Quarterly, 16,* 39–65.

Lammers, J. C. & Duggan, A. (2002). Bringing the physician back in: Communication predictors of physicians' satisfaction with managed care. *Health Communication, 14*(4), 493–513.

Lammers, J. & Geist, P. (1997). The transformation of caring in the light and shadow of managed care. *Health Communication, 9,* 45–60.

Lucas, K. & Fyke, J. P. (2013). Euphemisms and ethics: A language-centered analysis of Penn State's sexual abuse scandal. *Journal of Business Ethics,* 1–19.

Lupton, D. (1997). Psychoanalytic sociology and the medical encounter: Parsons and beyond. *Sociology of Health & Illness, 19*, 561–579.

Miller, K., Joseph, L., & Apker, J. (2000). Strategic ambiguity in the role development process. *Journal of Applied Communication Research, 28*, 193–214.

Minei, E. & Bisel, R. S. (2013). Negotiating the meaning of team expertise: A firefighter team's epistemic denial. *Small Group Research, 44*, 7–32.

Minogue, B. (2000). The two fundamental duties of the physician. *Academic Medicine, 75*, 431–442.

Morrison, E. W. & Milliken, F. J. (2000). Organizational silence: A barrier to change and development in a pluralistic world. *Academy of Management Review, 25*, 706–725.

Nembhard, I. M. & Edmondson, A. C. (2006). Making it safe: The effects of leader inclusiveness and professional status on psychological safety and improvement efforts in health care teams. *Journal of Organizational Behavior, 27*, 941–966.

Olufowote, J. O. (2011). A dialectical perspective on informed consent to treatment: An examination of radiologists' dilemmas and negotiations. *Qualitative Health Research, 21*, 839–852.

Ploeger, N. A., Kelley, K. M., & Bisel, R. S. (2011). Hierarchical mum effect: A new investigation of organizational ethics. *Southern Communication Journal, 76*, 465–481.

Pronovost, P. J. (2010). Learning accountability for patient outcomes. *JAMA, 304*, 204–205.

Real, K., Bramson, R., & Poole, M. (2009). The symbolic and material nature of physician identity: Implications for physician-patient communication. *Health Communication, 24*, 575–587.

Real, K. & Street, R. L. (2009). Doctor-patient communication from an organizational perspective. In D. E. Brashers (Ed.), *Communication to manage health and illness* (pp. 68–90). New York: Routledge.

Sonenshein, S. (2007). The role of construction, intuition, and justification in responding to ethical issues at work: The sensemaking-intuition model. *Academy of Management Review, 32*, 1022–1040.

Way, D. & Tracy, S. J. (2012). Conceptualizing compassion as recognizing, relating, and (re)acting: A qualitative study of compassionate communication at hospice. *Communication Monographs, 79*, 292–315.

Weick, K. E. & Sutcliffe, K. A. (2007). *Managing the unexpected: Resilient performance in an age of uncertainty* (2nd ed.). San Francisco, CA: John Wiley & Sons.

9

CONFLICT MANAGEMENT IN HEALTH CARE ORGANIZATIONS

Navigating the Intersection of Patients, Families, and Health Care Workers

Paula Hopeck

Conflict in health care organizations occurs at three levels: between members of the organization, between patients (and/or their families) and health care workers, and among families and patients using the health care organization. The focus of this chapter is on health care workers and how they manage conflict with and among patient families (see Wright and Nicotera, this volume, for a discussion of conflict between members within health care organizations).

Most health care workers do not receive training in conflict management processes but are often put in situations where conflict is present. Family conflict, particularly at the end of life, is likely to happen at the bedside of the patient (Breen, Abernethy, Abbott, & Tulsky, 2001), and hospital staff may not have much training in formal conflict resolution procedures (Haraway & Haraway, 2005). Most conflicts in the hospital, especially at the end of life, are resolved internally by the hospital (Bloche, 2005), and medical personnel can prevent long-term resentment between family members by resolving family tension (Boelk & Kramer, 2012).

Despite the prevalence of conflict in hospitals and other health care organizations, few health care organizations have implemented training programs for their employees or developed timely dispute resolution processes to help those engaged in conflict (Bloche, 2005; Bowman, 2000; Haraway & Haraway, 2005; Morreim, 2014). Conflict management resources would also facilitate understanding of the process of conflict, and help identify and manage it before it escalates. The goals of this chapter are to (1) review conflict and process models of conflict resolution; (2) to introduce strategies that health care workers currently use to resolve and manage conflict; and (3) to identify the necessary components for a conflict management system in health care, including potential benefits and barriers to implementation.

The Hypothetical Case of Mrs. Kalma

Before delving into different conflict models, an example is provided to help illustrate each of the models. The patient is Mrs. Kalma, who has dementia, but did not name a health care proxy.[1] Mrs. Kalma was brought to the emergency room by her older son (John) and daughter (Ann) after they found her unconscious in her home. John and Ann have families of their own. Both families are low-income, and live in a rural area 100 miles from the hospital. No member of the Kalma family has more than a high school education. John and Ann, up until a few years ago, were very close and relied on each other for help around the house, financially, and with childcare. Since their mother became ill, there has been resentment towards each other about their mother's care. Ann thinks their mother would be better off in an assisted living facility. John wants their mother to move in with Ann so she can be with family, and they can save money. Ann has a young family of her own and does not want to be overwhelmed. The two compromised, by hiring a part-time home health aide, and with Ann visiting their mother every day. After being revived in the emergency room, Mrs. Kalma was transferred to the ICU. John and Ann tell the physicians their mother's health history, although they do not disclose the details of their own decision about her living arrangements, or their resentment towards each other. The ICU can keep Mrs. Kalma alive, but not comfortable, on life support. The physicians recommend palliative care. Mrs. Kalma's children are unprepared for the diagnosis, and John wants more tests done. Ann has noticed a change in her mother over the past few months, and although not prepared for the palliative care recommendation, she tells John that maybe they should consider palliative care before making a decision. John refuses and becomes abrupt with his sister. Ann, out of frustration, accuses her brother of torturing their mother. John tells his sister that she is being selfish. This exchange has occurred in the ICU and many of the nurses, physicians, and aides have noticed.[2]

Conflict: Definitions and Models

Conflict refers to two or more parties who have (or perceive) differences in values, beliefs or goals. Individuals then respond communicatively, thus affecting working relationships and/or the work environment. Conflict occurs in a number of organizational situations. Organizational members have conflict over tasks, relationships, processes, status, or structures (Bendersky & Hays, 2012; Jameson, 1999; Jehn, 1995). Definitions of conflict assume that conflict is a process, not a fleeting event that is perceived, managed, and resolved at once. There are numerous prescriptive and descriptive models. For example, Pondy's (1967) seminal process model identified five phases of conflict. Kilmann and Thomas (1978) described process models as a reaction to events, whereas structural models assume that behavior is a result of an individual's condition. Kilmann and Thomas (1978) also note that conflict within the organization (internal perspective) should be handled differently from conflict that the organization has with an outside party (external perspective).

Beyond the basic perspectives of explaining causes of conflict, process models also assume that conflicts are not isolated incidents, and that individuals identify, manage, and resolve conflict through communication (Putnam, 2006). Communicative strategies may change over the course of the conflict, necessitating the need to distinguish between the different phases of conflict. Classifying the different phases of conflict allows practitioners to recognize and resolve conflict, and theorists to study patterns of strategies across situations.

In the above example, John and Ann appear to meet many of the criteria of a conflict. They perceive a difference in values or goals—they both want what is best for their mother, but disagree about what is "best". The siblings' relationship has been strained since the onset of their mother's illness. The disagreements of the past over her care are now resurfacing in the hospital environment. The medical care Mrs. Kalma receives is contingent on what John and Ann want, making this an organizational issue. Because aggressive care and palliative care are complete opposites, one or the other must be chosen. John and Ann disagree and are enacting their disagreement through accusations and personal attacks. The following paragraphs will review the basic tenets of the sequential contingency model of conflict and the situated model of conflict in social relations, and explain how they can resolve the conflict between Mrs. Kalma's children.

Sequential Contingency Model of Conflict

The sequential contingency model of conflict posits that conflict management depends on the individuals, their relationships, their experiences, and the nature of the conflict. The sequential contingency model assumes that conflict is a cyclical, not linear, process and expands the consequences of conflict beyond the parties involved, arguing that their actions cause reactions in the organization. John and Ann (individuals) are a brother and sister struggling to maintain the closeness they had in prior years (relationship). Ann has been caring for their mother more than John, although John is also concerned with finances and his mother's happiness (experience). In the initial conflict, the two compromised (conflict management style) on their mother's living situation, but neither John nor Ann are completely satisfied with the outcome.

As a result of their strained relationship, the past resolution of the conflict influences future resolution attempts. As noted above, this type of conflict cannot be resolved with a compromise. This conflict, while personal, can be extended to the organization, as their decision will affect the hospital staff, such that nurses or doctors may have to intervene in a family conflict, moving them outside of their normally prescribed organizational roles of health care delivery. If John or Ann is not satisfied with the outcome, they may enact the conflict towards each other in the hospital (upsetting other patients and families), direct their hostility toward the staff, file formal complaints, or, in the worst case, sue the hospital. Therefore, it is in the best interest of the hospital to resolve the conflict. Because the model also includes organizational reactions, it would also include how the staff responds to the family. Using process models in organizational conflict management allows individuals to examine the conflict and how it is managed at each phase to adjust for future interactions.

If Mrs. Kalma stays in the hospital, and her children visit regularly, hospital staff members face a number of challenges. First, they may have to settle more arguments between the siblings. Second, they may find themselves in the middle of a sibling conflict and serving as shuttle diplomats between the siblings to reach a solution about care. In an extreme case, if either sibling is unsatisfied with the final decision, they may file a grievance or a lawsuit against the hospital. Even if the conflict is resolved, the success of the process will influence how hospital staff members approach conflict in the future. They may become involved in family discussions earlier to prevent conflict from escalating, or pay closer attention to family dynamics when the patient is first admitted. They may also begin with asking more directed questions when presenting the diagnosis to get a sense of what the family wants.

The Situated Model of Conflict in Social Relations

The situated model of conflict in social relations can also be helpful in resolving the family conflict. The model includes goal interdependence, distribution of power, and the importance of relationships between parties, each of which can be placed on a continuum (i.e., between high and low). These three axes form a three-dimensional grid, referred to as "field" (Coleman, Kugler, Bui-Wrzosinska, Nowak, & Vallacher, 2012). Unlike the sequential contingency model, this model predicts that the combination of the three factors determines how the individual will approach the conflict. First, they will consider the extent to which the other person agrees with them with. Next, they consider their relative power. Then, the person considers how their goals are linked to the other party's, which determines the importance of the conflict and the relationship to them. The model also accounts for emotion, values, and experience playing a role in how the conflict is approached, which, when discussing the life and death of a relative, should not be excluded (a more in-depth review of emotion and conflict is below).

Referring back to the example of Mrs. Kalma and her children, the importance of this model can help hospital staff members focus on the reasons conflict is occurring. First, following the considerations each party takes, the hospital staff may discuss goals of care with John and Ann. John may want to keep his mother alive, while Ann wants to consider palliative care. Eventually, this may lead to the realization that they both want what is best and hospital staff may facilitate a discussion of what "best" means. Second, the hospital staff may pay attention to underlying power differences. Traditionally, it is assumed that John, as the older son, would have more power. However, the hospital staff may also see that Ann, who serves as the caregiver, may have more information about Mrs. Kalma's declining health. The hospital staff may use that knowledge to address the third consideration, goals of each party. Once again, the hospital staff can discuss John and Ann's goals for care, as well as orient them towards the outcome they want for their relationship.

Emotion in Conflict

Conflict scholars have argued that emotions are the reason for many conflicts (Bodtker & Jameson, 2001; Jones, 2000), and we can assume that this is also true for many patients and their families. Individuals tend to react more strongly to injustice than justice, as they perceive that they must defend themselves, causing emotional arousal (Bies & Tripp, 2002). Or, as Jones (2000, p. 91) noted, "to recognize that we are in conflict is to acknowledge that we have been triggered emotionally." In an atmosphere where emotions are prevalent, emotions may be much more influential in the enactment of conflict than in other organizations. One explanation is that emotions are tied to behaviors. Past emotions during conflict do not directly predict future behavior in conflict; however, what does matter is the individual's memory of the conflict (Kurt, Kugler, Coleman, & Liebovitch, 2014).

In our example above, both children feel resentment. John resents Ann for not wanting to take their mother into her home, and Ann resents John for not considering the strain this would place on the family. Although not explicitly mentioned, both parties care deeply for their mother, and are upset that she is dying. John responds by wanting to save his mother; Ann responds by considering what would make their mother the most comfortable. These two different responses also trigger memories of the past conflict. John recalls Ann being eager to put their mother in a nursing home, and is determined not to let Ann shirk her filial responsibility. Ann recalls that John seemed eager to upset her family's home and life, as well as place their mother in a potentially unsafe environment, in order to save a few dollars. The memories, accurate or not, affect the way that the siblings feel in the hospital.

Health Care Workers and Conflict Management: The 5 Rs

Health care workers are trained in patient care and medical practices (see Lammers, this volume, and Myers and Gaillard, this volume, for discussion of professionalization and organizational assimilation), but not necessarily conflict management. In the above example, hospital staff members have the skills to address the emotions that families are feeling during end of life for a loved one, although unprepared for resolving the conflict that is caused by them. Research into how members of health care organizations manage these types of conflicts identifies some of the strategies employed in conflict management. Data below are drawn from a larger study where individuals from nursing, social work, patient advocacy, and pastoral care (n = 72) were interviewed about their experiences managing conflict between family members. Analysis revealed that health care workers employ variations on one of five general conflict strategies: refocusing, reconciling, reflecting, reframing, and referring (Hopeck, 2013). While these styles may be used individually, many are also used in conjunction with each other.

First, health care workers "refocus" situations. Mostly, this involves bringing the attention of the family back to the patient and what they would want in that situation. Generally, refocusing is one way in which mediators use words strategically (Jacobs & Aakhus, 2002).

> Sheila, palliative care physician: I do the whole encounter as being some about the patient but also largely about the family and how they'll live with themselves and I think there was a phrase I heard: "I want you to feel like you know, you've been the best daughter—or wife or whatever the relationship is—that you can and what would it mean for you to be a good daughter in that situation?

In the above quote, Sheila refocuses the family member's attention by reminding them that they still want to be "the best" or "good" to their parent, but at this stage, that might be letting go, or letting them be at peace. It refocuses attention on the patient, but also refocuses the relationship of the patient to the family member.

Second, health care workers help "reconcile" relationships between family members, although reconciliation may not occur at the same time but instead as part of the grieving process.

> Frances, hospital chaplain: The way I see it in my head is you know those Elizabeth Kubler-Ross stages of acceptance and dying? So to me, there can be five different people in the room, they can each be in a different stage, so you know the patient might be in acceptance and the spouse might be in denial, so me, as a chaplain, I'm this, you know, somewhere it says in our literature that we should be a calm, non-anxious presence [chuckle] I can be like a mediator for the family and to help them accept

each other's point of view and to talk about it with each other may be my primary goal, but sometimes, like if I see the patient really needs to talk about it and the husband's not on the page, I'll wait for him to leave, and then I'll go in and meet with the patient.

Frances notes that sometimes discussing the state of the patients can help reconcile some of the relationship, without family members directly confronting each other. By waiting for the husband to leave for a discussion, she is able to help the patient address their concerns and talk about their illness. The husband may not have reached the acceptance level, but needs time to reach that level. When the chaplain speaks separately to each person, it alleviates the burden of them having to discuss the prognosis, and the frustration that may result when one person has accepted their illness and their spouse is not ready to discuss issues related to the death, such as funeral planning or what the spouse will do after their partner's death.

Next, health care workers "reflect" by considering their own perspectives, having a consciousness about their own behaviors when helping family members, considering the implications of their actions. Picard and Siltanen (2013) noted that understanding the emotions of the disputants may help mediators understand the conflict better itself. The patient advocate below, Olga, demonstrates the importance of understanding the emotions of the family member in terms of conflict management:

> Olga, patient advocate: I think what you have is you have several patients or clients when you're dealing with end-of-life issues, and that's how I teach others to consider it, that you're not only dealing with the dying person, who of course, is first and foremost in your mind, but you have to consider the people around that person who are losing that person to be equally as important in terms of interaction and I was always taught that you care for families, you know? So your care needs to extend beyond the individual in front of you and I think that gets lost and so I think when you're dealing with end-of-life issues, you really have to extend your breadth of work to the people surrounding the person dying.

Similar to Frances, Olga recognizes that family members are losing a significant part of their lives, and should be considered. As with Frances and Sheila, Olga openly reflects that work in this case must extend to the family and what they would need. She also notes that the family gets "lost" and it is important that health care workers reflect on the situation and ensure that they are doing the best possible work for the family.

Next, health care workers "reframe" situations by acting as translators for family members. Reframing allows health care workers to present information accessibly for them to ensure that everyone understands the circumstances of the patient. Based on their background, particularly if they are pastoral care workers, they can contextualize the doctor's words and suggestions in terms of the patient and family's faith.

> Nick, pastor: We talked a lot about what the doctors were saying they could do and the doctors had made it clear that what they could do was keep her body functioning and so we talked about quality of life versus longevity of life.

A theme that was echoed throughout the findings was the importance of quality versus quantity of life. Nick's patient had been given a diagnosis and was concerned that her medical decisions and the possible outcomes of those decisions would be acceptable based on her religious beliefs. Nick reframes the situation by discussing the medical side of the patient, but then translates what the implications of her decision would mean for living her life. He uses the phrase "keep her body functioning," indicating that the patient would be technically alive, although not *living*.

Finally, health care workers "refer" by acting as a network to help the family be at peace with their decision, knowing which individuals are best suited to handle particular problems.

> Sandra, nurse: We have a house supervisor who [is] put in that job because they're particularly skilled communicators, they deal with family conflict, so the house supervisor's a nurse who acts as a representative of the organization and they're just like a mediator and then I have the chaplain, which we have 24/7, and they are awesome because there's often a religious component to the issue, I have social workers if the conflict is related to financial issues and then we have an ethics committee where if we feel like there's only one person in the family that doesn't want, let's say Mom off the ventilator, then we can call the ethics committee and they can look at the evidence and the follow the evidence.

Sandra has the resources for conflict management, from the supervisor, to chaplains, to social workers, as well as the ethics committee. In her description, she discusses all of the many reasons that families may be in conflict, and for each of them she has someone that she can go to. Based on her positive descriptions of each of her colleagues, having the strong network of individuals is a benefit for health care workers when families are in conflict.

The above strategies reflect the sequential contingency model. First, the third parties are focused in resolving the conflict that repairs or preserves the relationship between the family members. Second, particularly in Sandra's response about referring third parties, family conflict often has consequences for the organization. The individuals who are working with the family can utilize their organizational resources to help families get the resources that they need. If the conflict process is cyclical, as predicted by sequential contingency model, this means that the way this conflict is resolved will impact the approach to the next type of conflict for both the family and the health care workers.

Additionally, the situated model assumes that the conflict is based on goals, power, and relationships. Many of the health care workers indicated that they draw on these parts of the model during their discussion. For example, Sheila emphasizes what it means to be a "good daughter," which addresses both goals and relationships of the party. Nick discusses quality versus quantity of life, which addresses goals. Both Frances and Olga address the need to see the goals and relationships of the family to ensure that the conflict is resolved. By incorporating the viewpoints of all family members, this reduces power that family members have over each other, as the health care workers try to redirect power towards the patient and their wishes. By allowing everyone to share their perspective, everyone has an equal voice.

Moreover, these strategies all share a concern for the patient, as well as the family, although it is unclear if these strategies are effective long term (a significant problem because health care workers rarely have contact with the family beyond the hospital experience). While health care workers can provide reasons and behaviors for managing conflict, implementing conflict resolution programs could provide more insight about the effectiveness of these techniques.

Developing and Implementing Conflict-Resolution Programs

Health care managers learn how to manage conflict through experience, not training, but they perceive that they have become better health care managers having gone through training (Nilsson & Furåker, 2012). Along with other forms of organizational support, conflict coaching is useful to nurses when handling specific conflict situations. For example, coaching can help socialize new organizational members on formal policies, as well as nurture potential leadership skills (Brinkert, 2011). Newer nurses also report higher levels of stress, and including managing conflict-related stress as part of the curriculum in nursing school may help alleviate this burden (Friedman, Tidd, Currall, & Tsai, 2000; Pines, et al, 2012). The models of conflict processes also demonstrate that individuals approach conflict based on a number of factors, and training in these types of models would provide a greater understanding about why the families are engaged in the conflict. They would be able to differentiate between when a conflict that needs mediating is occurring, and when family members are frustrated. One disadvantage to using the models is that, given the fast-paced environment of the hospital, health care workers may not have the time to go through each of the steps. In such cases staff may choose to "refer" patients and families to an organizational dispute resolution system. Individuals trained in dispute resolution could focus on helping the family understand why the conflict was occurring and work toward resolving the conflict. Two types of conflict resolution programs will be proposed below. The first entails hands-on training of health care workers, the second involves the implementation of formal systems in hospitals.

Training Programs

The first type of training program is conflict resolution sessions that can help individuals before conflict arises; the second is post-conflict analysis and discussion. First, an effective program should teach individuals to recognize issues that appear to be conflict, but are not. The reasons for engagement in conflict may stem from a number of issues that are unrelated to their hospital stay. These reasons could include frustration with the health care system that is directed at health care workers (Halpern, 2007), or preexisting tension in the family that surfaces when there is a family crisis (Kopelman, 2006). The cause of the conflict could be a result of miscommunication, perceived lack of support from health care workers, or emotional issues (Breen et al, 2001; von Gunten, Ferris, & Emanuel, 2000). Sometimes family members are overwhelmed and what appears to be conflict is an overreaction to the situation. In that case, cooling off and venting is often adequate enough to resolve the situation (Harrison, 2003, 2007). Training programs should also teach individuals how to recognize the differences between conflict that needs mediating or managing versus conflict that is based in stress and emotion that may resolve themselves through family members' venting.

However, not all conflict can be resolved by venting, and some employees (particularly new nurses) need more resources for dealing with conflict. Training programs could include reinforcing what the hospital's conflict resolution policy is—which could be that nurses are required to contact social work or human resources, or follow a specified protocol with the family. One type of resolution program that has been implemented is Schwartz Center Rounds. During Schwartz Center Rounds, a panel presents a case study and invites participants to reflect and share their thoughts on the matter. The discussion allows for sensemaking and emotional venting for caregivers (Schwartz Center Rounds, 2014). There are already many effective programs in place at hospitals around the United States. The key is to examine what has been successful for similar-type organizations and make sure that each solution is a good "match" for the organization. More importantly, conflict training should include skills to help individuals manage conflict directly, as critics of formal conflict resolution mechanisms argue that these forums tend to be biased. Individual hospitals and health care systems that have taken steps towards a policy of conflict resolution between physicians and family members may not have transparent policies. For example, when an impasse is reached, the policies tend to privilege the opinions of the physician and hospital representatives over those of the caregivers (Wojtasiewicz, 2006). Therefore, it is potentially better to have a formal system in place that consciously tries to avoid these problems inherent in standard policies.

Formal Conflict Resolution Systems

Alternative dispute resolution (ADR) involves systems that are found in many organizations, most notably in universities (Harrison, 2004, 2007) and corporations (Wagner, 2000). Utilizing ADR can reduce stress and improve work conditions (Haraway & Haraway, 2005), as well as reduce litigation costs (Lipsky & Seeber, 2006). ADR may provide any number of services, including (but not limited to) fact-finding, mediation, and arbitration (Rowe, 1995). While these services are distinct, fairness is consistently the most important factor in successful programs. Organizational fairness refers to three types of justice that organizational members may perceive: procedural, distributive, and interactional. Procedural refers to fairness of procedures in decision-making; distributive justice refers to the evaluation of decisions; and interactional justice refers to the behavior of the decision-maker. Interactional justice includes interpersonal sensitivity (the individual feels they were listened to) and informational justice, meaning they were able to voice their opinion (Korsgaard & Sapienza, 2002). Kulik and Holbrook (2002) examined patient complaints against their physician, and the fairness of the process. If patients perceive interactional fairness, this can lead to adherence to treatment plans because patients believe that the physician listened to them and addressed their concerns. In terms of conflict with family members, if family members perceive that they have been listened to, and have their concerns addressed, they may be more likely to reach a peaceful outcome.

Procedural justice scholarship indicates that when the process is fair, disputants tend to be satisfied with the outcome of the conflict (Eisenhardt, Kahwajy, &Bourgeois, 1997; Moorman, 1991; Szmania, Johnson, & Mulligan, 2008). There have been some critics that argue ADR tends to favor the organization and removes power from the disputant. These critiques have been noted in many types of organizations, but Wojtasiewicz (2006) addressed hospital policy specifically. For instance, African Americans have a long history of mistrusting the medical system. African-American populations tend to want more aggressive treatment at the end of life, although the hospital staff may perceive that aggressive treatment would not be effective for the patient. The disagreement may lead to the dispute being resolved at the institutional level, which may not represent what the family wants. By removing power from the family, this can create more distrust and make ADR less effective (Wojtaskiewicz, 2006).

One response to this problem is ombud offices. Ombud offices have been implemented in hospitals and nursing homes (Administration on Aging, 2014), and some researchers believe these ombud offices provide the only pure representation for residents in nursing homes (Arcus, 1999). Ombud offices are distinct from other forms of ADR because of the nature of their work. Their anonymity (no records are maintained of those who visit the office) presumes that they are also confidential, neutral, unbiased, and fair (Rowe, 1987, 1995; Wagner, 2000). Although ombuds report to the organization, they have no power to make a decision. Instead, ombuds make recommendations to those who seek their help. Compared to formal mediation sessions, ombuds can help a disputant without involving the other party. Often lawsuits occur because the family wants clarification, not because they perceive the physician was incompetent (Drill-Mellum, 2013; Huntington & Kuhn, 2003). Ombuds would be able to investigate the case for the family and take the time to explain what happened. The prevalence of ombuds also allows researchers numerous opportunities to study conflict resolution systems in health care.

Implementation Challenges

Leadership must support implementation—this includes following the steps that the chosen approach outlines and the transparency of the programs (Porter-O'Grady, 2004; Sirman, 2008). Leadership may also serve as a resource for identifying multiple barriers, as well as recommend how these barriers can be reduced given the cultural context of the hospital (Rosenbaum et al, 2004). One study found that administrators perceived more barriers to implementing a conflict resolution system than nurses or physicians (Rosenstein, 2002). Presumably, those in administrative levels have greater knowledge of interdepartmental hospital dynamics than staff who work in only one unit. So while nurses and physicians identify barriers in their own unit, administrators identify barriers in the entire hospital and with regulations and policies. Prior studies have examined the effects of implementing total quality management systems (Short & Rahim, 1995), and managed care (Miller & Apker, 2002). Findings from these studies indicate that administrators must address problems that they identify before implementation, including clarifying new responsibilities and roles that organizational staff will be expected to fulfill provided that there is a change.

Implications for Research

As with many projects that involve collaboration between researchers and practitioners, there are a number of problems assessing conflict resolution programs. Perhaps our greatest understanding of how to evaluate programs has emerged from ombud programs. As noted above, ombud programs are valued for what they offer nursing home residents (Arcus, 1999). Logically, this would be a first step for researchers who want to understand what a successful conflict resolution program entails. Prior researchers who have attempted to quantify and understand the success of programs have noted some of the challenges. Huber, Borders, Netting, and Nelson (2001) identified some of the problems inherent in collecting data in nursing homes related to this type of program. They analyzed data from six states—but for confidentiality reasons they were unable to reveal state names, making it difficult to identify how policy, laws, or other regulations influence nursing home care. The authors were interested in differences in types of complaints between race and gender. Due to the anonymous nature of ombuds programs (which makes them favorable), this data is often not recorded. Additionally, states record data differently depending on their regulations and political climate (Huber et al., 2001). Although conflict resolution programs may be distinct from ombuds programs, it does remind practitioners and theorists alike that state, local, and organizational politics may impede how data is collected and recorded. This may also affect assessing the implementation of programs, defining success rates, and making strong comparisons.

Huber et al. (2001) recommended that practitioners and researchers work together to recognize disparities across regions and overcome these issues. As found by Harrison (2004), success in ombuds processes means different things to different people. Having a clear definition of what it means to be successful, and to whom, will help ensure that outcomes are being met and processes followed. Beyond constraint of state regulation, many of the problems for hospitals also affect researchers. Aside from data collection, successful collaboration between researchers and practitioners depends on the relationship between the two. Macduff and Netting (2000) recommended that mutual respect between researchers and practitioners often result in successful partnerships. This suggests that researchers should not only make connections with practitioners, but communicate the expectations and outcomes of the respective projects (see Silk and Smith, this volume, for more on developing transdisciplinary collaborations).

Directions for the Future

There are many programs (mentioned throughout the above review) that have been tested and generally well received by those involved in the health care field. The changing demographics may also be more supportive of changing the old routines and making conflict resolution programs more accessible to all members of the hospital, and ones that will recognize diversity in the changing workplace. In addition, researchers should focus on specific elements of family dynamics and how they relate to conflict in medical and health care situations. Conflict resolution practitioners and scholars both have a strong foundation from which to work, and successful implementation in some systems may persuade skeptics to adopt a similar program for conflict management.

DISCUSSION QUESTIONS

1. This chapter barely scratched the surface of issues that affect implementation of a conflict resolution system—what other problems would a researcher/practitioner team encounter when implementing a system?
2. How can researchers balance confidentiality needs of disputants while also ensuring that specific needs of a health care organization are being met?
3. What components of a conflict resolution program would you like to see implemented in your organization?
4. Consider a conflict you had at your organization. How was it resolved? If it was not resolved effectively, why do you think that was? Could a conflict resolution program have helped improve the outcome? Why do you think that was?
5. Note that the conflict between John and Ann was not given a "resolution." Discuss the possible outcomes to their conflict. What do you think health care workers could do to help resolve the conflict effectively, and preserve the relationship between John and Ann?

Notes

1 Power of attorney laws differ by state—in some cases, the son would be recognized as next of kin; in others, the son and daughter would share the decision-making responsibilities. Even if the son does have decision-making power, interviews with medical staff found that most hospitals try to ensure that all family members accept the decision.
2 The example described above is not based on one specific instance of family conflict, but is based on a synthesis of staff members' experiences with family members during end-of-life.

Suggested Reading

Coleman, P. T., Kugler, K. G., Bui-Wrzosinska, L., Nowak, A., & Vallacher, R. (2012). Getting down to basics: A situated model of conflict in social relations. *Negotiation Journal, 28*, 7–43.

Porter-O'Grady, T. (2004). Constructing a conflict resolution program for health care. *Health Care Management Review, 29*, 278–283.

Speakman, J. & Ryals, L. (2010). A re-evaluation of conflict theory for the management of multiple, simultaneous conflict episodes. *International Journal of Conflict Management, 21*, 186–201.

References

Administration on Aging (2014). Outline of 2006 amendments to the Older Americans Act. Department of Health and Human Services. Retrieved from http://www.aoa.gov/.

Arcus, S. G. (1999). The long-term care ombudsman program. *Journal of Gerontological Social Work, 31*, 195–205.

Back, A. L. & Arnold, R. M. (2005). Dealing with conflict in caring for the seriously ill: "It was just out of the question." *JAMA, 293*, 1374–1381.

Bendersky, C. & Hays, N. A. (2012). Status conflict in groups. *Organization science, 23*, 323–340.

Bies, R. J. & Tripp, T. M. (2002). "Hot flashes, open wounds:" Injustice and the tyranny of its emotions. In S. W. Gilliland, D. D. Steiner, & D. P. Skarlicki (Eds.), *Emerging perspectives on managing organizational justice* (pp. 203–221). Greenwich, CT: Information Age Publishing.

Bloche, M. G. (2005). Managing conflict at the end of life. *The New England Journal of Medicine, 352*, 2371–2373.

Bodtker, A. M. & Jameson, J. K. (2001). Emotion in conflict formation and its transformation: Application to organizational conflict management. *The International Journal of Conflict Management, 12*, 259–275.

Boelk, A. Z. & Kramer, B. J. (2012). Advancing theory of family conflict at the end of life: A hospice case study. *Journal of Pain and Symptom Management, 44*, 655–670.

Breen, C. M., Abernethy, A. P., Abbott, K. H., & Tulsky, J. A. (2001). Conflict associated with decisions to limit life-sustaining treatment in intensive care units. *Journal of General Internal Medicine, 16*, 283–289.

Brinkert, R. (2011). Conflict coaching training for nurse managers: A case study of a two-hospital health system. *Journal of Nursing Management, 19*, 90–91.

Coleman, P. T., Kugler, K. G., Bui-Wrzosinska, L., Nowak, A., & Vallacher, R. (2012). Getting down to basics: A situated model of conflict in social relations. *Negotiation Journal, 28*, 7–43.

Drill-Mellum, L. (2013). Practicing medicine in an imperfect world: Five truths about preventing or surviving a lawsuit. *Minnesota Medicine*, 31–33.

Eisenhardt, K. M., Kahwajy, J. L., & Bourgeois, L. J., III. (1997). How management teams can have a good fight. *Harvard Business Review, 75*, 77–85.

Friedman, R. A., Tidd, S. T., Currall, S. C., & Tsai, J. C. (2000). What goes around comes around: The impact of personal conflict style on work conflict and stress. *The International Journal of Conflict Management, 11*, 32–55.

Halpern, J. (2007). Empathy and patient-physician conflicts. *Journal of General Internal Medicine, 22*, 696–700.

Haraway, D. L. & Haraway, W. M., III. (2005). Analysis of the effect of conflict-management and resolution training on employee stress at a healthcare organization. *Hospital Topics: Research and Perspective on Healthcare, 83*, 11–17.

Harrison, T. R. (2003). Victims, targets, protectors, and destroyers: Using disputant accounts to develop a grounded taxonomy of disputant orientations. *Conflict Resolution Quarterly, 20*, 307–329.

Harrison, T. R. (2004). What is success in ombuds processes? Evaluation of a university ombudsman. *Conflict Resolution Quarterly, 21*, 313–335.

Harrison, T. R. (2007). My professor is so unfair: Student attitudes and experiences of conflict with faculty. *Conflict Resolution Quarterly, 24*, 349–368.

Harrison, T. R. & Morrill, C. (2004). Ombuds processes and disputant reconciliation. *Journal of Applied Communication Research, 32*, 318–342.

Hopeck, P. (2013). End-of-life decisions: The intersection of health organizations, families, conflict, and policy (Unpublished doctoral dissertation). Purdue University, West Lafayette, IN.

Huber, R., Borders, K., Netting, F. E., & Nelson, H. W. (2001). Data from long-term care ombudsman programs in six states: The implications of collecting resident demographics. *The Gerontologist, 41*, 61–68.

Huntington, B. & Kuhn, N. (2003). Communication gaffes: A root cause of malpractice claims. *Baylor University Medical Center Proceedings, 16*, 157–161.

Jacobs, S. & Aakhus, M. (2002). What mediators do with words: Implementing three models of rational discussion in dispute mediation. *Conflict Resolution Quarterly, 20*, 177–203.

Jameson, J. K. (1999). Toward a comprehensive model for the assessment and management of intraorganizational conflict: Developing the framework. *The International Journal of Conflict Management, 10*, 268–294.

Jameson, J. K., Bodtker, A. M., & Linker, T. (2010). Facilitating conflict transformation: Mediator strategies for eliciting emotional communication in a workplace conflict. *Negotiation Journal, 26*, 25–48.

Jameson, J. K., Bodtker, A. M., Porch, D. M., & Jordan, W. J. (2009). Exploring the role of emotion in conflict transformation. *Conflict Resolution Quarterly, 27*, 167–192.

Jehn, K. A. (1995). A multimethod examination of the benefits of the benefits and detriments of intragroup conflict. *Administrative science quarterly, 40*, 256–282.

Jones, T. S. (2000). Emotional communication in conflict: Essence and impact. In W. Eadie & P. Nelson (Eds.). *The language of conflict and resolution.* Thousand Oaks, CA: Sage Publications.

Kesting, P., Smolinski, R., & Speakman, I. (2012). Conflict in organizations: The role of routine. *Problems and Perspectives in Management, 10*, 50–59.

Kilmann, R. H. & Thomas, K. W. (1978). Four perspectives on conflict management: An attributional framework for organizing descriptive and normative theory. *Academy of Management Review, 3*, 59–68.

Kopelman, A. E. (2006). Understanding, avoiding, and resolving end-of-life conflicts in the NICU. *The Mount Sinai Journal of Medicine, 73*, 580–586.

Korsgaard, M. A. & Sapienza, H. J. (2002). Economic and noneconomic mechanisms in interpersonal work relationships: Toward an integration of agency and procedural justice theories. In S. W. Gilliland, D. D. Steiner, & D. P. Skarlicki (Eds.), *Emerging perspectives on managing organizational justice* (pp. 3–33). Greenwich, CT: Information Age Publishing.

Kulik, C. T. & Holbrook, Jr., R. L. (2002). Patients and physicians as stakeholders: Justice in the medical context. In S. W. Gilliland, D. D. Steiner, & D. P. Skarlicki (Eds.), *Emerging perspectives on managing organizational justice* (pp. 77–101). Greenwich, CT: Information Age Publishing.

Kurt, L., Kugler, K. G., Coleman, P. T., & Liebovitch, L. S. (2014). Behavioral and emotional dynamics of two people struggling to reach consensus about a topic on which they disagree. *PLoS ONE 9*, 1–15.

Lipsky, D. B. & Seeber, R. L. (2006). Managing organizational conflicts. In J. G. Oetzel & S. Ting-Toomey (Eds.), *The SAGE handbook of conflict communication: Integrating theory, research, and practice* (pp. 359–390). Thousand Oaks, CA: Sage Publications.

Macduff, N. & Netting, F. E. (2000). Lessons learned from a practitioner-academician collaboration. *Nonprofit and Voluntary Sector Quarterly, 29*, 46–60.

Miller, K. I. & Apker, J. (2002). On the front lines of managed care: Professional changes and communicative dilemmas of hospital nurses. *Nursing Outlook, 50*, 154–159.

Moore, C. W. (2003). *The mediation process: Practical strategies for resolving conflict* (3rd ed.). San Francisco, CA: Jossey-Bass.

Moorman, R. H. (1991). Relationship between organizational justice and organizational citizenship behaviors: Do fairness perceptions influence employee citizenship? *Journal of Applied Psychology, 76*, 845–855.

Morreim, H. (2014). In-house conflict resolution processes: Health lawyers as problem-solvers. *Health Lawyer, 26*, 10–15.

Nilsson, K. & Furåker, C. (2012). Learning leadership through practice—healthcare managers' experience. *Leadership in Health Services, 25*, 106–122.

Picard, C. & Siltanen, J. (2013). Exploring the significance of emotion for mediation practice. *Conflict Resolution Quarterly, 31*, 31–55.

Pines, E. W., Rauschhuber, M. L., Norgan, G. H., Cook, J. D., Canchola, L., Richardson, C., Jones, M. E. (2012). Stress resiliency, psychological empowerment and conflict management styles among baccalaureate nursing students. *Journal of Advanced Nursing, 68*, 1482–1493.

Pondy, L. R. (1967). Organizational conflict: Concepts and models. *Administrative science quarterly, 12*, 296–320.

Porter-O'Grady, T. (2004). Constructing a conflict resolution program for health care. *Health Care Management Review, 29*, 278–283.

Putnam, L. L. (2006). Definitions and approaches to conflict and communication. In J. G. Oetzel & S. Ting-Toomey (Eds.), *The SAGE handbook of conflict communication: Integrating theory, research, and practice*. Thousand Oaks, CA: Sage Publications.

Rosenbaum, J. R., Bradley, E. H., Holmboe, E. S., Farrell, M. H., & Krumholz, H. M. (2004). Sources of ethical conflict in medical house staff training: A qualitative study. *The American Journal of Medicine, 116*, 402–407.

Rosenstein, A. H. (2002). Nurse-physician relationships: Impact on nurse satisfaction and retention. *American Journal of Nursing, 102*, 26–34.

Rowe, M. P. (1987). The corporate ombudsman: An overview and analysis. *Negotiation Journal*, 127–140.

Rowe, M. P. (1995). Options, functions, and skills: What an organizational ombudsman might want to know. *Negotiation Journal*, 11(2),103–114.

Schwartz Center Rounds (2014). The Schwartz Center for Compassionate Healthcare. Retrieved from www.theschwartzcenter.org.

Short, P. J. & Rahim, M. A. (1995). Total quality management in hospitals. *Total Quality Management, 6*, 255–264.

Sirman, R. (2008). Immunize your organization against superconflicts. *Employment Relations Today, 35*, 33–41.

Speakman, J. & Ryals, L. (2010). A re-evaluation of conflict theory for the management of multiple, simultaneous conflict episodes. *International Journal of Conflict Management, 21*, 186–201.

Szmania, S. J., Johnson, A. M., & Mulligan, M. (2008). Alternative dispute resolution in medical malpractice: A survey of emerging trends and practices. *Conflict Resolution Quarterly, 26*, 71–96.

von Gunten, C. F., Ferris, F. D., & Emanuel, L. L. (2000). Ensuring competency in end-of-life care: Communication and relational skills. *JAMA, 284*, 3051–3057.

Wagner, M. L. (2000). The organizational ombudsman as change agent. *Negotiation Journal, 16*, 99–114.

Wojtasiewicz, M. E. (2006). Damage compounded: Disparities, distrust, and disparate impact in end-of-life conflict resolution policies. *The American Journal of Bioethics, 6*, 8–12.

PART II

Work and Organizations' Effect on Individuals' Health

10

CONFLICT, SOCIAL SUPPORT, AND BURNOUT/TURNOVER AMONG HEALTH CARE WORKERS

A Review of Developments in Organizational Conflict Theory and Practice

Kevin B. Wright and Anne M. Nicotera

Effective communication is essential to building strong health care teams and organizations (Wright, Banas, Bessarabova, & Bernard, 2010; Wright, Sparks, & O'Hair, 2013). Quality communication among health care workers is at the core of health organizations, and it enhances patient care and furthers the goals of individual units and health care organizations. Communication problems can damage team relationships and organizational processes, impeding the accomplishment of organizational goals and compromising patient care (Canary & Lakey, 2006; Rouse, 2009). Poor communication in work-related conflict situations can create lower quality of work life, increase stress, and decrease job satisfaction, which often contributes to employee turnover, exacerbating the shortage of health care workers, depleting organizational efficiency, and ultimately increasing health care costs for consumers (Apker & Ray, 2003; Maslach, 2003; Nicotera & Mahon, 2013; Siefert, Jayaratne, & Chess, 1991; Wright et al., 2010). A variety of researchers, including communication scholars, have contributed to our understanding of these issues by examining how communication during conflict can impact health care workers and health care organizations in negative ways.

Specifically, poor conflict communication among workers (including health care workers) has been found to lead to higher stress and burnout (Fujiwara, Tsukishima, Tsutsumi, Kawakami, & Kishi, 2003; Montoro-Rodriguez & Small, 2006; Wright et al., 2010), both of which can contribute to mental and physical health issues such as substance abuse, depression, and stress–related diseases (Brown, Goske, & Johnson, 2009; Dunn, 2005; Schaufeli, Leiter, & Maslach, 2009), and they may ultimately influence a health care worker's decision to leave the organization. However, individual workers with high burnout who remain in the organization may begin to incur health care costs associated with stress-related illness (Maslach & Leiter, 2008). Moreover, health care organizations suffer financially from increased burnout and turnover among employees (Jones, 2008; Maslach & Leiter, 2008; Reid et al., 2010). One study found that the cost of recruiting, training, bringing new health care employees up to speed, and productivity loss represented a minimum of 5% of the annual operating costs for one health care organization, and this number can increase dramatically during times of high turnover (Waldman, Kelly, Aurora, & Smith, 2004). In addition, health care organizations pay a larger amount of money in health care costs to treat employees for problems such as substance abuse and stress-related disease in cases where worker burnout is high (Maslach & Leiter, 2008; Schaufeli et al., 2009).

However, conflict within health care organizations appears to be mediated by the enhancement of conflict management skills and social skills (such as helping people obtain social support inside and outside of the workplace) which can be a positive influence on reducing stress and burnout (Kim & Lee, 2009; Wright, Banas, Bessarabova, & Bernard, 2010; Firth, Mellor, Moore, & Loquet, 2004). Some communication researchers advocate training individuals to increase communication competencies or skills during conflict situations in an effort to improve organizational outcomes such as stress, burnout, and retention (Canary & Lakey, 2006; Maslach, 2003; Rancer, Kosberg, & Baukus, 1992). Other scholars have focused their attention on structures and situations within health care organizations that affect communication during conflict, health care worker dissatisfaction, stress, and burnout from a structurational divergence (SD) perspective (Nicotera & Mahon, 2013; Nicotera, Mahon, & Wright, 2014; Nicotera, Mahon, & Zhao, 2010). These researchers have found that members of health care organizations can be trained to identify these structures/situations and can improve situations that create or influence conflict through dialogue between various stakeholders within the health care organization.

This chapter explores literature related to the areas of health care worker conflict, social support, and the relationships among these variables and two key organizational outcomes: (1) employee burnout, and (2) employee turnover/retention in health care organizations. Toward that end, we provide an overview of conditions that often lead to conflict within health care organizations, a review of literature dealing with studies of the interrelationships among conflict, stress, social support, and burnout/retention among health care workers. We then discuss two broad approaches to conflict interventions regarding these variables within the literature: (1) communication competence approaches targeting individual health care workers, and (2) the structurational divergence theory approach. We provide a special emphasis on the latter since it is a relatively new intervention approach. Moreover, we provide an assessment of the strengths and limitations of these approaches to managing conflict within health care organizations. Finally, we discuss future directions for advancing theory, research, and communication-based interventions in this area.

Conflict, Stress, Burnout, and Retention Among Health Care Workers: Causes of Conflict in Health Care Organizations

Conflict among health care workers is inevitable given the multidisciplinary nature of health care organizations, and communication researchers have had a long history of focusing on conflict within health-related organizational contexts (see Nicotera & Dorsey, 2006). While conflict among health care workers is productive in many cases, negative forms of conflict have been found to contribute to health care worker stress, burnout, and retention (Aiken, Clarke, Sloan, Sochlaski, 2002; Lloyd, King, & Chenoweth, 2002; Wright et al., 2010). Conflict within health care organizations can occur due to a multitude of reasons. For example, health care workers often experience conflict between acting as patients' advocates representing their interests and the responsibility to ensure patients and their significant others are safe (see Hopeck, this volume, for a discussion on the influence of conflict with and among patients' family members). Moreover, competing values between administrators and health care workers have been identified as a source of stress and burnout (McLean & Andrew, 2000). Health care workers, such as nurses, often have little power or control in a physician-dominated authority structure. For example, nurses are often charged with the responsibility of discharging patients before they are ready to leave the hospital (due to organizational efforts to maintain costs). In such cases, a conflict between a nurse's desire to comfort the patient while simultaneously following the rules of the health care organization may emerge. Stress and burnout can also stem from role conflict, disagreement over best health care practices, lack of recognition, and restricted autonomy (Apker, Ford, & Fox, 2003; Apker, Propp, & Ford, 2005; Dorz, Novara, Sica, & Sanavio, 2010).

Ramanujam and Rousseau (2006) identify four unique features of the health care organization (HCO) context: (a) conflicting missions, (b) interaction of multiple professions, (c) multiple external stakeholders, and (d) an ambiguous and complex external environment. Ramanujam and Rousseau (2006) argue that this is not an exhaustive list of features of health care organizations that often lead to conflict, but they represent a group of common features found in empirical research findings.

First, hospitals have multiple and potentially *conflicting missions* such as patient care, community service, medical education, profit, health research, religious values, etc. Hence, assessment of mission achievement must be based on multiple dimensions. Second, a hospital's workforce is comprised of *multiple professions with a multitude of differing training and licensing requirements, salary structures, and power roles.* To complicate matters even more, these professionals have all been socialized in other organizational systems (see Myers & Gailliard, this volume, for a complete discussion on organizational socialization and identification of health care workers). According to Ramanujam and Rousseau (2006):

> The socialization of HCO professionals occurs pre-employment. . . . So dominant are institutionalized pre-employment processes that many HCOs attempt little or no socialization of their own workforce. Weak organization-based socialization means that individuals can have as many different professional practices and care-giving behaviors as the institutions that educated them. . . . The result is strong professional identification and weak organizational identification
>
> *(pp. 813–814)*

Third, hospitals typically face a complex *external environment with multiple stakeholders*. These stakeholders include third-party payers, consumers (households and employers), government, and multiple professional associations. Finally, the hospital *task environment is complex, ambiguous, dynamic, and local*—and subject to the simultaneous demands of standardization and flexibility. These four health care organization features amplify the administrative complexity of day-to-day tasks and seem to categorize the hospital as a unique organizational type.

Conflict and Burnout

Burnout among health care workers has been identified as a major problem in a variety of health care organizational settings (Aiken et al., 2002; Maslach, 2003; McManus, Winder, & Gordon, 2002; Siefert et al., 1991), often leading to absenteeism, reduced quality of health care delivery, and depersonalized feelings toward patients and coworkers. Burnout may take a personal toll on health care workers in the form of distress, substance abuse, and other stress-related physical, psychological, and relational problems, such as tiredness, headaches, eating problems, insomnia, irritability, emotional instability, and rigidity in relationships with other people (Brown, Goske, & Johnson, 2009; Schaufeli et al., 2009; Bakker, Le Blanc, & Schaufeli, 2005). Burnout is associated with a lower effectiveness at work, decreased job satisfaction, reduced organizational commitment, and turnover.

Maslach and colleagues (2001) described job burnout as a condition where meaningful and challenging work becomes unpleasant, unfulfilling, and meaningless. Although research offers various conceptualizations of burnout, it is typically conceptualized as having three dimensions: emotional exhaustion, depersonalization (or cynicism), and a sense of low personal accomplishment (Maslach, 2003; McManus et al., 2002).

Unproductive conflict among health care workers has been found to influence burnout. Poncet et al. (2007) found that perceived conflicts with patients and other staff members increased the risk of burnout syndrome among critical care nurses. Maslach, Schaufeli, and Leiter (2001) found that emotional exhaustion is a direct consequence of conflict among health care workers that often leads to depersonalization and to loss of a sense of personal accomplishment.

Social Support, Conflict, and Burnout/Retention in the Workplace

One variable that appears to mediate conflict, burnout, and retention among health care workers is social support. Workplace social support can be defined as the degree to which individuals perceive that their well-being is valued by workplace sources, such as coworkers and supervisors and the perception that these sources provide help to support this well-being (Dormann & Zapf, 1999; House, 1981; Kim & Lee, 2009). Workplace social support includes workplace interactions that lead to the provision of resources or that reinforce a particular type of role demand within the organization (Eisenberger, Singlhamber, Vandenberghe, Sucharski, & Rhoades, 2002). Employees who have greater access to workplace social support tend to gain access to workplace informational and instrumental resources over individuals who have less workplace support, and these resources often provide a buffer to workplace stress. In addition, workers who have strong workplace support networks tend to have greater emotional and psychological resources for coping with daily stressors that occur on the job (Dormann & Zapf, 1999).

In general, supportive relationships help to reduce uncertainty in organizational settings, increase worker job satisfaction, and decrease job burnout (Ray, 1987). The relationship between social support satisfaction and job burnout has received a great deal of attention from scholars (Aiken et al., 2002; Ellis & Miller, 1994; Maslach, 2003; Miller, Stiff, & Ellis, 1988). Social support satisfaction appears to play a crucial role in mitigating employees' perceived and real levels of stress and burnout (Firth, Mellor, Moore, & Loquet, 2004). Kalliath and Morris (2002) found that receiving satisfying social support from supervisors reduced the levels of nurses' burnout and indirectly reduced nurses' intention to quit. Conversely, failing to receive satisfying support from supervisors may lead to an increase in employee turnover (Hatton & Emerson, 1998).

Wright et al. (2010) examined how the relationship among communication competence and perceived job burnout is mediated by social support satisfaction and perceived stress in an attempt to empirically test and advance Kreps's (1988) Relational Health Communication Competence Model (RHCCM). Using a sample of health care workers from three Veterans Administration (VA) hospitals, the study found that perceived communication competence increases social support satisfaction and decreases stress. Furthermore, increased social support satisfaction with other employees predicted decreased perceptions of stress, which, in turn, predicted lower perceived job burnout.

Kim and Lee (2009) found that supportive supervisor communication predicted burnout and turnover intentions in a study of 200 health care workers in California. Specifically, these researchers found that supportive supervisor-employee communication had an indirect effect on burnout and turnover intention through its effect on perceived stress, whereas job-relevant communication had not only an indirect effect on burnout and turnover intention through its effect on stress, but also a direct effect on turnover intention. In addition, the results showed that upward communication between health care workers and supervisors moderated the relationship between stress and burnout.

Kim and Stoner (2008) examined the effects of role stress, job autonomy, and social support in predicting burnout and turnover intention among social workers in a large health care setting. Their analyses revealed that role stress had a positive direct effect on burnout. Social support and job autonomy had a negative direct effect on turnover intention, but not on burnout. Their results showed that job autonomy interacted with role stress in predicting burnout, while social support interacted with role stress in predicting turnover intention. These authors suggest that building supportive job conditions is needed to retain social workers who are experiencing high levels of role stress.

Communication Competence Approaches, Conflict Style, and Job Stress/Burnout

Much of the previous work in the communication discipline on conflict, stress, and burnout within organizations (including health care organizations) has approached conflict from an individually based, communication competency approach (Canary & Lakey, 2006; Canary & Spitzberg, 1987; Ting-Toomey & Oetzel, 2001; Wright et al., 2010). Communication competencies appear to influence the nature of conflict episodes (e.g., productive/unproductive conflict, duration of conflict, intensity of conflict, etc.) within organizations (Canary & Lakey, 2006). Communication competence has been conceptualized as a multidimensional construct that comprises a variety of communication skills and behaviors, including empathy, affiliation, behavioral flexibility, relaxation, and ability to adapt to changing situations (Canary & Lakey, 2006; Wiemann & Backland, 1980).

In terms of the relationship between communication competence and conflict, communication scholars have found that individuals who lack certain communication skills have a tendency to rely more on aggression or other negative forms of conflict (such as passive aggression or conflict avoidance) to achieve their goals (Canary, Spitzberg, & Semic, 1997; Canary & Spitzberg, 1987; 1989; Friedman, Tidd, Currall, & Tsai, 2000). This includes verbal and physical aggression and withdrawing behaviors during conflict situations. Such behaviors have been found to decrease relational satisfaction and undermine the stability of relationships (Gottman & Levenson, 1992). Other studies have found that having strong emotional reactions during conflict episodes is associated with reduced communication competence, increased aggression, and increased levels of communication apprehension (Hample, Dallinger, & Nelson, 1995). In comparison, competent conflict is typically a positive force in organizations, often leading to increased creativity, better decision-making, and the ability to move an organization beyond stagnation (Nicotera & Dorsey, 2006).

A variety of studies have examined the relationship between communication competence and conflict styles, such as cooperative, confrontational, and avoidance styles (Canary & Spitzberg, 1989; Putnum & Wilson, 1982; Rahim, 2002), including among health care workers (see Canary & Cupach, 1988; Canary, Cupach, & Serpe, 2001; Wright et al., 2010). From a communication competence perspective conflict style is viewed as a social skill in which people vary in terms of competency (Canary & Spitzberg, 1987). Competence-based interventions focus on helping employees in organizations achieve their goals in a way that is perceived as both appropriate and effective. Of course, conflict style is also influence by broader cultural influences (see Ting-Toomey & Oetzel, 2001). For example, many Asian cultures perceive obliging and compromising conflict styles as more competent than the U.S. norm of favoring integrating and compromising styles (Canary & Lakey, 2006). In general, within mainstream U.S. culture, dominating, obliging, and avoiding conflict styles are typically perceived as less competent compared to integrating and compromising styles. Moreover, in general, those conflict styles that are perceived as less competent tend to be predictive of higher stress and burnout. Yet, the research findings in this area are somewhat mixed.

For instance, Wright et al. (2010), in a study of 221 health care workers found that higher communication competence scores were predictive of integrating and obliging conflict styles while lower communication competence scores were predictive of dominating and avoiding conflict styles. Dominating and avoiding conflict styles were predictive of increased job stress and higher levels of burnout. Similarly, Montoro-Rodriguez and Small (2006) found that nurse who exhibited confrontational and avoiding conflict styles had lower workplace morale and higher burnout scores. However, Friedman, Tidd, Currall, and Tsai (2000) found that avoiding and obliging conflict styles were both predictive of higher worker stress while integrating and dominating conflict styles did not significantly predict stress.

One concern that several researchers have raised about communication competence (i.e., skills-based) approaches to managing conflict within organizations is that it places the responsibility for engaging in competent conflict on the individual while often ignoring institutional and cultural restraints within the organizational structure that lead to recurring conflict situations. For example, incompatible goals and role ambiguity (e.g., nurses who must simultaneously please physicians, administrators and patients who all desire different outcomes) and other sources of conflict are highly influenced by organizational structures, including the presence of incompatible rules between different types of health care workers embedded within the larger organizational culture.

Structurational Divergence Theory Approach to Conflict

An alternative perspective to the individual competency/skills perspective of conflict, stress, and burnout is the structurational divergence perspective. Structurational Divergence (SD) Theory explains how institutional factors can result in poor communication and conflict cycles. The theory has been developed in the nursing context, although it is applicable to all organizational settings (Nicotera & Mahon, 2013; Nicotera, Mahon, & Wright, 2014; Nicotera, Mahon, & Zhao, 2010; Nicotera, Zhao, Mahon, Kim & Conway-Morana, in press). SD is a particular type of recurrent conflict, rooted in incompatible social meaning structures. SD is characterized by a negative spiral of interaction—unresolved conflict, immobilization, and regressions in development—that serve to exacerbate the conflict. SD manifests in interpersonal conflict, but because its source is in meaning rather than oppositional goals, normal competent conflict management strategies often fail. Mahon and Nicotera (2013) found that cognitive communication competence (mindfully thinking about one's communication before, during, and after interaction) was positively correlated with SD, suggesting either that SD contributes to rumination over communication or that thinking about interaction deepens the SD conflict. Further, Nicotera et al. (in press) found that while undesirable conflict management styles (avoidance and controlling) were positively correlated with SD, desirable conflict style (solution-oriented) had no relationship at all, validating earlier conclusions that SD is not ordinary conflict. In addition, no conflict style mediated the impact of SD on job satisfaction or intentions to leave (Nicotera et al., in press). It is estimated that 12–15% of practicing nurses encounter a problematic level of SD (Nicotera & Mahon, 2013; Nicotera et al, in press). Given the difficulty in distinguishing SD from normal goals-based conflict, a relational approach to conflict and conflict management is highly recommended (Nicotera, Mahon & Wright, 2014). Health care researchers' information-focused approach to most worker conflict situations presumes that individual-level skill deficits are the main source of recurrent conflict and poor communication among workers. While improving individual-level skill is indeed a solution to recurrent conflict cycles, individual-level skill deficits are not necessarily a cause of recurring or intractable conflicts among health care workers. These cycles, rather, are often rooted in institutional and cultural constraints. Such conflicts have been termed structurational divergence.

Structuration is a sociological term that refers to the social and cognitive processes through which we draw upon cultural and societal rules and resources to understand and act appropriately in social situations (Giddens, 1984). Cultural/societal rules and resources tell us what things mean and what to do. Divergence refers to the intersection of multiple sets of rules/resources, beneath the level of individuals' awareness, that are in competition with one another. SD undermines personal and group efficacy. Because incompatible meaning structures are not apparent, the underlying sources of conflicts are unclear, making efforts to resolve

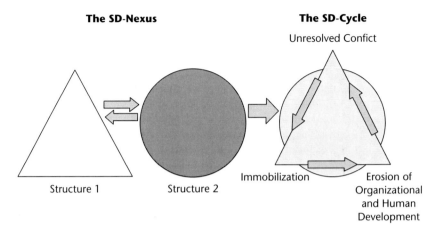

FIGURE 10.1   Structurational Divergence: The SD–Nexus and the SD–Cycle (Nicotera, Mahon, & Zhao, 2010).

them ineffective. As a result of these incompatible meaning structures, communication difficulties become entrenched in health care organizations. While SD theory has been pursued primarily in the nursing context, it is an institutional phenomenon.

There are two essential components of SD known as the *SD-nexus* and the *SD-cycle* (Nicotera, Mahon, & Zhao, 2010). See Figure 10.1. The *SD-nexus* is defined as an institutional positioning at the intersection of social structures characterized by simultaneous and equally compelling contradictory obligations. SD-nexuses result when institutional positioning crosses institutional and cultural boundaries. "Structure" in this case is defined sociologically as the rules and resources that both guide and are played out in social interaction (Giddens, 1984). Structure can be conceived as the connection between the institutional and the cognitive. In other words, structure tells us what things mean and how to act. These structures explain differences in the way we view things due to social and institutional variances, such as specialty training and practice, departmental norms, institutional roles (e.g., clinical, managerial, or financial), cultural background and experiences, and institutional histories. These variations provide individuals with differing lenses through which they understand the world and act in it. Socially navigating these variations is crucial to good teamwork. When these variations clash to the point where a recurrent conflict cycle occurs, SD can be diagnosed.

The *SD-cycle* refers to the negative spiral of communication resulting from an SD-nexus: unresolvable conflict, immobilization, and the erosion of development (individual, group, organizational, and/or institutional) that exacerbates unresolved conflicts. The hallmark symptom of SD is immobilization—not necessarily a lack of activity, but rather a frustrating lack of progress, feeling stuck in the same place, repeatedly facing the same problems, with no perceived end to the impasse. The individual feels futility and hopelessness. SD can be measured with a diagnostic self-report scale that identifies the three components of the cycle, as well as the cyclic connections among them (Nicotera, Mahon, & Zhao, 2010). When incompatible social structures bear on a situation, the clash creates unresolvable conflicts fueled by the simultaneous compulsion to fulfill irreconcilably oppositional obligations, creating a downward spiral of communication that can circle back to escalate the conflicts. SD renders the individual unable to act with efficacy because oppositional meanings make communication patterns incomprehensible or extremely challenging to transform. Because they must act, individuals must choose which structure to violate, suffering normative sanctions and escalating conflict.

Existing datasets contain excellent illustrations of SD, encompassed in Table 10.1. In each of these examples, SD theory points out how the problem appears to cause itself, with no rule/resource to prioritize one structure over the other (Nicotera & Mahon, 2013). Several studies have used the SD approach to improving situations that lead to unproductive conflict in health care organizations (Nicotera & Mahon, 2013; Nicotera, Mahon, & Wright, 2014; Nicotera, Mahon, & Zhao, 2010; Nicotera et al., in press). The nature of health care organizations frequently creates conditions in which SD is likely. First, for example, hospitals have multiple, potentially conflicting, missions (e.g., patient care, community service, medical education, profit, health research, religious values, etc.). Second, the workforce within most health care organizations consists of multiple professions with a wide variety of differing training and licensing requirements, salary structures, and power roles. In addition, these professionals have all been socialized in other organizational systems. Third, health care organizations exist in a complex environment with multiple stakeholders, including third-party payers, consumers (households and employers), government, and multiple professional associations. Fourth, the environment with most health care organizations is complex, ambiguous, dynamic, local, and subject to the simultaneous contrary demands of standardization and flexibility. Health care workers within this complex setting of intersecting incompatible meaning structures, makes SD an ever-present threat (Nicotera & Mahon, 2013; Nicotera, Mahon, & Wright, 2014).

SD interventions take a two-pronged approach: consciousness-raising and transformation. The first phase has two parts. To begin, participants are sensitized to the inevitability of conflict and to its potentially positive outcomes (critical thinking, innovation, development, etc.) and taught to view conflict itself as a normal part of human interaction. It is not conflict that is bad or good, but rather how it is managed. Then, participants are trained in conflict analysis using social science approaches to identify the root of conflict and discriminate goal opposition from meaning–structure opposition. The second phase, transformation, teaches negotiation skills for goals-based conflict and dialogue skills for SD. Dialogue skills are focused on finding common ground—understanding the other's way of seeing the world and accepting such differences. The goal of the

TABLE 10.1 Real Examples of SD From Existing Data

Description	SD-Nexus	SD-Cycle	Data Source
• Emergency Department (ED) transports patients to Geriatric Care (GC); pending admission, they require immediate care, then admitted to ICU. Record allows no documentation of GC labor • Management reviews credit care to ED and ICU • Negative impact (e.g., cost, time, and delayed care for others) results in GC performance sanctions • GC hesitant to provide care because of bureaucratic consequences • GC resentment for ED perpetuates conflict	Ethic for action: patient-centered vs. bureaucratic	**Unresolved Conflict:** ED vs. GC **Immobilization:** Reluctance to perform **Poor Development:** Unfair reviews	Nicotera & Clinkscales (2010)
• GC unable to accomplish scheduling • Frustrated nurses call in sick when unable to get reasonable day off (e.g., for a daughter's wedding) • Stress and confusion of short scheduling turnarounds causes tension between nurses and their managers	Decision-making: authoritative vs. collaborative	**Unresolved Conflict:** Scheduling problems **Immobilization:** Sick calls and turnover **Poor Development:** Staffing shortages	Nicotera & Clinkscales (2010)
• Supervisor for psychiatric student clinicals describes disconnect with clinical site • Program goal is to maximize patient contact • Site goal is to minimize patient contact (psychiatric inpatients with tendencies for harmful behavior)	Concern for students: learning vs. safety	**Unresolved Conflict:** Student role **Immobilization:** Unmet academic learning objectives **Poor Development:** Inadequate training	Nicotera, Mahon & Wright (2014)
• Unit achieves Magnet status • Nurses have less bedside time due to paperwork demand • Nurses see no benefit; requirements interfere • Feel ineffective, trapped, disloyal	Status "Excellence" vs. Care	**Unresolved Conflict:** "Excellence" status makes care difficult **Immobilization:** Magnet demands interfere with care **Poor Development:** Feeling ineffective	Nicotera, Mahon & Wright (2014)

transformation phase is to reframe the other from "opponent" to "colleague with whom I share a problem"—that problem being the SD conditions in which they must co-exist and collaborate. When dialogue cannot resolve the structural differences, the pair must cope with the stress of their differences. Teaching strategies for coping with stress is paramount.

Assessments of SD intervention effectiveness typically focus upon and measure negative conflict attitudes and behaviors, such as direct personalization, persecution feelings, negative relational effects, ambiguity intolerance, and triangulation (gossiping and complaining to uninvolved third parties). Assessment also targets important attitudes necessary for productive dialogue and conflict management: perceptions of positive relational effects, conflict liking, and positive beliefs about arguing. Previous work has found that, compared to non-participants, health care workers who have participated in SD-based interventions exhibit lower conflict persecution; higher recognition of positive relational effects; lower perceptions of negative relational effects; higher conflict liking; and lower ambiguity intolerance (Nicotera, Mahon, & Wright, 2014; Nicotera, Mahon, & Zhao, 2010). In addition, participants report having a better understanding of, and feeling more empowered to manage, workplace conflicts, and to sustain healthier workplace relationships. Such interventions can help health care workers develop tools to improve system-level function and build productive team relationships.

Nicotera et al. (2014) developed an intensive nine-hour workshop that provided training in conflict, SD analysis and dialogic conflict, and SD management in an intervention with 36 working nurses from a variety of settings. Quantitative pre- and post-tests were administered to both the intervention group and a comparison sample. The findings revealed that the course reduced measures of negative conflict attitudes and behaviors: direct personalization, persecution feelings, negative relational effects, ambiguity intolerance, and triangulation (gossiping and complaining to uninvolved third parties). The course also increased important attitudes necessary for productive dialogue and conflict management: perceptions of positive relational effects, conflict liking, and positive beliefs about arguing. Compared with nonparticipants, participant post-tests showed lower conflict persecution (as measured by Hample & Dalinger's, 1995, taking conflict personally scale); higher recognition of positive relational effects; lower perceptions of negative relational effects; higher conflict liking; lower ambiguity intolerance, and less triangulation.

Implications of Research Findings for Theory, Research, and Future Conflict Interventions Among Health Care Workers

This chapter examined two prominent approaches (individual competence approach and the structurational divergence approach) to studying health care worker stress, conflict, and social support, and the relationships among these variables and two key organizational outcomes: (1) employee burnout and

(2) employee turnover in health care organizations. This section explores the strengths and limitations of both the individual competence and the structurational divergence approaches in terms of designing interventions that target health care worker conflict, social support, burnout, and turnover issues. In addition, it discusses several areas within this topic that would benefit from future research.

Strengths and Limitations of Individual Competence and SD Approaches

Individual Competence Perspective

A considerable number of scholars take an individual competency approach to managing conflict situations among organizational workers, including health care workers (e.g., Canary & Lakey, 2006; Canary & Spitzberg, 1987; Montoro-Rodriguez & Small, 2006 Wright et al., 2010). Researchers from this perspective argue that conflict is the result of individuals interacting with one another, but also bring individual conflict style predispositions to the conflict situation (e.g., aggressive style, avoidant style, etc.), and this ultimately influences the quality of the interaction. In other words, from this conflict trait-like perspective, individual conflict styles are seen as the focal point a conflict intervention. Individual workers are assessed to determine each person's predominant conflict style, and the intervention targets behavior change among those individuals who have conflict styles that appear to lead to negative outcomes (e.g., verbal aggression; conflict avoidance) while simultaneously reinforcing "good" conflict styles (e.g., collaborating). One limitation of this approach is that current quantitative conflict style measures (e.g., Rahim. 1985) often ignore larger cultural variations in conflict style (See Ting-Toomey & Oetzel, 2001) as well as the influence of environmental/contextual factors (i.e., structure) that may lead to recurring unproductive conflict among health care workers. However, one advantage of this approach is that it is relatively easy to administer a questionnaire to health care workers that consists of a conflict style measure and other organizational variables of interest (e.g., social support, burnout, etc.). This can help determine which employee (or group of employees) is most at risk for engaging in unproductive conflict. Training these individuals is to manage conflict productively (and in some cases interventions include the creation of social support networks within the organization) may help workers to better manage conflict situations. However, given that this perspective does not focus on environmental/contextual variables that lead to unproductive conflict, it is possible that interventions fail to achieve sustainable outcomes (especially if the contextual factors persist for a long period of time).

SD Perspective

From the structurational divergence theory perspective, in terms of the causes of conflict, the shift of focus from individual health care workers to organizational structures implies that health care managers should cease blaming conflict and poor communication among workers based upon individual skill deficits and problem personalities. SD theory and research posits that the roots of intractable conflicts in health care environments are institutional constraints that require targeted intervention. In other words, from the SD perspective, future intervention work should aim at understanding the unique structural constraints of particular health care organizations that are facing high conflict, stress, burnout, and turnover situations as opposed to targeting individual skills when it comes to managing conflict situations (e.g., conflict styles, training, etc.).

Of course, the SD approach has shortcomings as well. SD interventions may be more time-consuming than individual competence-based interventions. However, recent work has found that SD interventions can be implemented over the course of a few days or a week-long workshop. In this sense, the amount of work required to conduct SD training among health care workers may not increase the length or the expense of the intervention. The main difference between the two intervention strategies is their focus on differing causes of conflict (i.e., individual competencies versus contextual/structural factors). Assessing structural factors that lead to conflict may vary from health organization to health organization, so the types of structures or situations in one organization will likely differ from another organization (although some similar patterns can be seen across organizations). This can lead to greater complexity when researchers make decisions on which of the structures that appear to lead to conflict they should focus on in a specific intervention. Gaining an understanding of the unique structures of organizations that are producing conflict may require a multi-methodological approach where researchers need to engage in qualitative research (e.g., interviews, ethnographic fieldwork) to better understand the specific health care organization culture. In addition, interviews with key stakeholders within the organization are required to assess perspectives of structures, conflicts, and views about oppositional forces within specific conflict situations. This type of research can lead to more labor-intensive work on the part of the researcher to uncover these themes.

In addition, findings that appear to be confined to a particular health care organization may be seen as having limited generalizability to researchers from the individual competency perspective who are interested in developing a more general framework (e.g., competency/conflict skills) that can be applied to a variety of health care organization conflict situations. SD has only examined the role of social support in conflict situations in a general way, although it has been found to be an important mediator of conflict, stress, burnout, and turnover in other approaches. Finally, another limitation to the SD approach is that it is a relatively new approach to managing conflict among health care workers. Additional research is needed to assess the theoretical assumptions behind the SD perspective as well as research that helps to improve the precision of this approach in terms of ameliorating organization conflict among health care workers.

Areas for Future Research

Future studies of conflict among health care workers and its relationship to burn-out and turnover should consider testing the individual (communication) competence approach and the structurational divergence (SD) approach to conflict resolution among health care workers. In addition, more elaborate interventions that take into account both individual traits and structural influences on conflict may help to draw upon the strengths found in both perspectives. However, individual competence approaches should recognize that organizational conflict stems well beyond the individual into rituals, practices, the organizational climate, and missions of health care organizations. Individual health care workers' conflict patterns appear to be influenced to a great degree by such structures, so future work should account for influences on conflict behaviors beyond the level of individual skills and traits. Given the heavy toll that conflict, burnout, and turnover take on both health care workers and health care organizations, it is important for health communication researchers to work at improving our understanding of conflict, social support, burnout and turnover, and other important variables within this context in the future.

DISCUSSION QUESTIONS

1. What are some of the major contributors to conflict among workers in health care organizations? Which variables related to individual characteristics can lead to unproductive conflict? Which variables related to the structure of the organization may influence conflict?
2. Of the individual (communication) competence approach to studying conflict in health care organizations or the structurational divergence (SD) approach, which do you think would be best for resolving conflict among health care workers? Why?
3. What are some of the implications of burnout and turnover in health organizations for the organization itself and patients? What is the role of social support in terms of its relationship to conflict, burnout, and turnover?

Suggested Reading

Canary, D. J. & Lakey, S. G. (2006). Managing conflict in a competent manner: A mindful look at events that matter. In J. G. Oetzel & S. Ting-Toomey (Eds), *The SAGE handbook of conflict management* (pp. 185–210). Thousand Oaks, CA: Sage.

Nicotera, A. M., Mahon, M. M., & Zhao, X. (2010). Conceptualization and measurement of structurational divergence in the healthcare setting. *Journal of Applied Communication Research, 38,* 362–385.

References

Aiken, L. H., Clarke, S. P., Sloan, D. M., Sochalski, J., & Silber, J. H. (2002). Hospital nurse staffing and patient mortality, nurse burnout, and job satisfaction. *JAMA, 288,* 1987–1993.

Apker, J., Ford, W. S. Z., & Fox, D. H. (2003). Predicting nurses' organizational and professional identification: The effect of nursing roles, professional autonomy, and supportive communication. *Nursing Economics, 21,* 226–232.

Apker, J., Propp, K. M., Ford, W. S. (2003). Negotiating status and identity tensions in healthcare team interactions: An exploration of nurse role dialectics. *Journal of Applied Communication Research, 33,* 93–115.

Apker, J. & Ray, E. B. (2003). Stress and social support in health care organizations. In T. L. Thompson, A. M. Dorsey, K. I. Miller, & R. Parrott (Eds.), *Handbook of health communication* (pp. 347–368). Mahwah, NJ: Lawrence Erlbaum Associates.

Bakker, A. B., Le Blanc, P. M., & Schaufeli, W. B. (2005). Burnout contagion among intensive care nurses. *Journal of Advanced Nursing, 51,* 276–287.

Brown, S. D., Goske, M. J., & Johnson, C. M. (2009). Beyond substance abuse: Stress, burnout, and depression as causes of physician impairment and disruptive behavior. *Journal of the American College of Radiology, 6,* 479–485.

Canary, D. J. & Cupach, W. R. (1988). Relational and episodic characteristics associated with conflict tactics. *Journal of Social and Personal Relationships, 5,* 305–325.

Canary, D. J., Cupach, W. R., & Serpe, R. (2001). A competence-based approach to examining interpersonal conflict: Test of a longitudinal model. *Communication Research, 28,* 127–150.

Canary, D. J. & Lakey, S. G. (2006). Managing conflict in a competent manner: A mindful look at events that matter. In J. G. Oetzel & S. Ting-Toomey (Eds), *The SAGE handbook of conflict management* (pp. 185–210). Thousand Oaks, CA: Sage.

Canary, D. J. & Spitzberg, B. H. (1987). Appropriateness and effectiveness perceptions of conflict strategies. *Human Communication Research, 14,* 93–118.

Canary, D. J. & Spitzberg, B. H. (1989). A model of the perceived competence of conflict strategies. *Human Communication Research, 15,* 630–649.

Canary, D. J., Spitzberg, B. H., & Semic, B. A. (1998). The experience and expression of anger in interpersonal settings. In P. A. Andersen & L. K. Guerrero (Eds.), *Handbook of communication and emotion: Theory, research, and applications* (pp. 189–213). San Diego, CA: Academic Press. Doi: 10.1016/b978-012057770-5/50009-6.

Dormann, C. & Zapf, D. (1999). Social support, social stressors at work, and depressive symptoms: Testing for main and moderating effects with structural equations in a three-wave longitudinal study. *Journal of Applied Psychology, 84,* 874–884.

Dorz, S., Novara, C., Sica, C., & Sanavio, E. (2010). Predicting burnout among HIV/AIDS and oncology health care workers. *Psychology & Health, 18,* 677–684.

Dunn, D. (2005). Substance abuse among nurses: Defining the issue. *AORN Journal, 82,* 572–596.

Eisenberger, R., Stinglhamber, F., Vandenberghe, C., Sucharski, I. L., & Rhoades, L. (2002). Perceived supervisor support: Contributions to perceived organizational support and employee retention. *Journal of Applied Psychology, 87,* 565–573.

Ellis, B. H. & Miller, K. I. (1994). Supportive communication among nurses: Effects on commitment, burnout, and retention. *Health Communication, 6,* 77–96.

Firth, L., Mellor, D. J., Moore, K. A., & Loquet, C. (2004). How can managers reduce employee intention to quit? *Journal of Managerial Psychology, 19,* 170–187.

Friedman, R. A., Tidd, S. T., Currall, S. C., & Tsai, J. C. (2000). What goes around comes around: The impact of personal conflict style on work conflict and stress. *The Journal of Conflict Management, 11*, 32–55.

Fujiwara, K., Tsukishima, E., Tsutsumi, A., Kawakami, N., & Kishi, R. (2003). Interpersonal conflict, social support, and burnout among home care workers in Japan. *Journal of Occupational Medicine, 5*, 313–330.

Giddens, A. (1984). *The Constitution of Society: Outline of the Theory of Structuration.* Berkeley, CA: University of California Press.

Gottman, J. M. & Levenson, R. W. (1992). Martial processes predictive of later dissolution: Behavior, physiology, and health. *Journal of Personality and Social Psychology, 63*, 221–233.

Hample, D. & Dallinger, J.M. (1995). A Lewinian perspective on taking conflict personally: Revision, refinement, and validation of the instrument. *Communication Quarterly, 43*, 297–319.

Hample, D., Dallinger, J. M., & Nelson, G. K. (1995). Aggressive, argumentative and maintenance arguing behaviors, and their relationship to taking conflict personally. In F. H. van Eemeren, R. Grootendorst, A. Blair & C. A. Willard (Eds.), *Reconstruction and application 3* (pp. 238–250). Amsterdam: SicSat.

Hatton, C. & Emerson, E. (1998). Organizational predictors of actual staff turnover in a service for people with multiple disabilities. *Journal of Applied Research in Intellectual Abilities, 11*, 166–171.

House, J. S. (1981). Work stress and social support. Reading, MA: Addison-Wesley.

Jones, C. B. (2008). Revisiting nurse turnover costs: Adjusting for inflation. *Journal of Nursing Administration, 38*, 11–18.

Kalliath, T. & Morris, R. (2002). Job satisfaction among nurses: A predictor of burnout levels. *Journal of Nursing Administration, 32*, 648–654.

Kim, H. & Lee, S. Y. (2009). Supervisory communication, burnout, and turnover intention among social workers in health care settings. *Social Work in Health Care, 48*, 364–385.

Kim, H. & Stoner, M. (2008). Burnout and turnover intention among social workers: Effects of role stress, job autonomy, and social support. *Administration in Social Work, 32*, 5–25.

Kreps, G. L. (1988). Relational communication in health care. *Southern Speech Communication Journal, 53*, 344–359.

Lloyd, C., King, R., & Chenoweth, L. (2002). Social work, stress and burnout: A review. *Journal of Mental Health, 11*, 255–26.

Maslach, C. (2003). Job burnout: New directions in research and intervention. *Current Directions in Psychological Science, 5*, 189–192.

Maslach, C. & Leiter, M. P. (2008). *The truth about burnout: How organizations cause personal stress and what to do about it.* Hoboken, NJ: John Wiley & Sons.

Maslach, C., Schaufeli, W. B., & Leiter, M. P. (2001). Job burnout. *Annual Review of Psychology, 52*, 397–422.

McClean, J. & Andrew, T. (2000). Commitment, satisfaction, stress, and control among social service managers and social service workers in the UK. *Administration in Social Work, 23*, 93–117.

McManus, I. C., Winder, B. C., & Gordon, D. (2002). The causal links between stress and burnout in a longitudinal study of UK doctors. *Lancet, 359*, 2089–2090.

Miller, K. I., Stiff, J. B., & Ellis, B. H. (1988). Communication and empathy as precursors to burnout among human service workers. *Communication Monographs, 55*, 250–265.

Montoro-Rodriguez, J. & Small, J. (2006). The role of conflict resolution styles on nursing staff morale, burnout, and job satisfaction in long-term care. *Journal of Aging and Health, 18*, 385–406.

Nicotera, A. M. & Clinkscales, M. C. (2010). Nurses at the nexus: A case study in structurational divergence. *Health Communication, 25*, 32–49.

Nicotera, A. M. & Dorsey, L. K. (2006). Individuals and interactive processes in organizational conflict. In J. G. Oetzel & S. Ting-Toomey (Eds.), *The SAGE handbook of conflict communication* (pp. 293–325). Thousand Oaks, CA: Sage.

Nicotera, A. M. & Mahon, M. M. (2013). Between rocks and hard places: Exploring the impact of structurational divergence in the nursing workplace. *Management Communication Quarterly, 27*, 90–120.

Nicotera, A. M., Mahon, M. M., & Wright, K. B. (2014). Communication that builds teams: Assessing a nursing conflict intervention. *Nursing Administration Quarterly, 38*, 248–260.

Nicotera, A. M., Mahon, M. M., & Zhao, X. (2010). Conceptualization and measurement of structurational divergence in the healthcare setting. *Journal of Applied Communication Research, 38*, 362–385.

Nicotera, A. M., Zhao, X., Mahon, M., Peterson, E., Kim, W., & Conway-Morana, P. (in press). Structurational divergence theory as explanation for troublesome outcomes in nursing communication. *Health Communication, 30*, 371–384. Doi: 10.1080/10410236.2013.863139.

Poncet, M., Toullic, P., Papazian, L., Kentish-Barnes, N., Timsit, J., & Pochard, F., et al. (2007). Burnout syndrome in critical care nursing staff. *American Journal of Respiratory Critical Care Medicine, 175*, 698–704.

Putnam, L. L. & Wilson, C. E. (1982). Communicative strategies in organizational conflicts: Reliability and validity of a measurement scale. In M. Burgoon (Ed.), *Communication yearbook 6* (pp. 629–652). Thousand Oaks, CA: Sage.

Rahim, M. A. (1985). A strategy for managing conflict in complex organizations. *Human Relations, 38*, 81–89.

Rahim, M. A. (2002). Toward a theory of managing organizational conflict. *International Journal of Conflict Management, 13*, 206–235.

Ramanujam, R. & Rousseau, D. M. (2006). The challenges are organizational not just clinical. *Journal of Organizational Behavior, 27*, 811–827.

Rancer, A. S., Kosberg, R. L., & Baukus R. A. (1992). Beliefs about arguing as predictors of trait argumentativeness: Implications for training in argument and conflict management. *Communication Education, 41*, 375–387.

Ray, E. B. (1987). Supportive relationships and occupational stress in the workplace. In T. L. Albrecht & M. B. Adelman (Eds.), *Communicating social support* (pp. 172–191). Newbury Park, CA: Sage.

Reid, R. J., Coleman, K., Johnson, E. A., Fishman, P. A., Hsu, C., Soman, M. P., . . . & Larson, E. B. (2010). The group health medical home at year two: Cost savings, higher patient satisfaction, and less burnout for providers. *Health Affairs, 29*, 835–843.

Rouse, R. A. (2009). Ineffective participation: Reactions to absentee and incompetent nurse leadership in an intensive care unit. *Journal of Nursing Management, 17*, 463–473.

Schaufeli, W. B., Leiter, M. P., & Maslach, C. (2009). Burnout: 35 years of research and practice. *Career Development International, 14*, 204–220.

Siefert, K., Jayaratne, S., & Chess, W. A. (1991). Job satisfaction, burnout, and turnover in health care social workers. *Health and Social Work, 16*, 193–202.

Ting-Toomey, S. & Oetzel, J. G. (2001). *Managing interpersonal conflict effectively*. Thousand Oaks, CA: Sage.

Waldman, J. D., Kelly, F., Aurora, S., & Smith, H. L. (2004). The shocking cost of turnover in health care. *Health Care Management Review, 29*, 2–7.

Wiemann, J. M. & Backlund, P. (1980). Current theory and research in communicative competence. *Review of Educational Research, 50*, 185–199.

Wright, K. B. (2011). A communication competence approach to healthcare worker conflict, job stress, job burnout, and job satisfaction. *Journal for Healthcare Quality, 33*, 7–14.

Wright, K. B., Banas, J., Bessarabova, E., & Bernard, D. R. (2010). A communication competence approach to examining healthcare worker social support, stress, and job burnout. *Health Communication, 25*, 375–382.

Wright, K. B., Sparks, L., & O'Hair, H. D. (2013). *Health communication in the 21st century* (2nd ed.). Malden, MA: Wiley-Blackwell.

11

WORKPLACE WELLNESS CAMPAIGNS

The Four Dimensions of a Whole-Person Approach

Jennifer A. Scarduzio and Patricia Geist-Martin

Workplace wellness campaigns are becoming more common as organizations try to create and sustain healthy work environments for employees (World Health Organization, 2010) and simultaneously meet requirements of the Patient Protection and Affordable Care Act (PPACA) (Colmer, Millea, & Wearne, 2013). In fact, the U.S. Department of Health and Human Services distributed $10 million in 2011 for grants to help companies develop wellness programs (Churchill, Gillespie, & Herbold, 2014). Organizations tend to encourage wellness program participation for several reasons. First, companies that help create healthy employees end up with workers who are motivated to work and ultimately use less sick time (Machen, Cuddihy, Reaburn, & Higgins, 2010). Second, organizations can gain financial benefit from government grants and from less employee turnover when employees are working well (Geist-Martin & Scarduzio, 2011). Third, organizations hope to decrease insurance premiums and chronic employee illness by encouraging healthy behaviors and providing incentives (Churchill et al., 2014). Yet despite the increasing prevalence of wellness programs and interest from organizations to develop programs, many current programs fail to address a multi-dimensional approach to health and wellness—frequently, emphasizing one facet of wellness, such as physical, and ignoring other facets, such as social and spiritual. The intent of this chapter is to describe and explain a whole-person approach (Geist-Martin, Ray, & Sharf, 2011) to workplace wellness campaigns.

First, we begin by defining the whole-person approach and explaining physical, psychological, social, and spiritual wellness. Second, we reveal why the whole-person approach to wellness is the preferred method for addressing workplace wellness and health issues in organizations. Third, we explicate specific ways that the whole-person approach can be translated into practice. Fourth, we explore various challenges and pitfalls that organizations may face as they implement a whole-person approach. Finally, we conclude by suggesting how positivity—including happiness, gratitude, and compassion—can be implemented into wellness campaigns through use of the whole-person approach (Mirivel, 2014).

Defining the Whole-Person Approach

The whole-person approach to wellness suggests that researchers consider the physical, psychological, social, and spiritual dimensions of wellness when crafting and creating wellness campaigns at work (Geist-Martin et al., 2011). Furthermore, the whole-person approach moves away from simply focusing on a scientific or biomedical approach, to wellness, and considers aspects of individuals' organizational experience that can contribute to their illness and disease. The four dimensions of wellness included in the whole-person approach are discussed below in more detail.

Physical Wellness

Physical wellness is defined as individual's biological and bodily health and fitness. Poor physical wellness encompasses chronic diseases and illnesses such as obesity, diabetes, and heart conditions, among others. Chronic diseases are responsible for more than 60% of deaths around the world (Malouf, 2011). Many chronic diseases are caused by individuals' level of stress. Occupational stress impacts individuals' physical wellness because many employees do not possess knowledge about effective coping mechanisms (Farrell & Geist-Martin, 2005). Instead, they rely on chemicals, such as alcohol or cigarettes, to cope with occupational stress (Ray & Miller, 1994). Additionally, employees' physical wellness could be impacted by their work environment. For example, environmental stressors such as improper equipment, lighting problems, temperature, and noise levels may negatively impact employees' physical wellness ("Overcoming Ergonomics Risks", 2012).

Psychological Wellness

Psychological wellness is defined as individuals' mental health and fitness. Anxiety, low self-esteem, depression, and boredom, among others, are all symptoms of poor psychological wellness (Farrell & Geist-Martin, 2005). Interestingly, one employee's depression can have ripple effects on other team members and the overall organizational culture of a company (Ramon, 2005). Indeed, it is important for businesses to understand how to help employees improve their psychological wellness. For example, psychological wellness is impacted by organizational change and perceived levels of autonomy and control (Loretto et al., 2005). Psychological wellness is also influenced by how much spillover employees have from work into their private lives (Loretto et al., 2005). Organizations that recognize what decreases psychological wellness, such as low levels of autonomy and high levels of spillover, can develop wellness campaigns to mitigate employee dis-ease (Hillier, Fewell, Cann, & Shephard, 2005).

Social Wellness

Social wellness is defined as individuals' relational health and fitness. In other words, social health is "the quality of an individual's networks of professional and personal relationships" (Farrell & Geist-Martin, 2005, p. 549). Social wellness can be improved through informal (e.g., lunch in the break room) and formal (e.g., company holiday party) practices. Furthermore, social wellness events can take place on-site and off-site (Farrell & Geist-Martin, 2005). In terms of the communication between employees, specific practices have been found to enhance social wellness. Nurses in a hospital setting had higher levels of retention and social wellness when they received social and grief support from coworkers (Medland, Howard-Ruben, & Whitaker, 2002). Also, organizations that communicate expectations and goals clearly to employees are likely to help them foster social wellness at work (Geist-Martin & Scarduzio, 2011).

Spiritual Wellness

Spiritual wellness is defined as individuals' sacred health (Pargament, 1999) and fulfillment. However, spirituality is not the same as religion. Remen (1993) suggests that spirituality is an essential human need. In her words, "The spiritual is inclusive. It is the deepest sense of belonging and participation. We all participate in the spiritual all the time, whether we know it or not" (p. 41). According to Ashar and Lane-Maher (2004), "when virtues, ethics, values, emotions, and intuition are part of the organization's behavior and policies, the organization is spiritually oriented" (p. 253). Spirituality for individuals in organizations is "an ongoing process of growth and nourishment; its quintessence is wisdom, connectedness, integration, independence and a holistic apprehending of organizational life" (Geist-Martin & Freiberg, 1992, p. 2). Religion on the other hand is described as a community or institution of spiritual belief (Koenig, 2008). Individuals' spiritual identity "includes a state of wholeness and health that is considered to be one's divine heritage" (Kline, 2011, p. 338). Organizations that consider employees' spiritual wellness can experience increased honesty and trust (Wagner-Marsh & Conely, 1999), higher levels of creativity (Freshman, 1999), and an elevated sense of employee personal fulfillment (Burack, 1999). Essentially, spirituality for individuals in organizations

> involves a desire to do purposeful work that serves others and to be part of a principled community. It involves a yearning for connectedness and

wholeness that can only be manifested when one is allowed to integrate his or her inner life with one's professional role in the service of a greater good.
(Ashar & Lane-Maher, 2004, p. 253)

Now that we have introduced the four dimensions of wellness, it is necessary to understand why the whole-person approach in organizations offers a valuable orientation toward individuals' work in organizations.

The Importance of the Whole-Person Approach

The whole-person approach helps employers communicate and interact with employees in terms of all dimensions of their personhood, not just in terms of the role they play or the function they serve in the organization. The unique contribution of the approach is that it reveals an entire picture of individuals' physical, social, psychological, and spiritual health. With this entire picture, employers and employees can assess trouble areas and address them accordingly. For example, an employee may seem perfectly healthy on the outside, but if they are experiencing social problems (e.g., divorce, social exclusion, bullying) they will not demonstrate wellness at work and will potentially be ineffective at their job. Companies work at "cross-purposes when, on the one hand, they offer programs which they believe will enhance the health of employees . . . but at the same time, do nothing to change the working conditions or organizational culture that are inherently stressful" (Geist-Martin & Scarduzio, 2011, p. 122). An employer who is able to recognize a health issue and address it accordingly can help foster a supportive and caring organizational culture (Williams & Bruno, 2007).

In order to be working well, employees need to create and sustain a health identity that includes a combination of all four dimensions of wellness. For instance, an effective health identity may include "a combination of all four health components, in varying degrees, at various times, over a week, month, or year in an organization" (Farrell & Geist-Martin, 2005, p. 576). Essentially, the four components of health may largely contribute to what individuals and the organization define as success—a sense of accomplishment, balance of work and family, and contributions to the community and colleagues (Asher & Lane-Maher, 2004). While the whole-person approach sounds good in theory, it is also relevant to discuss how to apply the approach in practice.

Translating the Whole-Person Approach Into Practice

First, to address physical wellness, campaigns could include exercise meetings, stress management programs, on-site fitness centers, health screenings (e.g., diabetes, heart disease, and other chronic diseases), and smoking cessation programs. For example, General Electric (GE) has a Healthymagination campaign that encourages employees to commit to one small change a day, such as walking to lunch (Healthymagination, 2014). In addition, they have a special division of human resources that is dedicated to enhancing their culture of health. At Accenture, employees receive incentives for reaching 10,000 steps a day (Accenture Wellness Centers, 2014).

Second, psychological wellness could be addressed through counseling services, bereavement services, mental health services, and alternative forms of psychological wellness such as meditation. At Bright Horizons, they take a whole-person approach to wellness by offering employees services such as legal assistance, growth and learning programs, and real-estate counseling (Family Resources, 2014). Additionally, Microsoft helps employees enhance psychological wellness by having an on-site pharmacy and counselors who will make house calls (Benefits, 2014).

Third, campaigns addressing social wellness might integrate holiday parties, spring picnics, monthly social gatherings (during work time), rewards for productivity that include social aspects such as lunches, break rooms that encourage socialization, and interior design elements that encourage open communication. Companies like Accenture offer intramural sports to increase social wellness and camaraderie. General Mills hosts Fitness Friday events such as dodgeball and Lumosity has a Culture Team dedicated to planning social events for employees (The 46 Healthiest Companies, 2014).

Fourth and finally, spiritual wellness aspects could include access to yoga, meditation, books, and materials that promote wisdom and learning. Employees could be encouraged to participate in complementary/integrative medicine (CIM) practices, if they desire, such as chiropractics and acupuncture. CIM includes a way of considering individuals' health that includes more than a focus on disease, biological health, and medical treatments (Sharf, Geist-Martin, & Moore, 2012) to include a focus on the whole person (Geist-Martin, Bollinger, Wiechert, Plump, & Sharf, In Press). Indeed, holistic medicine is based on all four components, and can be defined as "a wholeness of mind, body, and spirit, in contrast with the tendency toward reductive specialization in biomedicine" (Sharf, Geist-Martin, Cosgriff-Hernandez, & Moore, 2012, p. 434). Companies have attempted to address spiritual wellness through specific practices and offerings of CIM. For instance, Cisco offers employees acupuncture services and Hasbro has wellness workshops that teach employees about mindfulness and massage (The 46 Healthiest Companies, 2014). In addition to implementation into programs, wellness must be incorporated into the culture of the organization.

So, how can the four dimensions be integrated into workplace culture? As Churchill et al. (2014) claim, "the overall success of a program is strongly dependent on the ability of an organization to motivate employees to participate and create a culture of wellness" (p. 49). The first problem is that employees do not always want to participate in wellness campaigns. Indeed, research has found that lack of employee interest and low participation rates are common barriers for wellness campaigns (Churchill et al., 2014; Geist-Martin, Horsley, & Farrell, 2003). Employees have also cited lack of support from colleagues and supervisors, lack of time, and low funding (Malouf, 2011). Thus, there are specific ways that each dimension of wellness needs to be promoted.

Physical wellness can be promoted through monetary incentives for participation in health screenings and/or exercise programs. Research has determined that monetary and financial incentives are effective for health exams, and biometric and health screenings (Linnan et al., 2008). However, monetary incentives for smoking cessation and/or weight management programs are not as effective (Churchill et al., 2014).

Psychological wellness can be promoted through paid vacation and sick time as well as access to appropriate counseling and services if necessary. Additionally, employers can strive to create a culture where early self-referral to services is not viewed as a sign of "individual weakness" (Ramon, 2005, p. 315), but rather an appropriate response to stress and mental health issues. As aforementioned, a lack of perceived support can be a barrier for wellness campaigns. Thus, not surprisingly, research has found that perceived support—especially from leaders and managers— has a positive effect on employee psychological well-being (Loretto et al., 2005).

Social wellness can be promoted through the creation of a culture of camaraderie and compassion. Compassion communicated between work colleagues can increase productivity and strengthen connections (Dutton, Frost, Worline, Lilius, & Kanov, 2002; Frost, Dutton, Worline, & Wilson, 2000; Lilius et al., 2008). Indeed, when employees are the recipients of compassionate communication "it is thought to increase feelings of connection with one another, which in turn produces a variety of positive feelings" (Lilius et al., 2008, p. 196). As we discuss later in this chapter, compassion is one way to cultivate positivity at work and enhance employee experiences and affective commitment. In addition, companies can have social gatherings during work hours (on- and off-site) and encourage employees to get to know each other socially through Spring Picnics, holiday parties, and even mentoring.

Spiritual wellness can be promoted by encouraging employees to tap into their spiritual sides and providing opportunities for employees to share their spiritual experiences. Companies should avoid being fearful that spirituality is a risky topic (Lips-Wiersma & Mills, 2002). Moreover, companies should not commodify and regulate spiritual experiences through spiritual labor (see McGuire, 2009). Instead, spiritual wellness should not be based on the organization's spiritual beliefs—but rather, each employee should have the freedom to cultivate their own spiritual identity (Krishnakumar & Neck, 2002). Formative research needs to be conducted prior to the promotion of each of the dimensions of wellness and prior to the development of a company-specific wellness campaign.

Formative Research

There are a few issues that any company considering a whole-person approach to wellness should evaluate during formative research. First, the company should explore which dimensions of health the company already promotes effectively.

This can be accomplished through personal inventories and examining current practices. Second, the company should determine what dimensions need improvement in their services. Business can conduct employee interviews for feedback about current services. Third and finally, companies should define specific practices that each company can do to increase wellness within each dimension. For example, companies could look at current examples of wellness programs at other businesses for ideas. Despite the benefits of a whole-person approach, there are still various challenges and pitfalls of this perspective—an issue we turn to next

Challenges and Pitfalls of the Whole-Person Approach

There is no perfect approach to aid in the development of workplace wellness campaigns. With that said, we would be remiss to not mention the challenges and pitfalls of the whole-person approach. If companies are aware of the potential downsides of the whole-person approach, they can prepare accordingly for potential missteps.

The first challenge is that some organizations are not as well suited for the whole-person approach. Indeed, there are specific types of organizations where integration of the whole-person approach may be challenging. For example, highly competitive organizations, such as politicized business environments, would have a hard time integrating the whole-person approach because they typically also have high levels of bullying and cut-throat cultures (Salin, 2003). In addition, industries with a high degree of abuse, such as postal workers (Worsham, 1998), may also face challenges. When an organizational culture has become rampant with workplace bullying and emotional abuse (Lutgen-Sandvik & McDermott, 2008) or sexual harassment (Scarduzio & Geist-Martin, 2008, 2010), the wellness of employees may be extremely depleted. Thus, employees may need more critical intervention and support before implementing the whole-person approach.

A second challenge of the whole-person approach is the need to ensure that appropriate tailoring of each wellness campaign is specific to the considerations of each organization. For example, small businesses have different concerns than large corporations when implementing a wellness campaign. Wellness campaigns are prevalent in small businesses, with 65% offering at least one wellness benefit (Neely, 2012). Furthermore, specific implementation and participation practices have been found to be effective in small businesses, such as using data to design programs, helping people understand their health risks (e.g., health fairs), and providing people with incentives to decrease those risks (Neely, 2012). Space, context, culture, and employee motivation are also examples of factors to consider during wellness campaign tailoring.

There are two pitfalls to be avoided when integrating the whole-person approach to wellness campaigns. The first pitfall is providing service to one dimension of wellness (e.g., physical) while neglecting another dimension (e.g., spiritual). For instance, a wellness initiative may offer incentives for physical wellness and offer free health screenings but fail to provide any social activities and events for the employees. The second pitfall is espousing values of a whole-person approach, but not putting those values into action continuously. In other words, companies may claim to care about employees' wellness but fail to actually enact practices that address the four dimensions of wellness. Pitfalls can be avoided by taking a hands-on approach through frequent and consistent follow up with employees. Businesses should ask employees what they want and need in terms of each dimension of wellness. Additionally, as companies grow and change through mergers or cutbacks, business should also make changes to the wellness initiatives they offer.

Positivity and Wellness Campaigns

In this chapter, we have introduced the whole-person approach to wellness as an important method to employ when developing a workplace wellness campaign. We defined and explained the four dimensions of wellness, the importance of the whole-person approach, how to translate the approach into practice, and various challenges and pitfalls of the approach and how to avoid them. In the conclusion of this piece chapter, we briefly explain how a whole-person approach allows organizations to integrate positivity into their workplace cultures. We suggest that positivity be implemented into organizations through happiness, gratitude, and compassion.

Happiness at Work

Happiness research is split between those who view it as pleasant feelings and those who describe it as related to virtuous and moral behavior (Fisher, 2010). While happiness has been studied infrequently in organizational literature, numerous constructs have emerged that are related to positive affective experience. Concepts related to happiness include job satisfaction, affective commitment, mood at work, and dispositional affectivity (Fisher, 2010). Furthermore, people become happy because of something inside of them, something in the environment, and/or an interaction with another person. So what makes employees happy at work?

First, employees experience happiness when they can trust others in the workplace. According to The Great Place to Work Institute, people are happy at work when "they trust the people they work for, have pride in what they do, and enjoy the people they work with" (n.d.). Indeed, when employees feel a sense of equity with their coworkers and supervisors they are more likely to feel happy (Sirota, Mischkind, & Meltzer, 2005). Second, employees are happy when they have personal control, supportive supervision, environmental clarity, and opportunity for skill use (Warr, 2007). Thus, companies should strive to give employees support and also freedom to make some of their own decisions in order to enhance wellness.

Importantly, a culture of happiness can be created even if it does not currently exist. For example, in one study, financial sales employees participated in a cognitive-behavioral training program to help them adopt an optimistic style of thinking. Three months later, researchers found that the employees had increased job satisfaction and well-being (Proudfoot, Corr, Guest, & Dunn, 2009). Furthermore, at the end of two years the company had reduced employee turnover and higher levels of performance (Proudfoot et al., 2009).

Happiness can be implemented into considerations of physical wellness through offering employees external incentives and goal monitoring (Warr, 2007). In addition, by offering employees empowerment through feedback and job challenge, companies can enhance happiness and psychological wellness (Sirota et al., 2005). Camaraderie and equity among various coworkers helps employees feel happy at work while also increasing their social wellness. And finally, encouraging employees to express their individual spiritual beliefs may help employees feel enthusiastic and increase spiritual wellness at work. Besides pleasant feelings at work, employees work well when they feel appreciated.

Gratitude at Work

Gratitude is an expression of thanks or appreciation to another individual. It is defined as an "emotion which occurs after people receive aid which is perceived as costly, valuable, and altruistic" (Wood, Froh, & Geraghty, 2010, p. 890). When an individual feels gratitude they are more likely to repay a benefactor (Algoe & Haidt, 2009; Tsang, 2007) and also assist unrelated third party individuals in the future (Bartlett & DeSteno, 2006). In other words, a person who experiences a kind act from someone else is likely to repay that person in the future and also be kinder to other people in general. Thus, gratitude is not just an emotion experienced after someone helps an individual, it is "a producer of helping behavior" (Chang, Lin, & Chen, 2012, p. 762).

In the workplace, gratitude has a positive impact on wellness. Employees who experience gratitude have higher levels of corporate social responsibility toward societal and ethical issues (Andersson, Giacalone, & Jurkiewicz, 2007). Gratitude at work is a "life orientation towards noticing and appreciating the positive in the world" (Wood et al., 2010). Therefore, employees that communicate and experience gratitude are likely to have higher levels of wellness at work.

Companies should incorporate gratitude into their workplace cultures and wellness campaigns. Employees who improve their physical wellness can receive public praise and congratulations for their achievements. In addition, employees can be encouraged to look out for each other and refer others who may need assistance with their psychological wellness. Social wellness is enhanced when employees feel appreciated by their coworkers. Thus, companies may suggest that coworkers nominate each other for special awards or write each other thank you cards for their assistance. Employees could be encouraged to say thank you to others when they receive help. Finally, when employees experience gratitude they may in turn help others by creating an altruistic culture. A culture where everyone is helping each other will ultimately create higher levels of spiritual wellness. In addition to gratitude, the four dimensions of wellness can be developed when compassion is communicated.

Compassion at Work

Compassion has been defined and conceptualized in many ways. In communication research, Miller (2007) described the process of compassion as noticing, connecting, and responding. More recently, Way and Tracy (2012) conceptualized compassion as recognizing, relating, and (re)acting. The extension to the previous research suggested that compassion "can be proactive, prompting employees to recognize and relate in new ways" (Way & Tracy, 2012, p. 308). As aforementioned, compassion in the workplace has various positive effects too.

Compassion helps employees enhance their connections with coworkers and it may trigger additional feelings of positive emotion (Dutton et al., 2002). Compassion also helps employees find meaning during challenging life or work events (Lilius et al., 2008). At work, a compassionate response could include "gestures of emotional support, giving material goods, or providing a colleague with work flexibility" (Lilius et al., 2008, p. 195). Employees who feel and experience compassionate communication are likely to experience whole-person wellness.

In regard to physical wellness, compassion can be communicated to employees who have chronic diseases or health issues. Furthermore, employees experiencing psychological challenges would benefit from feelings of compassion from coworkers and management rather than judgment. If a culture of compassion exists, employees are likely to express empathy and social support with others which will increase social wellness. Lastly, employees that are compassionate and accepting of different spiritual beliefs may help to create a sense of spiritual wellness in the organization.

Communicating positivity at work through happiness, gratitude and compassion has various benefits for employees' wellness. At the same time, caution is recommended in that compassion can become a practice of organizational discipline and control (Simpson, Clegg, & Pitsis, 2014). As Simpson et al. (2014) point out, "organizational compassion is not invariably positive nor is it the universal good it is often presumed to be: We must always ask who benefits from what knowledge, what are its power effects and what types of subjects it constitutes" (p. 356). Furthermore, happiness can be faked during interaction (Fisher, 2010) and gratitude could be used to manipulate employees into acting certain ways (Andersson et al., 2007).

From a critical perspective, when organizations encourage participation in workplace wellness programs and/or positivity in the workplace there is a danger of encroaching too far into employees' lives (see May, this volume, for more on organizational control). As corporate colonization suggests, the "*content* of the spirit of capitalism is being *displaced* onto intimate life" (Hochschild, 2003, p. 24, emphasis in original). Furthermore, when organizations provide incentives for participation in wellness programs they covertly exert control over employees' private lives and behavior (Deetz, 1992). In other words, the expectations of wellness encouraged at work seeps into employees' private lives through discourse and practices. For example, if an employee is offered an incentive to wear a pedometer on a daily basis the organization's wellness program has seeped into non-work time. Thus, some may argue that workplace wellness programs and the potential incentives are just another way for organizations and managers to exert control over employees' lives.

In summary, this chapter started by defining the whole-person approach to wellness campaigns. We defined the four dimensions of health—physical, psychological, social, and spiritual—and explained why they are important. Next, we explained how the whole-person approach can be translated into practice by discussing various example wellness programs. Then, we explored various challenges of pitfalls of the whole-person approach and how to address these challenges. Finally, we ended by examining the relationship between positivity, especially happiness, gratitude, and compassion, and the whole-person approach. As people continue to spend more time at work, it is essential for organizations to consider a whole-person approach to their wellness campaigns for the success of the employees and of the organization as a whole.

DISCUSSION QUESTIONS

1. Which of the four components of the whole-person approach to workplace wellness have been emphasized most at a workplace where you have been employed?
2. Which of the four components of the whole-person approach have been most neglected at a workplace where you have been employed? Why do you think this is the case?
3. In what ways have you experienced happiness, gratitude, or compassion at work?
4. Do you believe that positivity and wellness campaigns can become manipulation and control? In what ways?
5. Do you see specific ways in which the whole-person approach might feel uncomfortable to you? If so, in what ways do you think employers and employees must communicate to negotiate boundaries between personal and professional lives?

Suggested Reading

Farrell, A. & Geist-Martin, P. (2005). Communicating social health: Perceptions of wellness at work. *Management Communication Quarterly, 18*, 543–592.

Geist-Martin, P. & Scarduzio, J. A. (in press). Workplace wellness as flourishing: Communicating life quality at work. In J. Yamasaki, P. Geist-Martin, & B. F. Sharf (Eds.), *Storied health and illness: Communicating personal, cultural, and political complexities.* Long Grove, IL: Waveland Press.

Mirivel, J. C. (2014). *The art of positive communication: Theory and practice.* New York, NY: Peter Lang.

Zoller, H. M. (2004). Manufacturing health: Employee perspectives on problematic outcomes in a workplace health promotion initiative. *Western Journal of Communication, 68*, 278–301.

References

Accenture Wellness Centers (2014) *Accenture wellness centers.* Retrieved from http://careers.accenture.com/in-en/your-future/rewards-benefits/Pages/wellness-resources.aspx.

Algoe, S. B. & Haidt, J. (2009). Witnessing excellence in action: The "other-praising" emotions of elevation, gratitude, and admiration. *The Journal of Positive Psychology, 4*, 105–127.

Andersson, L. M., Giacalone, R. A., & Jurkiewicz, C. L. (2007). On the relationship of hope and gratitude to corporate social responsibility. *Journal of Business Ethics, 70*, 401–409.

Ashar, H. & Lane-Maher, M. (2004). Success and spirituality in the new business paradigm. *Journal of Management Inquiry, 13*, 249–260.

Bartlett, M. Y. & DeSteno, D. (2006). Gratitude and prosocial behavior: Helping when it costs you. *Psychological Science, 17*, 319–325.

Benefits. (2014). *Microsoft benefits.* Retrieved from http://careers.microsoft.com/careers/en/us/benefits.aspx.

Burack, E. H. (1999). Spirituality in the workplace. *Journal of Organizational Change Management, 12*, 280–291.

Chang, Y.-P., Lin, Y.-C., & Chen, L.-H. (2012). Pay it forward: Gratitude in social networks. *Journal of Happiness Studies, 13*, 761–781.

Churchill, S. A., Gillespie, H., & Herbold, N. H. (2014). The desirability of wellness programs and incentive offerings for employees. *Benefits Quarterly, 30*, 48–57.

Colmer, V., Millea, C., & Wearne, N. (2013). Guidelines for improving workplace wellness. *Health Lawyer, 25*, 44–47.

Deetz, S. A. (1992). *Democracy in an age of corporate colonization: Developments in communication and the politics of everyday life.* Albany, NY: State University of New York Press.

Dutton, J. E., Frost, P. J., Worline, M. C., Lilius, J. M., & Kanov, J. (2002). Leading in times of trauma. *Harvard Business Review*, 54–61.

Family Resources (2014). *Bright Horizons family resources.* Retrieved from: http://www.brighthorizons.com/family-resources.

Farrell, A. & Geist-Martin, P. (2005). Communicating social health: Perceptions of wellness at work. *Management Communication Quarterly, 18*, 543–592.

Fisher, C. D. (2010). Happiness at work. *International Journal of Management Reviews, 12*, 384–412.

Freshman, B. (1999). An exploratory analysis of definitions and applications of spirituality in the workplace. *Journal of Organizational Change Management, 12*, 318–327.

Frost, P. J., Dutton, J. E., Worline, M. C., & Wilson, A. (2000). Narratives of compassion in organizations. In S. Fineman (Ed.), *Emotion in organizations* (pp. 25–45). Thousand Oaks, CA: Sage.

Geist-Martin, P., Bollinger, B., Wiechert, K. N., Plump, B., & Sharf, B. F. (in press: expected 2015). Challenging integration: Clinicians' perspectives of communicating collaboration in a center for integrative medicine. *Health Communication.*

Geist-Martin, P. & Freiberg, K. L. (1992, October). *The saving grace of organizational communication.* Paper presented at the annual convention of the Speech Communication Association, Chicago.

Geist-Martin, P., Horsley, K., & Farrell, A. (2003). Working well: Communicating individual and collective wellness initiatives. In T. L. Thompson, A. M. Dorsey, K. I. Miller, & R. Parrott (Eds.), *Handbook of health communication* (pp. 423–443). Mahwah, NJ: Erlbaum.

Geist-Martin, P., Ray, E. B., & Sharf, B. F. (2011). *Communicating health: Personal, cultural, and political complexities.* Long Grove, IL: Waveland.

Geist-Martin, P. & Scarduzio, J. A. (2011). Working well: Reconsidering health communication at work. In T. L. Thompson, R. Parrott, & J. F. Nussbaum (Ed.), *Handbook of health communication* (pp. 117–131). Mahweh, NJ: Erlbaum.

Healthymagination (2014). *Healthymagination at General Electric.* Retrieved from http://www.ge-healthahead.com/, http://www.ge.com/about-us/healthymagination.

Hillier, D., Fewell, F., Cann, W., & Shephard, V. (2005). Wellness at work: Enhancing the quality of our working lives. *International Review of Psychiatry, 17,* 419–431.

Hochschild, A. R. (2003). *The commercialization of intimate life: Notes from work and home.* Berkeley, CA: University of California Press.

Kline, S. L. (2011). Communicating spirituality in healthcare: A case study of the role of identity in religious health testimonies. *Journal of Applied Communication Research, 39,* 354–351.

Koenig, H. G. (2008). *Medicine, religion, and health: Where science and spirituality meet.* Conshohocken, PA: Templeton Foundation Press.

Krishnakumar, S. & Neck, C. P. (2002). The "what," "why," and "how" of spirituality in the workplace. *Journal of Managerial Psychology, 17,* 153–164.

Lilius, J. M., Worline, M. C., Maitlis, S., Kanov, J., Dutton, J. E., & Frost, P. (2008). The contours and consequences of compassion at work. *Journal of Organizational Behavior, 29,* 193–218.

Linnan, L., Bowling, M., Childress, J., Lindsay, G., Blakey, C., Pronk, S., Wieker, S., & Royall, P. (2008). Results of the 2004 national worksite health promotion survey. *American Journal of Public Health, 98,* 1503–1509.

Lips-Wiersma, M. & Mills, C. (2002). Coming out of the closet: Negotiating spiritual expression in the workplace. *Journal of Managerial Psychology, 17,* 183–202.

Loretto, W., Popham, F., Platt, S., Pavis, S., Hardy, G., MacLeod, L., & Gibbs, J. (2005). Assessing psychological well-being: A holistic investigation of NHS employees. *International Review of Psychiatry, 17,* 329–336.

Lutgen-Sandvik, P. & McDermott, V. (2008). The constitution of employee-abusive organizations: A communication flows theory. *Communication Theory, 18,* 304–333.

Machen, R., Cuddihy, T. F., Reaburn, P., & Higgins, H. (2010). Development of a workplace wellness promotion pilot framework: A case study of the blue care staff wellness program. *Asia-Pacific Journal of Health, Sport, and Physical Education, 1,* 13–20.

Malouf, M. (2011). Implementing a strategic approach to employee wellness: Globally and locally. *Benefits Quarterly, 27,* 13–16.

McGuire, T. (2009). From emotions to spirituality: "Spiritual labor" as the commodification, codification, and regulation of organizational members' spirituality. *Management Communication Quarterly, 24,* 74–103.

Medland, J., Howard-Ruben, J., & Whitaker, E. (2002). Fostering psychosocial wellness in oncology nurses: Addressing burnout and social support in the workplace. *Oncology Nursing Forum, 31,* 47–54.

Miller, K. I. (2007). Compassionate communication in the workplace: Exploring processes of noticing, connecting, and responding. *Journal of Applied Communication Research, 35,* 223–245.

Mirivel, J. C. (2014). *The art of positive communication: Theory and practice.* New York, NY: Peter Lang.

Neely, M. (2012). Wellness strategies for smaller businesses. *Benefits Quarterly, 28,* 16–19.

Overcoming Ergonomics Risks Improves Workplace Safety. (2012). *Professional Safety, 57*(9), 16.

Pargament, K. I. (1999). The psychology of religion and spirituality? Yes and no. *International Journal for the Psychology of Religion, 9,* 3–16.

Proudfoot, J. G., Corr, P. J., Guest, D. E., & Dunn, G. (2009). Cognitive–behavioral training to change attributional style improves employee well-being, job satisfaction, productivity, and turnover. *Personality & Individual Differences, 46,* 147–153.

Ramon, S. (2005). Promoting mental well-being in the workplace: International perspectives. *International Review of Psychiatry, 17,* 315–316.

Ray, E. B. & Miller, K. I. (1994). Social support, home/work stress, and burnout: Who can help? *Journal of Applied Behavioral Science, 30,* 357–373.

Remen, R. N. (1993, Autumn). On defining spirit. *Noetic Sciences Review, 27.*

Salin, D. (2003). Bullying and organizational politics in competitive and rapidly changing work environments. *International Journal of Management and Decision Making, 4,* 35–46.

Scarduzio, J. A. & Geist-Martin, P. (2008). Making sense of fractured identities: Male professors' narratives of sexual harassment. *Communication Monographs, 75,* 353–379.

Scarduzio, J. A. & Geist-Martin, P. (2010). Accounting for victimization: Male professors' ideological positioning in stories of sexual harassment. *Management Communication Quarterly, 24,* 419–445.

Sharf, B. F., Geist-Martin, P., Cosgriff-Hernandez, K-K., & Moore, J. (2012). Trailblazing healthcare: Institutionalizing and integrating complementary medicine. *Patient Education and Counseling, 89,* 434–438.

Sharf, B. F., Geist-Martin, P., & Moore, J. (2012). Communicating healing in a third space: Real and imagined forms of integrative medicine. In L. Harter, *Imagining new normals: A narrative framework for health communication* (pp. 125–147). Dubuque, IA: Kendall Hunt.

Simpson, A. V., Clegg, S., & Pitsis, T. (2014). "I used to care but things have changed": A genealogy of compassion in organizational theory. *Journal of Management Inquiry, 23,* 347–359.

Sirota, D., Mischkind, L. A., & Meltzer, M. I. (2005). *The enthusiastic employee.* Upper Saddle River, NJ: Wharton School Publishing.

The 46 Healthiest Companies. (2014). Greatist. Retrieved from http://greatist.com/health/healthiest-companies.

The Great Place to Work Institute. (n.d.). *Happiness at work.* Retrieved from http://www.greatplacetowork.com/.

Tsang, J.-A. (2007). Gratitude for small and large favors: A behavioral test. *The Journal of Positive Psychology, 2,* 157–167.

Vesley, R. (2012). Shaping up: Workplace wellness in the '80s & today. *Workforce Management, 28.*

Wagner-Marsh, F. & Conely, J. (1999). The fourth wave: The spiritually based firm. *Journal of Organizational Change Management, 12,* 292–301.

Warr, P. (2007). *Work, happiness, and unhappiness.* Mahwah, NJ: Erlbaum.

Way, D. & Tracy, S. J. (2012). Conceptualizing compassion as recognizing, relating, and (re)acting: A qualitative study of compassionate care at hospice. *Communication Monographs, 79*, 292–315.

Williams, S. & Bruno, A. (2007). Worksite wellness programs: What is working. *American Journal of Men's Health, 1*, 154–156.

Wood, A. M., Froh, J. J., & Geraghty, A. W. (2010). Gratitude and well-being: A review and theoretical integration. *Clinical Psychology Review, 30*, 890–905.

World Health Organization. (2010). Workplace health promotion. *Benefits.* Retrieved from http://www.who.int/ occupational_health/topics/workplace/en/index1.html.

Worsham, L. (1998). Going postal: Pedagogic violence and the schooling of emotion. *JAC: A Journal of Rhetoric, Culture, and Politics, 18*, 213–245.

12

CORPORATE SOCIAL RESPONSIBILITY AND EMPLOYEE HEALTH

Steven K. May

This chapter explores corporate social responsibility (CSR) as a set of organizing processes creating organizational environments directly impacting employee health and well-being. Typically, scholarship on CSR focuses on external stakeholders, such as consumers, suppliers, competitors, and regulatory agencies, among others (May, Cheney, & Roper, 2007). As such, many communication-based studies of CSR have examined it as a marketing or public relations practice. This chapter, by contrast, considers the ways organizational processes of CSR can enable (or constrain) the health and well-being of internal stakeholders such as employees (see also May & Roper, 2014).

The chapter begins with a theoretical overview of corporate social responsibility, with particular attention to its impact on the business/society relationship, in general, and healthy organizational environments, more specifically. Although most recent iterations of CSR focus on philanthropy, volunteerism, and community-based initiatives, among other programs, early iterations of the practice focused on the development and personal well-being of employees. It is important to consider how this emphasis shifted from employees to other sets of disparate stakeholders including, most recently, consumers who have become the focus of CSR-oriented marketing and advertising campaigns.

As an alternative to past theories of CSR, which largely ignored the impact of work on employee health, I draw upon the work of Michel Foucault to acknowledge and, hopefully, address many of the tensions inherent in business strategies to improve employee health. Specifically, I examine one of the most pervasive programs for employee health to date: employee assistance programs (EAPs). I review some of the more common practices of EAPs, their impact on employee health, and offer possible directions for future research and practice. Originally designed to help employees with drug and alcohol abuse, EAPs have now extended to the full range of other health-related concerns, both physical and mental. Such programs, as forms of corporate responsibility, raise interesting questions regarding the roles and responsibilities of organizations to strengthen employee health. Similarly, EAPs offer employees the opportunity to assess and improve their health, but do so within the context of organizational power dynamics and, therefore, also imply the possibility of organizational intervention into the health decisions of employees. At their most fundamental level, EAPs are often considered a money-saving device, given rising health care costs in the United States. Their use raises questions, therefore, regarding the tension between ethics and employee/organizational performance. While EAPs are fraught with challenges, they also offer employees a range of opportunities to manage their weight, quit smoking, handle substance abuse, and even find sources of counseling for physical and mental health. A Foucauldian approach to these seeming socially responsible programs complicates the motivations, practices, and outcomes of EAPs. Exploring these opportunities and challenges should offer a more realistic and, hopefully, constructive assessment of the current and future state of employee health, in light of the growth of CSR programs.

Theories of Corporate Social Responsibility

There have been many conceptualizations of CSR proposed in the last few decades. Archie Carroll (1999), often considered one of the most prominent scholars on the topic, noted CSR has been defined in a variety of ways within the academic literature. For example, the theory and research on CSR has ranged from narrow views of specific CSR strategies and practices to broader approaches exploring theories of the firm or the role of business in society. Similarly, the study of CSR has been increasingly widespread in a number of academic disciplines, such as business/management, economics, political science, sociology, environmental studies, and, more recently, communication studies. In the case of communication studies, the primary sub-areas addressing questions of CSR have been organizational communication (Kuhn & Deetz, 2008) and public relations (Roper, 2005), although scholars in rhetoric (Aune, 2007) and environmental communication (Peterson & Norton, 2007) have also begun to explore the topic recently. However, few scholars have sought to understand CSR as a set of practices that can (and should) be relevant to employee health and well-being. This chapter seeks to begin to fill that void. In a review article in the *SAGE Handbook of Organizational Communication*, Juliet Roper and I distinguish four strands of CSR research: 1) shareholder value theory; 2) corporate social performance; 3) corporate citizenship; and 4) stakeholder theory (May & Roper, 2014; see also Mele, 2008). Below, I briefly explain each of these scholarly strands and their implications for employee health, more specifically.

Shareholder value, a common theory of the firm, assumes the sole responsibility of businesses is to make a profit for shareholders and is described by many as fiduciary capitalism. According to this point of view, CSR programs are only deemed appropriate if they are "useful" to maximize shareholder value. Shareholder value, then, serves as a foundation for neoclassical economic theory and is focused on shareholder utility maximization. In a famous article in *The New York Times*, Milton Friedman argued against the popular CSR practices of the day and noted, "the only one responsibility of business towards society is the maximization of profits to the shareholders, within the legal framework and the ethical custom of the country" (1970).

As an extension of shareholder value, some scholars have adapted the theory to focus on "enlightened value maximization" that considers not just return on investment but also the long-term market value of the firm (Keim, 1978). As such, this strand of CSR research has focused on cause-related marketing (Smith & Higgins, 2000), corporate philanthropy (Porter & Kramer, 2006), and investments in the bottom of the economic pyramid (Prahalad, 2003) as means to balance social goods and economic value. A popular version of this perspective, "strategic CSR," has gained considerable traction as an opportunity to engage in community-based policies and programs while still supporting core business activities (Logsdon & Wood, 2002). CSR research is deemed valuable as a mechanism to conduct cost-benefit analyses of CSR initiatives (for a critique, see May, 2008). Corporate social responsibility, according to the main tenets of shareholder value theory, should only be pursued if and when corporate initiatives support the bottom line.

Not surprisingly, this approach to CSR tends to view employees as a means to an end—in this case, productivity and, in turn, profits. As such, investors are more likely to gain a return on their investment when employees stay healthy and productive. Employee health, from this perspective, is valued if, and only if, it contributes to the bottom line. In turn, it is no surprise employee health is likely to be seen as a cost by many advocates of this perspective. The result is that prevailing corporate assumptions regarding shareholder value produce a range of programs designed to improve employee health, but with a focus on those illnesses deemed most costly—either in terms of higher insurance or lowered productivity.

Corporate social performance (CSP), by contrast, tends to view business and society as interdependent. From this perspective, businesses have simultaneous economic and social responsibilities, creating at least a limited space for concerns over public health, in general, and employee health, specifically. Proponents of corporate social performance argue that, in addition to the creation of wealth for investors, businesses are responsible for any negative consequences they produce (Wartick & Cochran, 1985), which, presumably, would include workplace accidents, hazards, and stressors negatively affecting employee health. Donna Wood (1991), for example, defined CSR as "a business organization's configuration of principles of social responsibility, processes of social responsiveness, and policies, programs and observable outcomes as they relate to the firm's societal relationships" (p. 693). Authors from this point of view argue firms pay attention to societal expectations and, in particular, social needs at the time.

Given the rise in health care costs for employers and for the general public in the last few decades, this approach should account for health as a growing priority. Because businesses are expected to meet the current needs of the public, CSP is often referred to as a corporate responsiveness model (Ackerman & Bauer, 1976) of CSR which may be adaptive, anticipatory, or preventive (Sethi, 1975). From this perspective, CSR is necessarily linked to the general economic welfare of society and preserving shared human values. From this theoretical perspective, society necessarily grants legitimacy and power to businesses and, therefore, businesspersons must uphold those collective obligations. Although few scholars from this approach have made the connection between CSP and employee health, its assumptions are consistent with past work in health communication and ethics (Guttman & Thompson, 2011).

Corporate citizenship is a third theoretical perspective used by CSR scholars and it promotes common assumptions regarding appropriate citizenship in the business/society relationship. From this point of view, businesses should be "good corporate citizens" promoting human welfare in ways consistent not just with current laws, but also ethical standards and expectations of the day. As a result, scholars who draw upon notions of corporate citizenship have been interested in the philanthropic activities of businesses in the community, including donations and volunteerism (Crane & Matten, 2005). Some recent scholars (Birch, 2001) see CSR not so much as an external activity but instead as a core part of society. That is, business interests should not necessarily be separated from social interests in a society, as corporate citizenship is a metaphor for business participation in society (Moon et. al., 2005).

Scholars from this perspective, then, argue corporations, like individuals, are citizens of their communities (local, national and/or global) and, therefore, must attend to a diverse array of stakeholder interests, including community problems such as poverty, pollution, and racial discrimination, among others (Eilbert & Parker, 1973). Undoubtedly, corporate citizenship would also allow a place for considering human health and well-being as a broad-based citizen concern. Because of its early roots in Political Science, however, scholars of corporate citizenship have been more inclined to focus on corporate/government relations that are external rather than internal in nature. As a result, government and community-based efforts to improve the public's health may fall under its purview, but the more specific nature of employee health within the workplace has been largely ignored.

Stakeholder theory is an additional, widely-used approach to CSR research in the last couple of decades. From a stakeholder theory approach, scholars argue businesses should take into account individuals or groups who have a stake in their activities, particularly if the stakeholders are directly impacted by the business.

According to this perspective, "corporations have an obligation to constituent groups in society other than stockholders and beyond that prescribed by law or union contract" (Jones, 1980, pp. 59–60). In its early iterations, stakeholder theory was an alternative to traditional strategic management, with an emphasis on long-term financial success (Freeman, 1984). More recently, scholars have argued management has a moral duty to not only protect the fiduciary health of the business but to also negotiate the multiple claims of conflicting stakeholders (Evan & Freeman, 1988). So, although the survival of the firm is central to stakeholder theory, stakeholder scholars also assume the business should be managed for the benefit of all stakeholders, including customers, suppliers, owners, employees, and communities. As such, the role of employee health should be a consideration, according to the principles of stakeholder theory.

A normative version of stakeholder theory taking hold even more recently is the notion of *stakeholder engagement*. Stakeholder engagement focuses on the specific nature of the relationship with stakeholders and is oriented toward engaging them in dialogue and decision-making. "Partnering and engagement activities allow firms to build bridges with their stakeholders in the pursuit of common goals" (Andriof & Waddock, 2002, p. 36), such as when leaders tout efforts to improve health as a benefit to both employer and employee. From this approach, leaders are expected to coordinate activities and facilitate decision-making between stakeholders. This participative governance model leads to "more creativity, effecting new product development, greater efficiency and effectiveness in personal and organizational goal accomplishment, higher levels of mutual commitment, and great product and service customization" (Deetz, 2007, p. 276). In theory, stakeholder engagement should facilitate conversations regarding what constitutes employee health and who should have control regarding decisions related to it.

Reframing CSR: Employee Assistance and Health

I argue that, although some of the more recent iterations of CSR noted above offer more engaged and proactive approaches to employee health, CSR remains a largely externally-focused phenomenon. That is, CSR programs have focused almost exclusively on "external" stakeholders and a range of activities that, ultimately, ignore any direct responsibility to employees, in general, and employee health, more specifically. If CSR is to have any long-term benefit for society, attention must first be turned to corporate employees themselves because they, in the end, comprise the corporate culture which must reconstruct corporate strategy, operations, and decision-making to prioritize social issues. If the corporation has not developed embedded logics and practices to address difficult questions of social responsibility, it has no hope to participate in meaningful and constructive cultural change. Similarly, if the corporation has not been able to attend to its own employees, including their health, how can it be expected to address the social needs of diverse sets of stakeholders with a range of divergent interests?

The first test of responsibility, as a set of minimum specifications, must be the manner in which employees are treated at work. Unfortunately, however, recent theories of CSR, with their long-standing focus on external publics, have deterred any real consideration of employees' health and safety that may, ultimately, foster legitimate CSR. A viable test of a corporation's capacity for CSR, then, would be to first turn its attention inward and assess its ability to pursue ethical, responsible behavior towards, and among, its employees. In a global context of outsourcing, offshoring, and Third World labor, assessment of employees' well-being is complicated, although no less important. If anything, global labor and the immediacy of mediated networks have placed concerns about the conditions of work front and center.

How, then, have corporations focused on employee health? What are the specific programs and activities designed to improve employee health and well-being? What has been their impact? There is a range of complicated—and often competing—answers to these questions. Yet, the most long-standing and extensive set of programs designed to address employee health, employee assistance programs, can be understood as one of the first important turns in the conversation regarding corporate responsibilities towards employees. Before I discuss some of the specific practices of EAPs, though, they need to be understood in the context of past and current health care debates.

The current health care crisis in the United States has been a recurring source of discussion and disagreement among politicians, physicians, insurers, employers, and the general public. Over the last few years, the debate has raged over issues of health care access, quality, funding, and costs. While all four areas are significant sources of public concern, it is the latter issue—health care costs—seemingly driving the debate. In recent years, the Congressional Budget Office studied the health care problem and discovered higher prices, higher utilization rates, and higher population rates have all contributed to the spiraling cost of health care. Total national spending on health care services and supplies increased from 4.6% of GDP in calendar year 1960 to 9.5% in 1985 and to 16.2% in 2012.

Recent projections indicate health care costs will increase by more than 70% over the next 10 years and will continue thereafter to consume an increasingly greater portion of personal income (Social Security Advisory Board, 2014). For the roughly 60% of workers who receive some form of health care coverage from their employers, the cost of their health insurance premiums and out-of-pocket expenses have increased significantly faster than wages. Between 2000 and 2013, average health insurance premiums and out-of-pocket costs for deductibles, medications, and medical visits more than doubled while median wages increased by less than 3% during that period (Kaiser Family Foundation, 2013).

While these costs certainly impact all of us, my specific focus in this chapter is the consequence of these costs for corporations and, ultimately, their employees. For instance, by some estimates, health care costs have continued to escalate for employers, with expenditures doubling every five to six years (Baumol, 2012).

These costs for employers are directly attributed to health care provided for employees. However, corporations are also concerned with the less obvious link between employee health and lower productivity, as noted in my discussion of the theory of shareholder value. Corporate figures suggest the following costs in lost productivity:

- Alcoholism is costing U.S. companies more than $20.6 billion a year in lost productivity.
- The cost of lost productivity because of drug abuse is nearly $16.6 billion a year.
- Illness (both mental and physical) resulting from job stress accounted for $20 billion a year lost in productivity.

The total cost of alcohol, drug, and physical and mental health problems to corporations, then, surpasses $55 billion a year (Masi, 2012). As retired Surgeon General C. Everett Koop stated even as early as two decades ago, the nation's health care system is in "a crisis bordering on chaos," with corporations taking a large brunt of the "self-destructive whirlpool" of rising costs (Parker & Ure, 1991). From a corporate perspective drawing on notions of shareholder value, health care costs have eroded profits and, consequently, have motivated employers to be more aggressive in adopting cost containment strategies. One of the more recent proactive containment strategies has been the use of EAPs in the workplace. EAPs are commonly defined as "job-based programs operating within a work organization for purposes of identifying 'troubled workers,' motivating them to resolve their troubles, and providing access to counseling or treatment for those employees who need these services" (Sonnenstuhl & and Trice, 1986). EAPs are designed to identify, refer, and treat workers with alcohol and drug abuse, marital and family problems, financial difficulties, sexual dysfunction, as well as a variety of health and fitness problems. In effect, any worker's mental or physical problems, as identified by the employer or his or her coworkers, may fall under the rubric of an EAP. According to many proponents of EAPs, they represent an integration of employer and employee interests satisfying the business obligation to be responsible towards employees.

Although EAPs are still fairly new to the workplace, their growth has been significant and has followed, not surprisingly, the rise in health care costs. In 1970, there were fewer than 50 programs. By 1990, more than 12,000 programs existed in the United States, serving more than one third of the regular workforce (Blum & Roman, 2010). In each of the last 10 years, at least 500 new EAPs have been introduced, bringing the present total to over 16,000 (Sharar, Pompe, & Lennox, 2012). More specific estimates indicate approximately 80% of the Fortune 1000 companies and 75% of the Fortune 500 companies have instituted EAPs. Included among these companies are such well-known organizations as General Motors, Control Data Corporation, Chase Manhattan Bank, Westinghouse, Sheraton, McDonnell-Douglas, Honeywell, Lockheed, Marriott, Mobil Oil, in addition to many local, state, and federal agencies (including most universities).

Beyond the startling growth of EAPs, their impact has been significant as well. Under the auspices of EAPs, employees have been: fired for smoking off the job; fired for demonstrating "abnormal" homosexual tendencies; fired for being over-weight; fired for refusing to wear makeup; barred from engaging in risky leisure activities such as motorcycle riding, skydiving, surfing, and hang gliding; required to submit marital and sexual histories; and fined for scoring poorly on health screening tests including blood pressure readings and body-fat analyses (May, 1993). Ironically enough, the fines from health screenings were first introduced by Coors Brewing and Hershey's Foods. Although these examples are extreme, many more could be listed here. They are occurring with increasing frequency, as corporate health care costs have caused employers to focus more and more often upon what have traditionally been "private" areas of workers' health and well-being. More specifically, I argue that, under the principles of CSR and employee health, corporations are no longer merely a site for work but also a site for the surveillance of workers' bodies. EAPs produce a "political technology of the body," in which corporate power causes workers' bodies to be assessed, shaped, and improved—in effect, managed. This emphasis upon the body as a site of power occurs in at least two key realms within the EAP field: (1) fitness/wellness programs; and (2) health assessment/promotion programs.

Fitness and Wellness Programs

The first means by which the body has become a site of corporate power—fitness and wellness programs—have become quite common in today's work-place. Some organizations have on-site facilities for basketball, racquetball, weight-lifting, bicycling, and jogging. Other organizations offer a wide variety of corporate-sponsored team sports. Even for those companies without formal fitness or wellness programs, it is not uncommon to see workers use their lunch breaks for walking, running, biking, or lifting weights, among other activities.

In a range of publications devoted to EAP professionals, the value of such activities is strongly emphasized. For example, drawing on an article by the President's Council on Physical Fitness and Sports, one set of authors state "a fitness program should be recognized as an integral part of the job" (President's Council, 2011, p. 27). A commonly stated rationale for fitness and wellness pro-grams in the workplace is "not only will the health of the workers improve, but that the quality of their work will also be enhanced" (President's Council, 2011, p. 29). From this perspective, a healthy body is assumed to be a productive body. Similar statements regarding the mutual relationship between health and produc-tivity recur throughout other articles regarding fitness and wellness programs. According to another EAP professional, "good health *is* good business," since physically active employees "miss fewer workdays when they do get sick, are less vulnerable to accidents, have a higher overall work output, and suffer fewer emo-tional disorders and physical disabilities" (Watkins, 1981, p. 5). Even the need to stay competitive in the global economy may be attributed to the worker's body, from this point of view. The President's Council (2011) notes, for example, "the competitive edge will go increasingly to organizations whose employees are the most loyal, stable, *productive, fit, and healthy* [emphasis added]" (p. 47).

While the overall value of these benefits should not be overlooked, it is important to recognize whose interests are served by them. Not surprisingly, advantages for the employer appear to supersede advantages for the employee. Only improved leisure enjoyment and quality of life are primarily related to sole benefits for the employee. The rest of the benefits are accrued economically, either directly or indirectly, by the company. For instance, the employer benefits by reducing health care costs, lowering absenteeism, increasing energy level of employees, and reducing accidents. Again, it is important to note employees also benefit, although it is unlikely corporations would show such an interest in employee health were there no economic benefits. Trade publications touting EAPs also note physical fitness is not viewed as an activity to be developed only during workers' leisure time; these programs "can give employees the chance to develop physical fitness on the job" (Osborne & Wiechetek, 1991, p. 41). The worker's improved physical body will not only benefit the company, but it may also occur under the space and time of the company—under the company's direct or indirect supervision.

In contrast to the assumption of physical fitness programs that humans require activity, wellness programs assume employees typically lack healthy bodies because they are "uninformed." Although in some cases wellness programs may include fitness activities, their primary focus is on "health awareness" at the workplace (see Scarduzio and Geist-Martin, this volume, for a prescriptive approach to wellness programs). The goal is to educate workers about "how to pay attention to their bodies," as well as "how to detect and treat physical illnesses," assuming "it is cheaper to keep an employee healthy and on the job than it is to pay the costs of ill health, rehabilitation, and replacement" (Renner, 1987, p. 49).

Typically, a wellness program begins with participants being given a series of physical tests in order to determine their physical condition and "specific exercises are then prescribed based on the test results" (President's Council, 2011, p. 30). Beyond the "prescribed" exercises based on the company's "determination" of the worker's physical condition, wellness programs frequently include illness assessment and detection programs. Not surprisingly, the illnesses assessed and detected are determined by the company's insurance costs. Given criteria for inclusion, heart disease and lower back pain are two of the most common illnesses covered in wellness programs. Other examples include nutrition counseling, weight control, breast and colon cancer screening, smoking cessation, and hypertension and cholesterol testing.

Although not necessarily a new phenomenon in the workplace (industrial welfare programs had similar practices at the turn of the century), wellness programs do further legitimate medical terminology and practice in the workplace. With the introduction of wellness programs, the workplace is viewed not only as a place to labor but also as a place to improve one's body. In fact, some EAP professionals argue health assessment programs are actually better suited to the workplace than to the doctor's office. As one author notes, "the worksite is a cost-effective and convenient place for teaching employees healthier habits" (Brennan, 1985, p. 29). Wellness programs in the workplace are more convenient and accessible than the doctor's office. They also "have the potential for making health activities a part of one's normal routine" within the workplace (Renner, 1987, p. 51). As such, some authors argue wellness programs could be easily integrated into the organizational routine as well as into the company's policies. Such integration into the workplace is beneficial since employees' health status can be "evaluated and monitored over a long period of time" (Renner, 1987, p. 51).

Furthermore, EAP professionals argue health awareness can easily be generated at the worksite through existing communication channels. According to one EAP professional, "in-house communication organs can create program visibility, disseminate health news, and act as a *subtle reinforcement* [emphasis added] to participants" (Brennan, 1985, p. 30). Finally, the most significant advantage, according to many EAP professionals, is that on-site treatment of illnesses is more cost-effective than community care. As is typical with EAP programs in general, however, the benefits are couched as being equal for both employer and employee: "Business has the leadership to make preventive medicine in the workplace a common practice—one that can improve employee health and morale and *the bottom line* [emphasis added]. It conceivably will be an everyone wins situation" (Parcell, 1985, p. 22).

Health Assessment Programs

Health promotion has also been a prevailing concern for EAP professionals from its early emergence as an apparent form of corporate social responsibility. As one prominent author of EAP research notes, "health promotion is a social movement of major proportions" (Chamber Study, 1981, p. 12). The increased interest in the health movement can be attributed to "rapidly rising health care costs and to concern that health status in general is not improving even though an increasing number of dollars are being spent for health care." (Chamber Study, 1981, p. 12) Additionally, the article also suggests "it has become more and more apparent that inappropriate lifestyle and negative health habits are associated with a decrease in the health status of many Americans" (Chamber Study, 1981, p. 12).

Given the presumed problems of "inappropriate lifestyle and negative health habits" of workers, the author concludes the workplace is, "the setting particularly well-suited to effective and widespread health promotion" (Stay Well, 1985, p. 12) lacking in society in general. Through such programs, it is argued, companies "can help employees and their families achieve and maintain better health" by moving "from a passive to an active role in health care involvement" and "from support of expensive treatment-oriented health care to promotion of less costly, prevention-oriented programs" (Stay Well, 1985, p. 12).

Health assessment and disease prevention programs are an option for corporations when workers do not recognize their own need for physical activity or assessment of their bodies. In such cases, the EAP is expected to take an active role. According to more health care professionals, preventive programs in general are being lauded as the "future of the health care system" (Oss, 1991, p. 36). Before considering what many believe to be the inherent benefits of such a program, however, one should consider what preventive health care in the workplace might look like. One proposed model is "health engineers" who engage in individualistic health assessments of employees. Such health assessments "could draw on both a systematic analysis of health information about individuals . . . and on the application of epidemiological studies of health problems" (Parcell, 1985, p. 20). This particular model of health care prevention would require a precise assessment of each worker's body and its physical problems. According to practitioners in the EAP field, this assessment could develop along two lines. The first form of assessment would be based upon an ongoing and detailed documentation of the worker's medical and psychological history. This assessment would verify past individual health problems. The second form of assessment, on the other hand, would serve to predict future individual health problems. Through epidemiological studies of health problems "involving variables such as age, sex, ethnicity, socio-economic status, and geographical location," a worker's future propensity to develop illnesses could be determined (Parcell, 1985, p. 22).

EAPs and the Productive Body

These examples suggest the corporate body is directly involved in a political field. That is, power relations have an immediate hold on the body; "they invest it, mark it, train it, torture it, force it to carry out its tasks, to perform ceremonies to emit signs" (Foucault, 1979, p. 25). This "political technology of the body" is invested not only in the physical make-up of the human form but also in its economic use, as is evident in the importance of "cost-effectiveness" with regards to the body. The body, in its economic application, must be both manageable and productive. Workers who participate in EAPs oriented toward the "healthy body" are only made to be productive once they have been "caught up in a system of subjection (in which need is also a political instrument meticulously prepared, calculated, and used); the body becomes a useful force only if it is both a productive body and a subjected body" (Foucault, 1979, p. 26).

The convergence of the productive and the subjected body develops through strategies of "bio-power," which are designed to increase the ordering of all realms of human life under the guise of improving the welfare of the population. Foucault suggests bio-power emerged as a coherent political technology in the Classical Age. During this period, the growth, care, and evaluation of populations became a central governmental concern. Bio-power in the seventeenth century brought human life into the realm of science, such that explicit calculations were made to improve the well-being of the populace. Knowledge/power immersed the human body in order to transform human life.

The potential transformation of human life coalesced around two poles. The first pole was organized around the reproductive possibilities of the human species. For perhaps the first time in history, scientific categories, such as species and population, rather than juridical ones became the object of political attention (Dreyfus & Rabinow, 1983, p. 134). The government, for instance, became increasingly interested in statistical studies of population. The population, studied under the discipline of demography, was approached as a topic to be known, controlled, taken care of, and made to flourish. It became necessary to "analyze the birthrate, the age of marriage, the legitimate and illegitimate births, the precocity and frequency of sexual relations, the ways of making them sterile or fertile, the effects of unmarried life or of the prohibitions, the impacts of contraceptive practices" (Foucault, 1980, p. 25). The reproductive body became an object of observation for science as well as for the state, as in previous centuries. The ultimate aim here is control of the species.

The second pole of bio-power revolves more specifically around control of the body as an object to be manipulated. According to Foucault, the goal of this latter emphasis has been to produce "docile bodies." As noted earlier, the body in this sense must be simultaneously subjected and productive. The body must be malleable but in such a way that it "works" economically. Docile bodies were developed and perfected in workshops, prisons, military barracks, and hospitals. In each of these institutions, the body was "managed" and manipulated in order to be more useful. It was not enough to have a body; one had to use the body, produce with the body.

As in the case of EAPs, however, the economic importance of the productive body is often couched in terms of welfare that will meet workers' needs and, therefore, increase their personal well-being. This interest in the body and its relation to human welfare is not necessarily a new phenomenon. In fact, the desire to improve the body has been a common goal to which governments have dedicated themselves even before the Classical Age. More recently, however, the needs of the body are no longer considered as ends in and of themselves. The human need (desire) to physically improve the body is now an instrumental means to an economic end. As a result, the welfare of the human body has become a concern for EAPs largely because of its economic benefits (increased productivity or reduced insurance costs) for the corporation, thereby reaffirming traditional arguments regarding the primacy of shareholder value theories of CSR.

Through EAPs, workers' bodies can be medically tested and examined for various maladies such as cancer, heart disease, high blood pressure, diabetes, and so on—all for the seeming benefit of the worker. The effect for the company is insurance costs will be reduced. In addition, workers' bodies are exercised in order to increase their productive capabilities but are again gauged in terms of health, fitness, and athletics. The effect for the company is reduced absenteeism as well as stronger, more physically fit employees. In this sense, EAPs focusing upon both health prevention and wellness programs, for example, produce an intensification of the body as a site for health-oriented techniques for maximizing life. Through such EAPs, the body has become another site to be examined, studied, understood, and managed by the corporation. Even outside of work time and place, the body is to be continually and actively managed through a growing field of "leisure" activities provided (or, at the least, proposed) by the corporation. From the corporate perspective, maximizing one's life is maximizing one's work. The two are inseparable.

Implications and Directions for Future Research

EAPs raise a number of challenging questions regarding a company's social responsibility for the health and well-being its employees. As I have noted in this chapter, CSR programs have historically focused on external stakeholders, in general, and shareholders, more specifically. Although seemingly altruistic, the goal of CSR programs has primarily been to strengthen a company's reputation and legitimacy. To date, such programs have focused on philanthropy, volunteerism, and community initiatives tending to provide a return on investment. I have suggested CSR programs have typically overlooked the needs of other stakeholder groups, such as employees. When relevant employee-based programs do exist, such as EAPs, the emphasis has been instrumental, with a focus on minimizing the health care costs of employees. As I have noted, EAPs do offer an opportunity for employees to improve their mental and physical health via fitness/wellness and health assessment/ promotion programs. Yet, the intent of EAPs has been to "manage" employee behaviors in such a way to minimize company expenditures on employees and their dependents. As a result, EAPs are fraught with a range of ethical considerations including risks of "profiling" unhealthy employees, engaging in surveillance of employee behavior, and encroaching on private realms of employees' lives.

Further theorizing is needed which takes into account both the challenges and opportunities of CSR and health, in general, and EAPs, more specifically. In terms of CSR, scholars and practitioners would benefit from studies examining the range of corporate responsibilities employers have towards their employees, including providing a work environment promoting—rather than diminishing— mental and physical health. Increasingly, scholars have begun to account for the physical and emotional work environment not just in industrialized countries but also in emerging economies, as well. More specifically, we also need to consider the extent to which communicative practices within organizations produce/reproduce such healthy/unhealthy work conditions. To what extent, for example, might greater transparency, candor, and voice regarding the nature and impact of work on employees transform future work practices? Even in cases where CSR efforts are directed outwards to other stakeholders, it is important to evaluate their overall impact on employee well-being, as well.

In terms of EAPs, research is needed that further explores the ethical dilemmas inherent in the tensions between bottom line economic interests of companies and the health needs of employees. For example, what are the decision-making logics and practices used to negotiate the balance between profits vs. people in most corporate settings? In what ways do EAPs programs enable and/or constrain the health potential of employees? Scholars should begin to conduct empirical research seeking to better understand the health outcomes of EAPs and other related programs designed to provide "employee assistance." Finally, scholarship is needed that begins to address fundamental questions regarding what actually constitutes assistance to employees with regard to their health. What, if any, role should companies play in answering such questions? That is, how do we begin to understand when/where/how the employers' interests end and the employees' interests begin? Answering such questions, I believe, will move scholars and practitioners closer to what might constitute constructive CSR and, in turn, also create both healthy and productive lifestyles for employees.

DISCUSSION QUESTIONS

1. Given the continued rise in health insurance costs for companies, employers are likely to be increasingly interested in the health of employees. To what extent is employee health an individual concern versus an organizational issue? How does the prevailing focus on shareholder value impact the kinds of decisions organizations make about employee health?
2. To what extent should CSR programs focus on the well-being of "internal" stakeholders, such as employees? In your opinion, what are the opportunities and challenges of doing so? How, if at all, should organizations balance their need for economic viability with employees' desire for privacy, in terms of EAPs? How do organizational power dynamics impact how, when, and for whom employee assistance services are provided to employees?
3. What are some specific strategies employers and employees could implement to strengthen employee health in ways that are both productive and humane, and responsive and responsible?

Suggested Reading

Ihlen, O., Bartlett, J., & May, S. (Eds.). (2011). *Handbook of communication and corporate social responsibility*. Boston, MA: Wiley-Blackwell.
May, S. K. & Roper, J. (2014). Corporate social responsibility and ethics. In L. Putman & D. Mumby (Eds.), *The SAGE handbook of organizational communication: Advances in theory, research, and methods* (pp. 767–789). Thousand Oaks, CA: Sage.

References

Ackerman, R. W. & Bauer, R. (1976). *Corporate social responsiveness*. Reston, VA: Reston Publishing Co.

Andriof, J. & Waddock, S. (2002). Unfolding stakeholder engagement. In J. Andriof, S. Waddock, B. Husted & S. Sutherland Rahman (Eds.), *Unfolding stakeholder thinking* (pp. 19–42). Sheffield, UK: Greenleaf Publishing.

Aune, J. (2007). How to read Milton Friedman: Corporate social responsibility in today's capitalisms. In S. May, G. Cheney & J. Roper (Eds.), *The debate over corporate social responsibility* (pp. 207–218). New York: Oxford University Press.

Baumol, W. J. (2012). *The cost disease*. New Haven, CT: Yale University Press.

Birch, D. (2001). Corporate citizenship: Rethinking business beyond social responsibility. In M. McIntosh (Ed.), *Perspectives on corporate citizenship* (pp. 53–65). Sheffield: Greenleaf.

Blum, T. C. & Roman, P. (1986). Alcohol, drugs and EAPs: New data from a national survey. *ALMACAN, 16*, 33–36.

Blum, T. C. & Roman, P. (2010). The social transformation of an alcoholism intervention: Comparisons of job attitudes and performance of recovered alcoholics and non-alcoholics. *Journal of Health and Social Behavior, 26*, 365–78.

Brennan, D. (November/December, 1985). Health and fitness boom moves into corporate America. *EAP Digest, 5*(6), 29–33.

Carroll, A. B. (1999). Corporate social responsibility: Evolution of a definitional construct. *Business and Society, 38*, 268–295.

Congressional Budget Office (2014). *The 2014 long-term budget outlook*. Washington, DC: U.S. Congress.

Crane, A. & Matten, D. (2005). Corporate citizenship: Missing the point or missing the boat? A reply to van Oosterhout. *Academy of Management Review, 30*, 681–684.

Deetz, S. (2007). Corporate governance, corporate social responsibility, and communication. In S. May, G. Cheney, & J. Roper (Eds.), *The debate over corporate social responsibility* (pp. 267–278). New York: Oxford University Press.

Dreyfus, H. L. & Rabinow, P. (1983). *Michel Foucault: Beyond structuralism and hermeneutics*. Chicago, IL: University of Chicago Press.

Eilbert, H. & Parker, I. R. (1973). The current status of corporate social responsibility. *Business Horizons, 16*, 5–14.

Evan, W. M. & Freeman, R. E. (1988). A stakeholder theory of the modern corporation: Kantian capitalism. In T. Beauchamp & N. Bowie (Eds.), *Ethical theory and business* (pp. 75–93). Englewood Cliffs, NJ: Prentice Hall.

Foucault, M. (1979). *Discipline and punish: The birth of the prison*. (A. Sheridan, Trans.). New York: Vintage Books.

Foucault, M. (1980). *The history of sexuality. Volume 1: An introduction*. New York: Vintage Books.

Freeman, R. E. (1984). *Strategic management: A stakeholder approach*. Boston, MA: Pitman.

Friedman, M. (1970, September 13). The social responsibility of business is to increase its profits. *The New York Times Magazine*, pp. 32–33, 122, 126.

Gerstein, G. H. & Bayer, G.A. (2011). Fitness and work. *EAP Digest, 11*(1), 27–47.

Guttman, N. & Thompson, T. L. (2011). Ethics in health communication. In Cheney, G., May, S. K., & Munshi, D. (Eds.), *Handbook of communication ethics* (pp. 293–308). New York: Routledge.

Jones, T. M. (1980). Corporate social responsibility revisited, redefined. *California Management Review, 22*(2), 59–67.

Kaiser Family Foundation (2013). *Survey of employer sponsored health benefits 2000–2013.* Washington, DC. The Kaiser Family Foundation and Health Research and Educational Trust.

Keim, G. D. (1978). Corporate social responsibility: An assessment of the enlightened self-interest model. *Academy of Management Review, 3,* 32–40.

Kuhn, T. & Deetz, S. (2008). Critical theory and corporate social responsibility: Can/should we get beyond cynical reasoning? In A. Crane, A. McWilliams, D. Matten, J. Moon, & D. Siegel (Eds.), *The Oxford Handbook of Corporate Social Responsibility* (pp. 173–196). New York: Oxford University Press.

Logsdon, J. M. & Wood, D. J. (2005). Global business citizenship and voluntary codes of ethical conduct. *Journal of Business Ethics, 59,* 55–67.

Masi, D. A. (2012). *Designing employee assistance programs.* New York: American Management Associates.

May, S. (2008). Reconsidering strategic corporate social responsibility: Public relations and ethical engagement of employees in a global economy. In A. Zerfass, B. van Ruler, & K. Sriramesh (Eds.), *Public relations research: European and international perspectives and innovations* (pp. 365–383). Wiesbaden, Germany: VS Verlag fur Sozialwissenschaften.

May, S. (1993). *Employee assistance programs and the troubled worker: A discursive study of knowledge, power, and subjectivity.* (Unpublished doctoral dissertation). Salt Lake City, UT: University of Utah.

May, S., Cheney, G., & Roper, J. (Eds.). (2007). *The debate over corporate social responsibility.* New York: Oxford University Press.

May, S. & Roper, J. (2014). Corporate social responsibility and ethics. In L. Putman & D. Mumby (Eds.), *The SAGE handbook of organizational communication: Advances in theory, research, and methods* (pp. 767–789). Thousand Oaks, CA: Sage.

Mele, D. (2008). Corporate social responsibility theories. In A. Crane, A. McWilliams, D. Matten, J. Moon, & D. Siegel (Eds.), *The Oxford handbook of corporate social responsibility* (pp. 47–82). New York: Oxford University Press.

Moon, J., Crane, A., & Matten, D. (2005). Can corporations be citizens? Corporate citizenship as a metaphor for business participation in society. *Business Ethics Quarterly, 15*(3), 429–453.

Osborne, J. & Wiechetek, W. (1991). The supervisor's role in fitness for duty exams. *EAP Digest, 12,* 41–44.

Oss, M. (1991). Managed behavioral health benefits: Trends in buying, packaging, and delivery. *EAP Digest, 11*(5), 36–40.

Parcell, C. (1985). Wellness vs. illness: Which road are we taking? *EAP Digest, 4*(2), 22–325.

Parker, D. L. & Ure, J. (24 May, 1991). Koop sees insurance for all in 10 years. *Salt Lake Tribune,* sec. B, p. 1.

Peterson, T. R. & Norton, T. (2007). Discourses of sustainability in today's public sphere. In S. May, G. Cheney, & J. Roper (Eds.), *The debate over corporate social responsibility* (pp. 351–364). New York: Oxford University Press.

Porter, M. E. & Kramer, M. R. (2006, December). Strategy and society: The link between competitive advantage and corporate social responsibility. *Harvard Business Review,* 78–92.

Prahalad, C. K. (2003). Strategies for the bottom of the economic pyramid: India as a source of innovation. *Reflections: The SOL Journal, 3,* 6–18.

Renner, J. (1987). Wellness programs: An investment in cost containment. *EAP Digest, 7*(2), 31–33.

Roper, J. (2005). Symmetrical communication: Excellent public relations or a strategy for hegemony? *Journal of Public Relations Research, 17*, 69–86.

Sethi, S. P. (1975). Dimensions of corporate social performance: An analytical framework. *California Management Review, 17*, 58–64.

Sharar, D. Pompe, J., & Lennox, R. (2012). Evaluating the workplace effects of EAP counseling. *Journal of Health and Productivity, 6*(2), 5–14.

Smith, W. & Higgins, M. (2000). Cause-related marketing: Ethics and the ecstatic. *Business and Society 39*, 304–322.

Social Security Advisory Board (2014). *The unsustainable cost of health care*. Washington, DC: Social Security Administration.

Sonnenstuhl, W. J. & Trice, H. M. (1986). *Strategies for employee assistance programs: The crucial balance*. Ithaca, NY: ILR Press.

U.S. Chamber of Commerce (1981). Chamber study urges business to focus on prevention and health promotion. *EAP Digest 1*(1), 12–16.

Wartick, S. L. & Cochran, P. L. (1985). The evolution of the corporate social performance model. *The Academy of Management Review, 10*, 758–769.

Watkins, G. T. (1981). In house. *EAP Digest, 1*(6), 5–8.

Wood, D. J. (1991). Corporate social performance revisited. *Academy of Management Review, 16*, 691–718.

13

DO I FEEL LIKE I'M A PART OF THIS ORGANIZATION? ORGANIZATIONAL IDENTIFICATION AND USING TECHNOLOGY TO COMMUNICATE ABOUT HEALTH

Keri K. Stephens and Yaguang Zhu

> I know everyone at my barbershop. Last time I got my hair cut I noticed a flyer on the wall that said, "Did you eat your vegetables today? Tweet about it!"

> I love my job, and my workplace just announced that I can meet with a registered dietician through a web-conference any day next week.

Health messages are popping up everywhere. While at first glance, some of these examples might seem like odd places to talk about health, these types of social interactions in diverse types of organizations are having some interesting successes. With the rising cost of health care in the US and the growing need to reach a dispersed population with health information, it is important that we find novel ways to disseminate information and impact health behaviors and decisions. Thus far, most of the research about organizational health dissemination has focused on pragmatic issues like reach, access, and finding captive audiences (Krueter, Alcaraz, Pfeiffer, & Christopher, 2008). But we now have research suggesting that organizations like beauty shops (Johnson, Ralston, & Jones, 2010), nonprofit organizations (Boyle, Donald, Dean, Conrad, & Mutch, 2007) and employers (Farrell & Geist-Martin, 2005; Kirby, 2006; Zoller, 2003; 2004; Stephens, Goins, & Dailey, 2014) can be a key source of health information. Yet the findings surrounding the organization's role in the positive promotion of health behavior are mixed.

This chapter centers on the role that organizations—and the connections that people feel—play in technology-infused health communication practices. We begin with a review of two perspectives on how organizations might be helpful in disseminating health information. First, organizations function as metachannels (Stephens, Rimal, & Flora, 2004) because they often have access to many members and diverse information and communication technologies (ICTs) to share information. Health information is often disseminated through these organizations using programs like workplace health promotions and organizational information sharing. Our chapter examines theory-driven organizational interventions and models of organizational wellness programs (e.g., Farrell & Geist-Martin, 2005) that further substantiate the value organizations can have when communicating about health. In addition, we include research that critiques employer involvement in their employees' health practices (Zoller, 2003; 2004).

Our second perspective on why organizations can be helpful in health information dissemination focuses on theoretical explanations for why some of these organizations are more successful in disseminating health information than others. We use social identity theory and organizational identification (e.g., Ashforth & Mael, 1989; Scott & Stephens, 2009) to provide solid explanations for how organizational members interpret and implement health practices (Stephens, Goins, & Dailey, 2014a; Stephens, Pastorek, Crook, Mackert, Donnovan-Kicken, & Shalev, 2015). Furthermore, when people feel connected to an organization that provides them with health information, that connection affects how they subsequently share this information with others (Crook, Stephens, Pastorek, Mackert, & Donovan, in press; Stephens et al., 2015).

In this chapter, we also address the growth of using communication technology as an integral part of these organizational health interventions (e.g., Stephens et al., 2014). With the rise in communication technologies—e.g., social media and intranets—being used to disseminate health information, and the role human resource departments play in this process (Stephens, Waters, & Sinclair, 2014), there are new opportunities to engage organizational members and positively influence their health attitudes and behaviors. Finally, we provide an agenda for future research that builds on past studies and establishes parameters for how organizations might best be used to promote health.

An Organizational Communication Approach to Health Communication

When organizational scholars examine communication phenomena, we tend to focus on organizations as being more than simply a channel to reach members (Kirby, 2006a; Stephens et al., 2014, Stephens et al., 2015; Zoller, 2003, 2004). Organizations provide people with opportunities to share, discuss, and engage in sensemaking—all vital processes to facilitate communicating about health (Apker, 2012). Furthermore, organizations themselves can influence the processes involved in communicating about health (Harrison et al., 2011; Kirby, 2006a; Stephens et al., 2014; Stephens et al., 2015), including having negative influences (Kirby, 2006b; Zoller, 2003, 2004). Organizational health communication can be considered multifaceted, because it not only examines individual and collective communicative behaviors (i.e., improving or enabling health within organizations from either a physical or mental perspective), but it can also examine more macro-level impacts of organizations and organizing processes on communicating health issues. In their model of Working Well, Farrell and Geist-Martin (2005) capture an organizational communication perspective on health communication by saying, "health communication must be conceived not only in terms of channels, such as mass media or interpersonal channels, but also in terms of a system" (p. 580). Scarduzio and Geist-Martin (this volume) further elaborate on the whole-person approach and provide solid suggestions for how organizations can motivate employees to participate in employee assistance programs, workplace wellness initiatives, and work–life balance.

Even though organizations are more than simply channels, they are clearly related to the concept of communication channels because they can function as vehicles for information dissemination. Organizations have been considered metachannels (Stephens et al., 2004) because they contain a multitude of channels like email, bulletin boards, and social media networks. For this reason, we begin this chapter by examining the research on workplace health promotions (WHP), a common organizational practice for disseminating health information in work organizations, and then we move to examining theoretical reasons why many types of organizations might be particularly useful health dissemination vehicles.

Workplace Health Promotions as a Health Dissemination Practice

Workplaces, one of the most common organizations disseminating health information today, share health information with their members in health and wellness "areas once considered to be private, including cardiovascular health, nutrition, weight loss, smoking cessation, hypertension control, stress management, and fitness levels" (Zoller, 2003, p. 174). In addition to concerns for their employee's health, employers have business-related reasons to participate in health dissemination. Business practices are affected by poor employee health and it may lead to missed work, reduced productivity, increased insurance and workers compensation costs, and reduced organizational profitability (Cancelliere, Cassidy, Ammendolia, & Cote, 2011; Henke Goetzel, McHugh, & Issac, 2011; Robroek, van den Berg, Plat, & Burdorf, 2011; Zoller, 2003).

Workplaces also serve as opportune settings for health promotion due to the presence of natural social networks, infrastructure support (Chu, Driscoll, & Dwyer, 1997), access to a larger group of people (i.e., employees), and the amount of time employees spend at work (Dishman, Oldenburg, O'Neal, & Shephard, 1998; Hutchinson & Wilson, 2012). Beyond that, WHP programs can contribute to the reduction of health inequalities in organizations, as programs can be tailored to meet the specific needs of minority groups in the workforce (Baron et al., 2014).

Most WHP programs have a dual purpose: improve employees' health and help the organization accomplish its work objectives. These programs often share a common set of organizational goals including (1) controlling insurance costs, (2) boosting workplace productivity, (3) improving organizational commitment, (4) lowering absenteeism, and (5) decreasing employee turnover (Dejoy & Wilson, 2003). Previous systematic reviews of literature have shown that WHP programs can improve overall organizational health (Hutchinson & Wilson, 2012), increase physical activity (Proper et al., 2003; Conn, Hafdahl, Cooper, Brown, & Lusk, 2009), control employee obesity (Anderson et al., 2009), and positively influence employees' dietary behavior (Ni Mhurchu, Aston, & Jebb, 2010). In addition to directly impacting employee health, other studies have shown that WHP programs may decrease the rate of absenteeism due to sickness (Conn et al., 2009; Proper et al., 2003; Kuoppala, Lamminpaa, & Husman, 2008) and increase productivity at work (Kuoppala et al., 2008).

Yet there are also critiques of WHP programs because they can be driven primarily by profit motives and they can pressure employees to get involved in issues many people regard as private (Geist-Martin, Horsley, & Farrell, 2003; May, this volume; Murphy, Hurrell, & Quick, 1992). Historically, many for-profit organizations have followed a financial model equating business health to sound financial health (Shanbhag, 2010). In her work linking public health and organizational health, Zoller (2010) posits that organizing public health practices in organizations is continuously in conflict with business interests. Additionally, some WHP programs are more of a covert approach to getting employees to care and improve their health (Kirby, 2006b).

Community and Nonprofit Organizations as Health Dissemination Vehicles

In addition to workplaces, there are many other types of organizations that can function as health dissemination vehicles. Community-based health promotion programs have been recognized as a clear strategy for achieving population-level change in risk behaviors and health (Merzel & D'Afflitti, 2003). Navarro and his colleagues (2007) found that community-level changes can foster and sustain health behavioral change. Health-related nonprofit organizations (NPOs) also play a role in health promotions. Boyle and his colleagues (2007) investigated the contributions made by NPOs to mental health and well-being. They found NPOs that embrace the ideas of mental health promotion are in a central position to enhance resiliency in a wide cross-section of activities. NPOs collectively direct their activities to a diverse range of groups experiencing a variety of health and social problems (Boyle et al., 2007). Similarly, religious organizations have also begun promoting health. These groups can reach a broad population and they have great potential for reducing health disparities and influencing members' health behaviors at multiple levels (Campbell et al., 2007).

But what is it about the community, nonprofit, and work organizations that make some of these health interventions successful? Thus far, much of this research has justified the focus on using organizations as channels because of practical dissemination reasons like proximity, reach, and access (Krueter et al., 2008). While there is value in establishing practical reasons to use organizations as dissemination tools, there are also theoretical reasons that organizations can help improve health. In the next section we focus on social identity and organizational identification as core theoretical reasons that explain how some organizations might be better health dissemination vehicles than other organizations.

Social Identity and Organizational Identification

Social identity is a key constituent of human agency. As such, it is important to understand how people's identities in organizations are constructed in response to navigating individual, organizational, and social contexts. Social identity theory (SIT) was originally formulated to explain intergroup behavior (Tajfel & Turner, 1979; Tajfel & Turner, 1986). It refers to the portion of an individual's self-concept derived from participating in social collectives and the perceived significance of group membership (Ashforth, Harrison, & Corley, 2008). A core concept of SIT is that the "extent to which people identify with a particular social group determines their inclination to behave in terms of their group membership" (Ellemers, Kortekaas, & Ouwerkerk, 1999, p. 372). For example, Myers and Gaillard (this volume) also discuss the role social identity plays in forming the professional identity of health care workers. Much of the research in this area suggests that people who feel a part of a group are more likely to behave like other group members.

People tend to classify themselves and others into many social categories, including their organizational memberships (Ashforth & Mael, 1989). In this way, SIT provides the theoretical basis for the concept of organizational identification, a communicative bond formed between organizations and their members (Mael, & Ashforth, 1992; Scott, Corman, & Cheney, 1998). Mael and Ashforth (1992) define organizational identification as "the perception of oneness with or belongingness to an organization, where the individual defines him- or herself in terms of the organization to which he or she is a member" (p.104). Organizational identification is the process that teaches people the norms, values, and behaviors of an organization in ways that ultimately produce a new social identity (Scott et al., 1998).

Organizational identification is often considered a mutually beneficial relationship between an organization and its members (see Gossett, 2002 for a divergent opinion). Furthermore, a positive and distinct organizational identity can "attract the recognition, support, and loyalty of not only organizational members but other key constituents" (Ashforth & Mael, 1989, p. 28). Miller, Allen, Casey, and Johnson (2000) argue that organizations desire identified employees because then those employees are more likely to act responsibly in achieving their organizational goals, representing the organization during interactions with non-employees, and separating themselves from others who have contradictory values and goals with the organization. These identified members "adopt the defining characteristics of the organization as defining characteristics of themselves" (Dutton, Dukerich, & Harquail, 1994, p. 242).

Yet some organizations have been slow to recognize that in addition to financial profits, organizational identification, emotional satisfaction, and employee physical well-being are also important factors in boosting organizational performance and productivity (Shanbhag, 2010). Several studies have shown that organizations' and employees' sense of identification mutually influence one another. As suggested by Geist-Martin and Scarduzio (2011), an employee's sense of identification is "influenced by the ways health and wellness are communicated in the organization" (p. 118). Organizations influence an employee's sense of identification through the creation of policies (Kirby & Krone, 2002), the perceptions of wellness at work (Farrell & Geist-Martin, 2005), and the expectations developed by the organization (Newton, 1995). Meanwhile, organizations benefit from employees' strong sense of identification including organizational social responsibilities (Dukerich, Golden, & Shortell, 2002), participation in organizational activities (Mael & Ashforth, 1992), greater cooperation at work (Bartel, 2001), and member adaptions (Carmeli, Gilat, & Waldman, 2007). Next, we focus specifically on connecting social identity with issues related to organizational health communication.

Identity and Health Promotion

Since many workplace health promotion programs are built around the idea of getting members to participate in healthy activities as a group, it follows that researchers have started examining how social identity and organizational identification function in disseminating health information (Farrell & Geist-Martin, 2005; Harris, Cameron, & Lang, 2011; Stephens et al., 2014; Stephens et al., 2015). In addition to studies specifically mentioning these theoretical frameworks, there are several related studies that suggest identity is important (Miller, Birkholt, Scott, & Stage, 1995; Zoller 2003, 2004). Across all these studies, identity and identification are clearly linked to health outcomes. As illustrated above, the process of integrating WHP programs or new health-related values into an organization requires deeper insight into how members formulate identification with an organization, alongside its mission, belief, and values. To summarize the theories, methods, contexts, and findings from these core studies centered around the theoretical concepts of social identity, see Table 13.1.

TABLE 13.1 Social Identity–Related Studies From Organizational and Health Communication

Authors	Journal	Subjects	Context	Theory	Method	Findings Related to Outcomes and Controls
Farrell & Geist-Martin (2005)	*Management Communication Quarterly*	Employers & employees	Wellness & stress	Social identity	Qualitative observations & interviews	The Model of Working Well—integrates individual and organizational health identities; talking to peers; challenges with supervisors; family
Harris, Cameron, & Lang (2011)	*Journal of Community and Applied Social Psychology*	Community-based organizations	HIV/AIDS	Social identity Hope Self-efficacy	Survey	Organizational identification plays a role in the persistence and self-perceived competence of HIV community-based agencies; in-group effects mediate turnover intentions; in-group ties mediate general self-efficacy; hope is unrelated to social identification
James, Lovato, & Khoo (1994)	*Academy of Management Journal*	Minority employees	Blood pressure	Social identity	Survey	Minority employees' identities influence their physical health outcomes
Miller et al. (1995)	*Communication Research*	Health care organizations	Caregiving	Social identity	Qualitative observations & interviews	Job involvement, organizational role, and attitude about service recipients are all part of burnout in human services organizations
Stephens et al. HITs (2014a)	*Health Communication*	University community	Skin cancer	Social identity Multiple ICTs	3x2 Experiment	Identification mediator, health knowledge, message attitude, overload

Author (Year)	Journal	Population	Topic	Theory	Method	Findings
Stephens et al. (2015)	*Health Communication*	Employers and health clinics	Healthy heart	Social identity Multiple identification	Experiment	Health literacy, intention to share info interpersonally and with coworkers, behavioral intent, identification
Verdonk, Seesing & de Rijk (2010)	*BMC Public Health*	Employees	Workplace physical activity	Social identity Gender theory	Qualitative observations & interviews	Masculine identity influences workplace physical activity. Workplace health promotion programs, including workplace physical activity, may benefit from the tensions between health behaviors and masculinity
Zoller (2004)	*Western Journal of Communication*	Employers & employees	Workplace health promotion	Critical ideology	Qualitative observations & interviews	Implementation of WHP influences employee perceptions; WHP can alienate employees; WHP can be positive
Zoller (2003)	*Management Communication Quarterly*	Employers & employees	Workplace health promotion	Critical ideology	Qualitative observations & interviews	Interrelationships between health promotion discourse and managerial ideology, employee's perceptions of health and personal identity, employee resistance

Nuanced Perspectives on Social Identity and Organizational Health Communication

The studies summarized in Table 13.1 provide evidence that social identity can help as scholars expand their work into organizational health issues. The core findings from these studies suggest that organizational identification (a) is linked to persuasion goals, (b) is associated with health information sharing at work, (c) helps community groups reduce turnover, (d) is related to emotion labor in health care contexts, and (e) can work along with information and communication technologies (ICTs) to influence health outcomes.

Persuasion and Attitude

A person's attitude toward messages is frequently measured in persuasion and communication research studies (Chaiken, 1987; Petty & Cacioppo, 1986), and it is typically regarded as a precursor to behavior change. Organizational identification plays a key role in shaping attitudes and behaviors, including affect, involvement, satisfaction, and commitment to the organization (Ashforth et al., 2008). Along with behavioral intentions, which refer to people's self-reported intent to conduct the desired behavior, message attitude—people's attitudes toward specific message content—can provide significant evidence for behavior change. Stephens et al. (2014a) found that when organizations disseminate health information, the relationship variable—i.e., organizational identification—functions in conjunction with cognitive variables, like message attitude, to help achieve persuasion goals.

Information Sharing

Information sharing is important in health communication because conversations about health messages can lead to positive outcomes such as improved esteem, opinion verification, and obtaining personal goals (Southwell & Yzer, 2009; see Harrison, this volume, for a counterpoint on the possible complications of conversations about health messages). Furthermore, when information sharers acquire new information that matches the information needs of others, the sharer can pass that information on (Rioux, 2005). Two studies in Table 13.1 found evidence linking social identities and willingness to share information. Farrell and Geist-Martin's (2005) Model of Working Well integrates individual and organizational health identities and finds that talking to peers is a central part of what creates this integrated system approach to studying organizational health. Stephens and her colleagues (2015) used a cross-organizational sample of over 100 different employers and found that when people strongly identify with their employer they have a higher intention to share health information with coworkers than employees with lower organizational identification.

Reduce Turnover

Prior research on organizational identification in work and volunteer contexts has found that people who identify strongly with their organization are less likely to report intentions of leaving that organization (Ashforth & Mael, 1999; Scott et al., 1999; Scott & Stephens, 2009). In community-based health organizations, like the HIV/AIDS agency studied by Harris and colleagues (2011) organizational identification (defined as agency organization in their study, but measured in a manner similar to organizational identification) kept this HIV support group together and reduced their turnover intentions.

Emotion Labor

Several researchers, such as Miller and colleagues (1995), have examined caregivers and the emotion labor integral to the job of being a health care or human services worker. In their study examining human services organizations, they found that job involvement, organizational role, and attitude about service recipients, all contributed to burnout (Miller et al., 1995). While they relied on several theoretical perspectives to guide their work, social identity was used to justify the inclusion of job involvement in their overall model.

To summarize, research relying on social identity concepts is beginning to create a base of findings suggesting that the relationships people have with their organizations can influence their interpretation and behavioral intentions with organizational health information. Next, we delve into the role technology plays in understanding social identity and organizational health communication.

ICT Use and Organizational Health Communication

Organizations are increasingly using information and communication technologies (ICTs) for activities like communicating with employees and members (D'Urso & Pierce, 2009), and customers (Kaplan & Haenlein, 2010). ICTs are concerned with the storage, retrieval, manipulation, transmission, or receipt of digital media through communication devices or applications (e.g., television, mobile phones, and network hardware and software), as well as the various services and applications associated with them (Stephens, Sørnes, Rice, Browning, & Sætre, 2008b). Workers use a wide variety of over 20 different ICTs, with 88% of people using email at work, 85% using an Intranet (D'Urso & Pierce, 2009), and a rising number (15%) using newer tools such as Twitter (Smith & Brenner, 2012).

One group of ICTs that have received recent attention in organizational health contexts is social media (e.g., Stephens et al., 2014a). Social media provide organizations, organizational members, and health care professionals with additional opportunities to collect, manage, and share health information in a more public forum. These technologies can serve as unique channels for organizations to harness member identification and effectively disseminate health information (Stephens et al., 2014a).

There is some evidence that social identity might work along with ICTs to guide organizations in how they can use technology to communicate about health information with their members. In their study on using the social medium of Facebook to disseminate health messages, Stephens and her colleagues (2014a) found that if an organization has highly identified members, it can successfully use social media for health information dissemination. Their study found that a social medium makes organizational membership more salient through the use of identity cues like logos and other members' comments. These highly identified members had more positive attitudes toward the health message and they reported being less overloaded than organizational members who were not as highly identified. These authors speculate that when people have a strong sense of organizational identification they might view health messages coming from their organization as more important and, thus, they read them and find them helpful instead of a waste of time. Furthermore, the findings regarding information overload suggest that "identification buffers the overload individuals experience when they consume health information" (p. 406). This is particularly important since uncertainty is often associated with health information because it contains medical jargon and ambiguity concerning health (Thompson et al., 2011). However, the authors caution that their study used the health context of skin cancer and other more stigmatized illnesses might not have similar results due to the public nature of social media.

According to SIT, people define themselves partly in terms of salient organizational memberships (Ashforth & Mael, 1989), so it seems plausible that identification is linked to certain ICTs. In social networking sites such as Facebook and Twitter, organizational membership can appear more public because many other organizational members can view and share the comments and information. Based on a structurational perspective of organizational identification (Scott et al., 1998), these online social interactions offer a multilevel influential structure for individuals to collaborate and express their organizational membership (Stephens et al., 2014a). Individuals incorporate those organizational membership cues into their construction of personal and social identity, which ultimately influence their attitudes and behavior (Larson & Pepper, 2003). These public reminders of organizational identity are likely different than a more interpersonal approach that uses email to send individualized health messages to people.

Organizational Digital Divides and Health

Despite the growth in ICTs, one of the biggest challenges organizations face concerning distributing health information to their members is that not all employees have access to the internet or intranet-based health resources (Stephens et al., 2015).

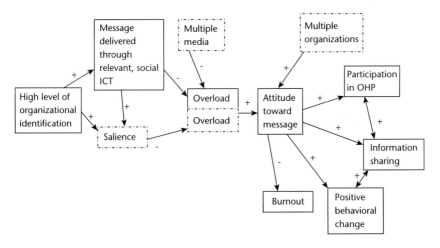

FIGURE 13.1   Organizational Identification, ICTs, and Health Outcomes.

For example, employees in knowledge-worker positions have computers on their desks, but labor workers have much less access to computers and the internet at work and at home (Stephens et al., 2008a). This can result in a new organizational digital divide based on access to health information. These opportunities and challenges lead researchers in new directions that can influence organizations and their members' health.

Directions for Research in Organizational Identification and Health

This review of literature focused on organizations, identity, and health paints a picture for how some key variables operate as we try to promote health behaviors. Figure 13.1 compiles the reviewed literature into a visual representation of the empirical relationships found in the existing literature. While we know that this model might not apply for every type of health information, we provide it to guide thinking and additional empirical research. We use solid boxes to represent the existing findings and dashed boxes to represent the most promising areas for future research. We discuss the model and each of these four major directions next.

This model focuses on the role that higher levels of organizational identification have on changing health behaviors. We combine the findings that higher levels of identification, combined with organizations delivering messages through ICTs that enhance the salience of that identification, will have an influence on health behavior. Next we include the effect that identification has in reducing overload. This communication process increases people's attitude toward the health message, increasing the likelihood they will participate in an organizational health program, share information, and ultimately change their behavior.

You will notice that we also added a direct arrow between attitude and behavior change because it is possible that making people aware of health messages does not also require them to be involved with an organizational health promotion program to change their behavior.

Salience

The first variable we added to this model that is important for future research is salience. Much of the health communication research, including the Health Belief Model (Rosenstock, 1974) is premised on the assumption that people must view the particular health message as relevant and salient for them to attend to the message. In our model, we suggest that organizational identification might have an impact on making a health message salient, but we also acknowledge that salience may come from messages received outside of an organization.

Multiple Media

The second area for future research is examining how health messages sent through multiple media affect desirable health outcomes. Studies suggest that workplace health promotions are most effective when they combine media with interpersonal channels to disseminate messages (Morgan, 2009). We further justify examining this variable because recent persuasion research has shown that using two media with different properties can obscure the overload from a redundant message, improve attitude, and positively affect behavioral intentions (Stephens & Rains, 2011). While people tend to be less overloaded from messages received from an organization where they are highly identified (Stephens et al., 2014a), we have no data concerning peoples' perceptions of receiving multiple messages about the same health topic.

Multiple and Collaborating Sources

The third area for future research focuses both on redundant messages and receiving similar messages from multiple organizations. People can be attached and feel a part of multiple organizations, a term called multiple identification (Scott et al., 1999). While most of the existing research on multiple identifications has not addressed health issues (Larson & Pepper, 2003; Scott et al., 1999; Scott & Fontenot, 1999; Scott & Stephens, 2009), these studies provide evidence that attachment to organizations is fleeting and that people can have multiple attachments (Scott et al., 1999). If multiple organizations collaborate on health promotions, they might boost the positive health benefits. Feeley and O'Mally (this volume) provide several examples of how NPOs have partnered with for-profit organizations to achieve better health dissemination outcomes in organ donation campaigns. Harrison and colleagues (2011) summarize these relationships well in their research on organ donation campaigns by demonstrating how "the physical, social, and information structures of organizations" (p. 535) are different between organizations. The combination of hearing a health message from two different organizations might positively influence health and make both programs more successful.

Overload

The final area for future research is to better understand how we overload people with health information and how relationship variables might reduce peoples' perception of overload. There is some empirical evidence that positive identification reduces overload (Stephens et al., 2014a), but we should combine this variable with issues of health literacy to learn how to craft messages that can be read and perceived by multiple audiences. People are bombarded with messages through multiple media today and if health communicators want their messages seen, they need to find ways to rise above the noise that people experience in their everyday lives. Exploring the variable of overload could offer some guidance in this challenging problem.

Conclusion

People are social. It seems natural that social and relationship variables, like identity, should play a key role in how we attend to messages, make decisions to share information, and change our behaviors. This chapter provided a summary of the current empirical literature on social identity, organizational identification, organizational health promotions, and ICT use. As we continue to strive and improve the health of people around the world, we cannot forget that *people* must make these health decisions, and even when they are part of an organization, *people* are social.

DISCUSSION QUESTIONS

1. What organizations do you believe are likely to have strongly identified members?
2. In addition to social media, which other ICTs could be used to heighten the salience of member identification?
3. What specific health conditions or concerns are most likely to benefit from the identification people feel with their organizations?
4. What types of organizations should consider partnering to maximize their health message redundancy without overloading their members with information?
5. What aspects of social identity theory are most applicable when organizations decide to disseminate health messages?

Suggested Reading

Stephens, K. K., Goins, E. S., & Dailey, S. L. (2014). Organizations disseminating health messages: The roles of organizational identification and HITs. *Health Communication, 29*, 398–409.

Stephens, K. K., Pastorek, A., Crook, B., Mackert, M., Donovan-Kicken, E., & Shalev, H. (2015). Boosting employer-sponsored health dissemination efforts: Identification and information sharing intentions. Manuscript accepted for publication at *Health Communication*.

References

Andersen, P. A., Buller, D. B., Voeks, J. H., Walkosz, B. J., Scott, M. D., & Cutter, G. R. (2008). Testing the long term effects of the Go Sun Smart worksite sun protection program: A group-randomized experimental study. *Journal of Communication, 58*, 447–471.

Anderson, L. M., Quinn, T. A., Glanz, K., Ramirez, G., Kahwati, L. C., Johnson, D. B., . . . Katz, D. L. (2009). The effectiveness of worksite nutrition and physical activity interventions for controlling employee overweight and obesity. *American Journal of Preventative Medicine, 37*, 340–357.

Apker, J. (2012). *Communication in health organizations*. Polity Press: Malden, MA.

Ashforth, B. E., Harrison, S. H., & Corley, K. G. (2008). Identification in organizations: An examination of four fundamental questions. *Journal of Management, 34*, 325–374.

Ashforth, B. E. & Mael, F. (1989). Social identity theory and the organization. *Academy of Management Review, 14*, 20–39.

Baron, S. L., Beard S., Davis, L. K., Delp., L., Forst, L., Kidd-Taylor, A., . . . Welch, L., S. (2014). Promoting integrated approaches to reducing health inequities among low-income workers: Applying a social ecological framework. *American Journal of Industrial Medicine, 57*, 539–556.

Bartel, C. A. (2001). Social comparisons in boundary-spanning work: Effects of community outreach on members' organizational identity and identification. *Administrative Science Quarterly, 46*, 379–413.

Boyle, F. M., Donald, M., Dean, J. H., Conrad, S., & Mutch, A. J. (2007). Mental health promotion and non-profit health organizations. *Health & Social Care in the Community, 15*, 553–560.

Campbell, M. K., Hudson, M. A., Resnicow, K., Blakeney, N., Paxton, A., & Baskin, M. (2007). Church based health promotion interventions: Evidence and lessons learned. *Annual Review of Public Health, 28*, 213–234.

Cancelliere, C., Cassidy, J. D., Ammendolia, C., & Cote, P. (2011). Are workplace health promotion programs effective at improving presenteeism in workers? A systematic review and best evidence synthesis of the literature. *BMC Public Health, 11*, 395–406.

Carmeli, A., Gilat, G., & Waldman, D. A. (2007). The role of perceived organizational performance in organizational identification, adjustment and job performance. *Journal of Management Studies, 44*, 972–992.

Chaiken, S. (1987). The heuristic model of persuasion. In M. P. Zanna, J. M. Olson, & C. P. Herman (Eds.), *Social influence: The Ontario Symposium* (Vol. 5, pp. 3–39). Hillsdane, NJ: Lawrence Erlbaum.

Chu, C., Driscoll, T., & Dwyer, S. (1997). The health-promoting workplace: An integrative perspective. *The Australian and New Zealand Journal of Public Health, 21*, 391–397.

Conn, V. S., Hafdahl, A. R., Cooper, P. S., Brown, L. M., Lusk, S. L. (2009). Meta-analysis of workplace physical activity interventions. *American Journal Preventive Medicine, 37*, 330 –339.

Crook, B., Stephens, K. K., Pastorek, A. E., Mackert, M., & Donovan, E. E. (in press). Sharing health information and influencing behavioral intentions: The role of health literacy, information overload, and the web in the diffusion of healthy heart information. Manuscript accepted for publication at *Health Communication*.

DeJoy, D. M. & Wilson, M. G. (2003). Organizational health promotion: Broadening the horizon of workplace health promotion. *American Journal of Health Promotion, 17*, 337–341.

Dishman, R. K., Oldenburg, B., O'Neal, H., & Shephard, R. J. (1998). Worksite physical activity interventions. *American Journal Preventive Medicine, 5*, 344–361.

Dukerich, J. M., Golden, B. R., & Shortell, S. M. (2002). Beauty is in the eye of the beholder: The impact of organizational identification, identity, and image on the cooperative behaviors of physicians. *Administrative Science Quarterly, 47*, 507–533.

Dutton, J., Dukerich, J., & Harquail, C. (1994). Organizational images and member identification. *Administrative Science Quarterly, 39*, 293–363.

D'Urso, S. C. & Pierce, K. M. (2009). Connected to the organization: A survey of communication technologies in the modern organizational landscape. *Communication Research Reports, 26*, 75–81.

Ellemers, N., Kortekaas, P. & Ouwerkerk, J. (1999). Self-categorisation, commitment to the group and group self-esteem as related but distinct aspects of social identity. *European Journal of Social Psychology, 29*, 371–389.

Farrell, A. & Geist-Martin, P. (2005). Communicating social health: Perceptions of wellness at work. *Management Communication Quarterly, 18*, 543–592.

Geist-Martin, P., Horsley, K., & Farrell, A. (2003). Working well: Communicating individual and collective wellness initiatives. In T. L. Thompson, A. M. Dorsey, K. I. Miller, & R. Parrott (Eds.), *Handbook of health communication* (pp. 423–443). Mahwah, NJ: Lawrence Erlbaum.

Geist-Martin, P. & Scarduzio, J. A. (2011). Working well: Reconsidering health communication at work. In T. L. Thompson, R. Parrott, & J. F. Nussbaum (Eds.), *The Routledge handbook of health communication* (pp. 117–131). New York: Routledge.

Gossett, L. M. (2002). Kept at arm's length: Questioning the organizational desirability of member identification. *Communication Monographs, 69*, 385–404.

Harris, G. E., Cameron, J. E., & Lang, J. (2011). Identification with community-based HIV agencies as a correlate of turnover intentions and general self-efficacy. *Journal of Community and Applied Social Psychology, 21*, 41–54.

Harrison, T. R., Morgan, S., Chewning, L., Williams, E., Barbour, J., DiCorcia, M., & Davis, L. (2011). Revisiting the worksite in worksite health campaigns: Evidence from a multisite organ donation campaign. *Journal of Communication, 61*, 535–555.

Hutchinson, A. D. & Wilson, C. (2012). Improving nutrition and physical activity in the workplace: A meta-analysis of intervention studies. *Health Promotion International, 27*, 238–249.

James, K., Lovato, C., & Khoo, G. (1994). Social identity correlates of minority workers' health. *Academy of Management Journal, 37*(2), 383–396.

Johnson, L. T., Ralston, P. A., & Jones, E. (2010). Beauty salon health intervention increases fruit and vegetable consumption in African-American women. *Journal of the American Dietetic Association, 110*, 941–945.

Kaplan, A. M. & Haenlein, M. (2010). Users of the world, unite! The challenges and opportunities of social media. *Business Horizons, 53*, 59–68.

Kirby, E. L. & Krone, K. J. (2002). The policy exists but you can't really use it: Communication and the structuration of work-family policies. *Journal of Applied Communication Research, 30*, 50–77.

Kirby, E. L. (2006a). Helping you make room in your life for your needs: When organizations appropriate family roles. *Communication Monographs, 73*, 474–480.

Kirby, E. L. (2006b). Your attitude determines your altitude: Reflecting on a company-sponsored mountain climb. In J. Keyton & P. Shockley-Zalabak (Eds.), *Organizational communication: Understanding communication processes* (2nd ed., pp. 99–108). Los Angeles, CA: Roxbury.

Krueter, M. W., Alcaraz, K. I., Pfeiffer, D., & Christopher, K. (2008). Using dissemination research to identify optimal community setting for tailored breast cancer information kiosks. *Journal of Public Health Management and Practice, 14*, 160–169.

Kuoppala, J., Lamminpaa, A., & Husman, P. (2008). Work health promotion, job well-being, and sickness absences: A systematic review and meta-analysis. *Journal of Occupational and Environmental Medicine, 50*, 1216 –1227.

Larson, G. S. & Pepper, G. L. (2003). Strategies for managing multiple organizational identifications: A case of competing identities. *Management Communication Quarterly, 16*, 528–557.

Mael, F. & Ashforth, B. E. (1992). Alumni and their alma mater: A partial test of the reformulated model of organizational identification. *Journal of Organizational Behavior, 13*, 103–123.

Merzel, C. & D'Afflitti, J. (2003). Reconsidering community-based health promotion: Promise, performance, and potential. *American Journal of Public Health, 93*, 557–574.

Miller, K., Birkholt, M., Scott, C., & Stage, C. (1995). Empathy and burnout in human service work: An extension of a communication model. *Communication Research, 22*, 123–147.

Miller, V. D, Allen, M., Casey, M. K., & Johnson, J. R. (2000). Reconsidering the organizational identification questionnaire. *Management Communication Quarterly, 13*, 626–658.

Morgan, S. E. (2009). The intersection of conversation, cognitions, and campaigns: The social representation of organ donation. *Communication Theory, 19*, 29–48.

Murphy, L. R., Hurrell, J. J., & Quick, J. C. (1992). Work and well-being: Where do we go from here? In J. C. Quick, L. R. Murphy, & J. J. Hurrell, Jr. (Eds.), *Stress and well-being at work: Assessments and interventions for occupational mental health* (pp. 331–347). Washington, DC: American Psychological Association.

Navarro, A., Voetsch, K. P., Liburd, L.C., Giles, W., & Collins, J. L. (2007). Charting the future of community health promotion: Recommendations from the national expert panel on community health promotion. *Preventive Chronic Diseases, 4*, 1–7.

Newton, T. (1995). *"Managing" Stress: Emotion and power at work.* London: Sage.

Ni Mhurchu, C., Aston, L. M., & Jebb, S. A. (2010). Effects of worksite health promotion interventions on employee diets: A systematic review. *BMC Public Health, 10*, 62–74.

Petty, R. E. & Cacioppo, J. T. (1986). *Communication and persuasion: Central and peripheral routes to attitude change.* New York: Springer-Verlag.

Proper, K. I., Koning, M., Van der Beek, A .J., Hildebrandt, V. H., Bosscher, R. J., & van Mechelen, W. (2003). The effectiveness of worksite physical activity programs on physical activity, physical fitness, and health. *Clinical Journal of Sport Medicine, 13*, 106–117.

Rioux, K. (2005). Information acquiring-and-sharing. In K. E. Fisher, S. Erdelez, & L. McKechnie (Eds.), *Theories of information behavior* (pp. 169–173). Medford, NJ: Information Today.

Robroek, S. J., van den Berg, T. I., Plat, J. F., & Burdorf A. (2011). The role of obesity and lifestyle behaviours in a productive workforce. *Occupational and Environmental Medicine, 68*, 134–139.

Rosenstock, I. M. (1974). The health belief model and preventive health behavior. *Health Education Monographs, 2*, 354–385.

Scott, C. R., Corman, S. R., & Cheney, G. (1998). Development of a situated-action theory of identification in the organization. *Communication Theory, 8*, 298–336.

Scott, C. R., Connaughton, S. L., Diaz-Saenz, Maguire, K., Ramirez, R., Richardson, B., . . . Morgon, D. (1999). The impacts of communication and multiple identifications on intent to leave: A multimethodological exploration. *Management Communication Quarterly, 12*, 400–435.

Scott, C. R. & Fontenot, J. (1999). Multiple identifications during team meetings: A comparison of conventional and computer-supported interactions. *Communication Reports, 12*, 91–100.

Scott, C. R. & Stephens, K. K. (2009). It depends on who you're talking to . . . : Predictors and outcomes of situated measures of organizational identification. *Western Journal of Communication, 73*, 370–394.

Shanbhag, S. M. (2010). The healthy workplace initiative. *Indian Journal of Occupational and Environmental Medicine, 14*, 29–30.

Smith, A. & Brenner, J. (2012). Twitter use 2012. *Pew Internet.org*. Retrieved from: http://www.pewinternet.org/Reports/2012/Twitter-Use-2012.aspx.

Southwell, B. G. & Yzer, M. C. (2009). When (and why) interpersonal talk matters for campaigns. *Communication Theory, 19*, 1–8.

Stephens, K. K. et al. (2008a). Communication practices in university operations. The University of Texas: Austin, TX. Retrieved from http://www.utexas.edu/operations/files/University OperationsReport_1109_details.pdf.

Stephens, K. K., Goins, E. S., & Dailey, S. L. (2014a). Organizations disseminating health messages: The roles of organizational identification and HITs. *Health Communication, 29*, 398–409.

Stephens, K. K., Pastorek, A., Crook, B., Mackert, M., Donovan-Kicken, E., & Shalev, H. (2015). Boosting employer-sponsored health dissemination efforts: Identification and information sharing intentions. *Health Communication, 30*, 209–220.

Stephens, K. K. & Rains, S. A. (2011). Information and communication technology sequences and message repetition in interpersonal interaction. *Communication Research, 38*, 101–122.

Stephens, K. K., Rimal, R. N., & Flora, J. (2004). Expanding the reach of health campaigns: Community organizations as metachannels for the dissemination of health information. *Journal of Health Communication, 9*, 97–111.

Stephens, K. K., Sørnes, J. O, Rice, R. E., Browning, L. D., & Sætre, A. S. (2008b). Discrete, sequential, and follow-up use of information and communication technology by managerial knowledge workers. *Management Communication Quarterly, 22*, 197–231.

Stephens, K. K., Waters, E. D., & Sinclair, C. (2014). Media management: The integration of HR, technology, and people. In M. E. Gordon & V. D. Miller (Eds). *Meeting the challenge of human resource management: A communication perspective* (pp. 215–226). New York: Routledge.

Tajfel, H. & Turner, J. C. (1979). An integrative theory of intergroup conflict. In W. G. Austin & S. Worchel (Eds.), *The social psychology of intergroup relations* (pp. 33–47). Monterey, CA: Brooks/Cole.

Tajfel, H. & Turner, J. C. (1986). The social identity theory of intergroup behaviour. In S. Worchel & W. G. Austin (Eds.), *Psychology of intergroup relations* (pp. 7–24). Chicago, IL: Nelson-Hall.

Thompson, T. L., Parrott, R., & Nussbaum, J. F. (2011). *The Routledge handbook of health communication*. New York: Routledge.

Verdonk, P., Seesing, H., & De Rijk, A. (2010). Doing masculinity, not doing health? A qualitative study among Dutch male employees about health beliefs and company exercise. *BMC Public Health, 10*, 712–726.

Zoller, H. M. (2003). Working out: Managerialism in workplace health promotion. *Management Communication Quarterly, 17*, 171–205.

Zoller, H. M. (2004). Manufacturing health: Employee perspectives on problematic outcomes in a workplace health promotion initiative. *Western Journal of Communication, 68*, 278–301.

Zoller, H. M. (2010). What are health organizations? Public health and organizational communication. *Management Communication Quarterly, 24*, 482–490.

14

THE SOCIAL DIFFUSION OF HEALTH MESSAGES IN ORGANIZATIONS

Tyler R. Harrison

Organizations have become places where health issues are commonly addressed. There are numerous types of health campaigns and programs that occur in organizations. They can be broken down roughly as follows: (a) health campaigns designed to increase employee health (e.g., the Working Well Trial, Wiener, Lewis, & Linnan, 2009; five-a-day for better health, Buller et al., 1999; obesity, Pratt, Lemon, Fernandez et al., 2007, and physical activity, Hopkins, Glenn, Cole, McCarthy, & Yancey, 2012); (b) campaigns to get employees to participate in health related programs or initiatives that benefit themselves or others (e.g., University of Miami's Dolphin Cycling Challenge to raise funds for cancer, eVeritas, 2013; blood drives, Smith, Matthews, & Fiddler, 2011; organ donation campaigns, Morgan, Miller, & Arasaratnam, 2002; Morgan, Harrison, Chewning, DiCorcia, & Davis, 2010); and (c) campaigns that occur at organizations but may also target consumers (e.g., DMVs for organ donation, Harrison, Morgan, & DiCorcia, 2008; Harrison et al., 2010; King, Williams, Harrison, Morgan & Havermahl, 2012; sunscreen at ski resorts, Walkosz et al., 2014).

One key reason to utilize organizations for health promotion has to do with what Harrison (2012) identifies as the law of large numbers. Many community health organizations rely on public outreach at health fairs and related events. These cater to people actively searching for a specific piece of health information, and the reach is correspondingly low. However, organizations provide an often much larger and essentially captive audience for health messages. Large organizations that have tens of thousands of employees offer a kind of economy of scale when it comes to health promotion. Additionally, when consumers or clients who interact with or enter the organization are considered, that number can reach into the millions (for example, all individuals in a state who wish to drive or have an identification card must go through the DMV—essentially providing reach to all adults in the state). As such, working with (and within) organizations to promote health change provides a much more efficient use of resources than many health fairs and other general community outreach events that reach only small numbers of individuals who are already predisposed to a given health concern.

The Social Diffusion of Health Messages

Health campaigns in organizations are not just influenced by campaign messages, but by social processes as well. Most of us would take it as a given that effective health communication campaigns require persuasive messages. Health campaigns in general, and worksite health campaigns in particular, have often operated under the model that messages should be directed to individuals in order to change unhealthy behaviors. This hypodermic needle model of influence processes fails to explain why health campaigns that work well in some organizations are less successful in others. Work by Hornik and Yanovitsky (2003) and others (Morgan, 2009; Southwell & Yzer, 2009) challenges the individual message model and argues that messages are mediated through social diffusion processes; these same processes occur in organizations (Harrison, Morgan, Chewning et al., 2011). In other words, to understand how health messages work in organizational contexts, we have to understand how the social nature of organizations influences the use and processing of health messages. While we have many theories to help us develop persuasive, audience-centered content, we have much less theorizing that explains how those messages are transformed once people start to talk about them.

While historically many health interventions focused on individual exposure, there has been a move toward examining social processes in health campaigns; the goal of these health campaigns is for individuals to talk and share information about health in a social manner (e.g., Bull, Levine, Black, Schmiege, & Santelli, 2012). The assumption behind this approach is that as individuals converse about health messages they are persuading others to engage in positive health behaviors. Morgan and colleagues (2010) used narratives of organizational members who have been touched by organ donation as one way to spur positive conversations about donation and transplantation in their worksite campaigns, which resulted in positive behavior change (increased donor registrations). Peer educators have also been used to create positive health behavior change in worksite campaigns (Buller et al., 1999). The assumption of positive behavior change results from conversation was also evidenced by a requirement by the Division of Transplantation in the 1990s and early 2000s that specified that family discussion was a mandatory outcome of funded grant proposals. But, while positive behavior change based on social interaction is the ideal, it does not always happen. The Division of Transplantation changed the requirement of family discussion in part due to research that showed that when family members discussed organ donation a significant number of nondonors persuaded their loved ones not to be potential donors (Morgan, Harrison, Long, Afifi, & Stephenson, 2008).

While this is one example that demonstrates how conversations can produce a boomerang effect, research in worksite health campaigns shows other complexities that can arise in the social diffusion of messages. The Workplace Partnership for Life (WPFL) campaign provides an excellent illustration. The campaign was designed to encourage people to become organ donors; it used multiple means of message dissemination (posters, voicemails, newsletters, table tents) and also utilized the narratives of employees touched by organ donation (Harrison, Morgan, Chewing et al., 2011; Morgan et al., 2010). The campaign was conducted in 46 organizations across a wide variety of industries, including hospitals, universities, service and manufacturing, city governments, pharmaceuticals, and smaller community based organizations, using three experimental conditions. While the message strategies were all very similar across intervention organizations, the outcomes were very different. It appears that the nature of work and social processes in hospitals, pharmaceutical corporations, and service and manufacturing organizations may help to explain variations in the social diffusion of messages in this campaign and helps explain some of the disparate outcomes.

For example, people who work in hospitals tend to be very mobile during work. Nurses have central stations but move from patient room to patient room. Doctors make rounds, often with residents. As part of this movement there is talk. While much of the talk is patient-centered (see Barbour, Gill, & Dean this volume for more on physician and nurse discourses), members also talk about other issues, as we would expect in any organization. In addition, hospitals are places of medical expertise, and as such, members tend to respect the opinion of other hospital employees about medical and health issues. This combination of a social environment combined with medical expertise should provide an excellent example of how social diffusion of messages related to a health campaign could have a positive influence. While hospital employees did report significant levels of peer influence and frequency of conversation, these conversations did not translate into increased knowledge about organ donation. In part, this is because hospital employees not directly involved in organ donation share similar levels of knowledge and attitudes toward organ donation as the general public (e.g., Sque, Payne, & Vlachonikolis, 2000). Given the levels of respect afforded to medical professionals, though, the negative stories associated with many organ donation myths are likely to carry significant weight. In this case, then, social diffusion of the messages did not have the positive outcome desired.

In contrast, employees in big pharma headquarters tend to work in very different ways than hospital employees. They are more likely to work individually or in small teams and are more likely to work in front of a computer or lab equipment. While there is respect among employees for their colleagues, there is no expectation that they are experts on a specific medical issue such as organ donation. As such, employees reported lower levels of peer influence and less frequency of conversation about organ donation than did hospital employees, but they reported greater levels of knowledge change about the issue. This suggests they relied more on the campaign messages and less on the social diffusion of those messages in making their assessments of organ donation. As one might expect, employees in manufacturing and service-based jobs also engage in work in very different ways from both hospital employees and pharmaceutical companies. Workers talk with each other on assembly lines or as they pass each other in warehouses; they are not confined to offices in the way those in big pharma are. But, they also have no reason to expect that their fellow employees are experts in organ donation. As such, employees in these types of organizations reported the second highest frequency of conversation but the lowest levels of peer influence. This means that decisions about organ donation were made based on campaign messages or on outside influences such as media messages or family.

While this campaign was based on the organ donor model (Morgan, Miller, & Arasaratnam, 2002), the theory could only explain part of the effects on attitude, knowledge, and behavior. What these stories of work and talk demonstrate is the need to think more carefully about how the structure of the organization and the nature and materiality of work influence the social diffusion of campaign messages that are based on traditional behavior change theories. Diffusion of innovations provides a starting point for examining some of these issues, and Harrison's Model of Interaction Environments for Health Interventions in Organizations (MIE) presented later in this chapter provides additional ways of examining organizational and work features, especially as they relate to health interventions and messages. While the MIE explores how organizational structures influence communication and decisions about health messages, there are other bodies of work that complement this approach and together provide for a more complete and sophisticated approach. Work on peer educators in organizational health campaigns (e.g., Morrill, Buller, Buller, & Larkey, 1999) have specifically utilized social processes to influence health-related behaviors. Each of these processes is explored in more detail in the following sections.

Lessons From Diffusion of Innovations

Literature on diffusion processes typically focus on diffusion of innovations. Greenhalgh, Robert, Macfarlane, Bate, and Kyriakidou (2004) in their systematic meta-review of the literature on diffusion in health service organizations distinguish between dissemination (active and planned efforts to persuade target groups) and diffusion (passive spread). In tracing the disciplinary traditions, Greenhalgh et al. (2004) show how Everett Rogers' initial conceptions of innovations included ideas or practices seen as new; diffusion involved the spreading of these ideas through imitation. In the communication discipline, they argue, we see innovations as new information, and the spread of innovations occurs through mediated or interpersonal channels.

Health interventions in organizational contexts that adopt a diffusion of innovation perspective tend to focus more on processes of organizational (rather than individual) adoption and implementation. In other words, campaign organizers focus on processes involved with convincing organizations to adopt the campaign and how well organizations actually implement the program. This approach can be seen in recent work on skin cancer prevention where Buller and colleagues (2012) adopt a diffusion of innovations approach for persuading ski resorts to adopt the Go Sun Smart campaign. Similarly, Hopkins and colleagues (2012) used a diffusion of innovations framework to conduct an evaluation of adoption and implementation of the WORKING program to increase physical activity in organizations. Consistent with Rogers' (2003) Diffusion of Innovations model, both programs maintain that successful implementation depends on organizational level factors, change agents, the nature of the innovation, and the larger context within which organizations are nested.

While organizational adoption is one element related to diffusion of innovations, individual adoption of the health behavior by organizational members is another. For health campaigns in organizations, we can conceive of health messages as including ideas or practices we want individuals to engage in, and we often include new information as part of this approach. However, most health campaigns focus on dissemination of messages and information (including whether the individual received the message), but ignore diffusion processes that focus on the social elements that influence adoption

Since early conceptions that focused primarily on organizational adoption, a more recent range of approaches adds insight into the social nature of diffusion. For example, researchers have examined issues of culture, climate, and social relationships, as well as social networks and their influence on collaboration. Additionally, structural influences such as size, and functional differentiation have been explored (see Greenhalgh et al., 2004, for a full review of these literatures). Ultimately, if we think about health campaigns in organizations as an innovation we are attempting to disseminate, "mass media and other impersonal channels may create awareness of an innovation, [but] interpersonal influence through social networks [. . .] is the dominant mechanism for diffusion" (Greenhalgh et al. 2004, p. 601).

Key components related to the social component of diffusions of innovations include network structure, homophily, opinion leaders, champions, as well as formal dissemination programs (Greenhalgh et al. 2004). Network structure is related to group types with horizontal network structures being better at spreading peer influence. Individuals are more likely to adopt innovations if they share similar characteristics (homophily) with current users. There are several types of opinion leaders: experts who influence through their knowledge and position and peers who influence through their representativeness and credibility; opinion leaders who can have a positive or a negative effect on dissemination and adoption efforts; and champions who provide support for adoption either through a bending of the rules, transformational leadership, buffering the organization, or facilitating the network. Formal dissemination programs need to create appropriate, persuasive, tailored messages, delivered through appropriate channels, and be rigorously evaluated.

These social elements all impact the diffusion of innovations in health service organizations, including health campaigns. However, Greenhalgh and colleagues (2004) caution against the assumption that these processes function in the same ways across organizations. Not only are social processes different from organization to organization, certain structural features of organizations can vary as well.

A few key structural features related to diffusion of innovation that have been found to have positive effects include complexity (differentiation and specialization), involvement in extra organizational professional activities, communication among units, managerial attitude toward change, professionalism, slack resource (unallocated or extra resources that can be redirected to new projects), and technical capacity. Overall, though, these variables account for less than 15% of the variation among comparable organizations (Greenhalgh et al., 2004). One problem, though, is that this type of research has had a strict variable analytical approach, and recent studies suggest that these features may interact in complex and unpredictable ways (e.g., Ferlie & Shortell, 2001).

Greenhalgh and colleagues (2004) present a very complex model that encompasses these elements in addition to issues such as system readiness, adopter needs, assimilation processes, system antecedents, and specific outer organizational contexts. While many of these are relevant for specific types of innovations and are less useful for helping us understand the role of organizations and social processes for health messages and behaviors, there are a couple of exceptions. First, messages must to take into account adopter needs, motivations, goals, learning styles, and social networks. Second, at a larger scale, system antecedents for readiness for innovation may be important. If we want to create a worksite intervention to increase physical activity at work, for example, we need to understand the structure of the organization and its capacity for making this type of change. This issue will be addressed more in depth in discussions about design, space, and materiality.

While studies of diffusion of innovations in health services organizations do not necessarily address worksite campaigns and interventions to improve or change health behaviors specifically, the processes of diffusion provide insight into how messages work in organizational contexts. While not adopting a specific diffusion of innovations framework, a number of organizational campaigns and interventions follow similar approaches, focusing on both social processes and organizational features in message processing.

Organizational Interaction Environments

All organizations have unique interaction environments that influence the social diffusion of health promotion and campaign messages. Harrison, Morgan,

Chewning, and colleagues (2011) move beyond a strict focus on social interaction to advance a general theory of organizational features that influence organizational health campaigns. This approach accounts for the complex nature of interaction between structural features of an organization and social interaction processes in an attempt to understand what elements make certain campaigns or certain organizations better and more effective places for health behavior change. These organizational features collectively constitute the interaction environment of the organization, and consist of physical structures (size, density, collective gathering areas, etc.), social structures (individually created and organizationally fostered social relationships and interactions), and information structures (the number and types of ways in which information is disseminated in organizations—including traditional paper and pencil type channels as well as new ICT channels; see also Stephens & Zhu, this volume, for more on ICTs and health messages). Each organization has a unique interaction environment, and collectively and individually the structures that make up the interaction environment can influence knowledge, communication with peers and peer influence, and behaviors/decisions about health and health information. In testing this model in their worksite organ donation campaign, the interaction environment accounted for a 12% reduction of variance in knowledge change, an 11% reduction of variance in conversation frequency, and a 46% reduction of variance in peer influence, showing that organizational features do play a role in the effectiveness of worksite health campaigns.

In their initial theorizing, Harrison, Morgan, Chewning et al. (2011) advanced three features of organizations (physical, social, and information) that they posited influenced the effectiveness of health interventions in organizations. However, the stories presented earlier in the chapter about campaigns and interaction in hospitals, big pharma, and service and manufacturing environments suggest that the nature and materiality of work being performed by members of the organization need to be added to the model as an additional feature of interaction environments. While these four elements (physical structure, social structure, information structure, and nature and materiality of work) form the interaction environment of the organization, their influence on health decisions and behaviors are mediated by issues such as individual epistemological orientations (e.g., preferences for research-based messages versus interpersonal interaction) and barriers to adoption (e.g., the availability of gym facilities if the organization encourages exercise at lunch time). The addition of these elements is represented in the Model of Interaction Environments for Health Interventions in Organizations presented in Figure 14.1.

Elements of the Model of Interaction Environments for Health Interventions in Organizations

There are four elements that comprise the interaction environment of the organization, the physical structure, social structure, information structure, and nature

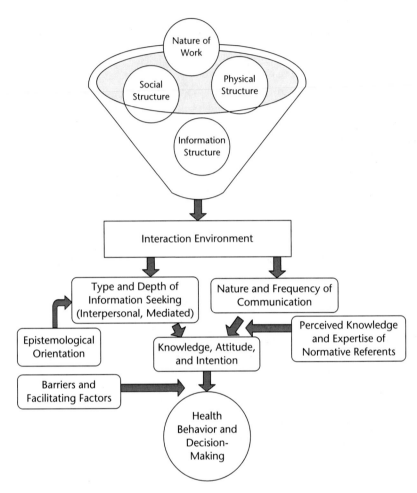

FIGURE 14.1   The Model of Interaction Environments (MIE) for Health
Interventions in Organizations.

of work. *Physical structure* consists of the size of the organization, density, collective gathering areas and other features that influence when and how employees interact with each other. *Social structures* are individually created and organizationally fostered social relationships and interactions. Individual relationships between organizational members are formed through interaction, but are relationships of individual choosing, and can be measured using measures of liking and respect and frequency of interaction. Organizationally fostered relationships occur through organizational events such as meetings, parties, and picnics. *Information structures* consist of the number and types of ways in which information is disseminated in organizations—including traditional paper and pencil type channels as well as new ICT (information and communication technology) channels. Initial measurement of these items simply consists of a checklist of their existence within an organization, with more channels representing more opportunities for dissemination of information. Future measurement should also focus on how the different channels are utilized by organizational members, and this may also inform the nature and materiality of work. *Nature and materiality of work* was not measured in the initial study (Harrison, Morgan & Chewning et al., 2011). Assessments of the nature and materiality of work need to be established and may include frequency of individual versus group or team based work, time spent using technology (computers, lab equipment, machinery) and how these factors influence processes of interaction and information seeking, and the content or production of work.

This new model posits that the interaction environment influences the social diffusion of campaign messages through processes of *information seeking* and through the *nature and frequency of interaction*. Research within hospitals, big pharma, and manufacturing and service suggests, that there are individual preferences for how information is sought, shared, and evaluated as individuals process health related messages. Employees in big pharma, for example, might be more inclined to seek information electronically, engage in less frequent conversation, and be less influenced by their peers because of evaluation of their expertise. Understanding the nature of their work, which involves more isolation than work in hospitals, and pharmaceutical researchers' reliance on computers and scientific methods might provide insight into their *epistemological orientations*; for example, we might expect them to rely on the science and facts of health messages, rather than the personal stories told by colleagues, whose level of *expertise* they would likely judge. Through this process the campaign messages are influenced by interaction environments and help shape attitudes, knowledge, and intention toward the health behavior.

Finally, implementation of health behaviors is influenced by *barriers to adoption* or by factors that *facilitate adoption*. A simple example of a facilitating factor for healthy eating is the availability of inexpensive, healthy meals that are subsidized by the organization. If these are present and processed food that is high in sugar and fat is not offered, this is a facilitating factor that makes behavior change easier. An example of a barrier to adoption in relation to an organizational campaign toward physical activity would be the lack of a walking area or easy access to other types of physical fitness equipment and space. These facilitating factors and barriers should be taken into consideration during the design of the health intervention. They remind us there is only so much a health communication intervention can accomplish – structural barriers must also be taken into consideration.

While many elements of the MIE have been tested, this model presents significant revisions from the early conceptions of interaction environments (Harrison, Morgan, Chewing et al., 2011; Harrison, Morgan, & Williams, 2012). As such, relationships between variables need to be tested. Additionally, alternate approaches and measures to social relationships and diffusion need to be considered as part of the model. One such area that may enhance the value of peer influence in the consideration of formally selected and trained peer educators as opposed to the naturally occurring social relationships currently specified.

The Role of Peer Educators in Social Diffusion in Organizations

The Model of Interaction Environments recognizes that social relationships and judgments of peer expertise will influence how much peer influence occurs. While the initial conceptualization of the model relied on naturally occurring relationships, another common approach in health campaigns is the use of peer educators.

Peer educators have been used extensively in health promotion. Using network analysis to select peer educators is a relatively common approach, but is not without issues and complications. Leaders may be most central and most frequently nominated organizational members, but they also may tend toward upholding the status quo, while early adopters or innovators may be social isolates. Similarly, the measurement of social relations is complicated—friendship is subjective, but eating lunch together is objective. Valente (2012) presents an excellent discussion of the problems and issues in using networks for interventions. Additionally, network analysis is time-consuming, complicated, and costly; thus, most campaigns are not sophisticated in their selection of peers. Some examples of selection process include surveys asking for individuals to rate themselves and others on characteristics corresponding to the network roles of persuaders, connectors, or mavens (de Souza et al., 2014). While social capital and tenure are a few items mentioned as preferred characteristics among peer educators or program champions, identifying individuals with these characteristics can be very challenging; many campaign organizers use simpler methods of selection such as self-referral or coworker recommendation, even though the success of an intervention is heavily dependent on the skills and qualities of the peer educators (e.g., Hopkins, Glenn, Cole, McCarthy, & Yancey, 2012). While Hopkins and colleagues (2012) focus primarily on implementation processes, they do note that success was influenced by worksite layout and social climate, with organizations having one physical location with frequent opportunities for employee interaction being more successful than those with multiple locations and fewer opportunities for interaction.

One of the more sophisticated approaches to selecting peer educators was used by Buller and colleagues (Buller et al., 1999; Morrill et al., 1999; Larkey et al., 1999) in an intervention for 93 intact workgroups for the five-a-day Fruits and Vegetables campaign in the mid-'90s. Their intervention focused specifically on the social nature of diffusion processes. By conducting extensive network analysis (asking all members of intact workgroups to rate their interactions with all other members of the workgroup on a variety of items) they were able to identify central members of each network and recruit them to be peer educators. These individuals were chosen based on in-degree ratings on characteristics like frequency of interaction, frequency of lunch, liking, and so on. In other words, other individuals in the group identified them as the person they trusted and were most likely to interact with. While not a diffusion study, the study uses several of the social components of diffusion of innovations identified by Greenhalgh and colleagues (2004), focusing specifically on horizontal social networks, and peer educators (opinion leaders or program champions). Additionally, the workgroups had a fair degree of homophily (largely Hispanic, similar SES, in the same workgroup), and the intervention dissemination was planned to help meet the goals and values of the targeted population. This intervention was successful in increasing the consumption of fruits and vegetables.

The diffusion of innovations framework, the Model of Interaction Environments, and the use of peer educators all have interaction with others as a central component of their theorizing. Diffusion of innovations depends on champions and opinion leaders; the Model of Interaction Environments relies on naturally existing relationships with colleagues; peer educators are specified individuals who meet some desired criteria. All of these conceptualizations work well within the Model of Interaction Environments and are likely to have an impact on the nature and frequency of conversations, and organizational members' evaluations of their expertise will influence knowledge, attitude, and intentions relevant to a given behavior change. Future research should focus on comparing the planned use of significant opinion leaders and peer educators versus naturally and spontaneously occurring peer influence, and under what conditions which approaches work best. Additionally, future research should focus on comparing systematically selected peer educators versus self or other referred, versus natural opinion leaders. Finally, future research should also compare methods of selecting peer educators; peer influence occurs in health campaigns and understanding when it leads to positive outcomes will help us refine and improve our interventions.

Using Communication Design to Situate Health Campaigns in Interaction Environments

Campaign creation and implementation is a process of design, which should incorporate specific health and behavior change theories appropriate for a given interaction environment and health issue. Organizations are unique, and health interventions must move beyond simple approaches of creating and disseminating "one-size-fits-all" messages and assuming they will work simply by reaching individuals. Social diffusion processes and the Model of Interaction Environments do not provide explicit recommendations on how to adapt an individual campaign to an individual organization, but suggest ways in which these considerations can be used. Putting the model into practice is largely a matter of communication design, which can help situate campaigns to specific sites of intervention and enhance traditional health and behavior change theories (Harrison, 2014).

Translating theoretical constructs into practice requires assessment of the organization. This includes interviews with people in Human Resources who can provide insight into basic elements of the organization, and a walk through of the organization to check for physical elements such as gathering spaces, bulletin boards, break rooms, and offices. Harrison, Morgan, and Williams (2012) present a checklist for assessing the organizational interaction environment. Additionally, formative research should focus on knowledge and attitudes toward the issue, as well as the nature of intraorganizational relationships, trust, and interaction with colleagues. Understanding how messages are shared within the organization, how and where people interact, and how they view their relationship with organizational colleagues provides insight into both the types of messages needed, and the best ways to disseminate those messages.

Refining and Improving Theory and Practice While Avoiding Pitfalls

There is a great deal of room for refinement and improvement of theories related to organizational interaction environments and social diffusion processes. Additionally, there are many pitfalls associated with diffusion processes that need to be mitigated.

Space and Place

While these approaches demonstrate the social nature of message processes, additional theorizing about issues of space and place has the potential to inform how we think about health campaigns in organizations. Theorizing on space and place as they relate to organizational social interactions, collaboration, and work processes can provide additional insight into how organizational space can be used or transformed as part of health interventions. While physical space is important in the model of interaction environments, space in that model focuses primarily on the physical layout and how it influences opportunities for interaction. This is an important conception of space, but space "is not just about the arrangement of the organization's built environment, but about how organizations relate to each other and to the wider social world of which they are a fundamental part" (Dale & Burrell, 2008, p. xiii; see also Aakhus and Harrison, this volume, for more on the relationship between built environments and the social world). Space is a physical location, but place is the pause where we feel at rest. We assign meaning and emotions to places (Dale & Burrell, 2008), and that is likely to influence our perceptions and processing of messages. If we can transform spaces into places such that they incorporate the association of health messages into other pleasant memories and associations, the willingness to engage messages in positive social interactions should be enhanced as well.

One example of a health intervention that utilized these notions of space to relate to the wider social world was the Tell Us Now organ donation campaign in drivers license facilities in Michigan (Harrison et al., 2010; Harrison, Morgan, King, & Williams, 2011; King, Williams, Harrison, Morgan, & Havermahl, 2012). While not using the full interaction model as its foundation, space was extremely important in the design of this intervention. The Michigan Secretary of State (SOS) offices are designed primarily for licensing individuals to drive and for licensing their automobiles and watercraft. The goal of the campaign was to increase the number of organ donor registrations during driver's license issuance.

The interaction space within the branch offices was focused exclusively on the business of licensing, and discussion of organ donation registration had to be initiated by individuals, not the clerks who would perform the registration. As such, the design process involved analysis of how space affected interaction, and how space could be used to facilitate a shift in the interaction space to include "dialogue" about organ donation. The design focused on unique patterns of movement through the space of the SOS office and the interactions that occurred at various locations during the process. Materials and messages were developed to allow customers to initiate a conversation about joining the organ donor registry. These materials include items such as "counter cards" that told stories of donation and transplantation on one side and a simple statement, "Tell us now that you want to be an organ donor" on the other. In addition to posters and prompts at each station, the clerks for the final interaction wore stickers that said "Tell Me Now" and also had a bumper sticker size message on the counter where paperwork was filled out, which provided a reiteration of the message.

While it is unclear if this turned a space into a place, space was essential to the design of the campaign, and registration rates increased by an average of 200–300%. Future research should continue to focus on how we can shift notions of space and place to be more conducive to incorporating health into organizational practices. Part of this shift may be dependent on our messages such that we help employees develop new scripts and schemas for organizational space. Additionally, consistent and dedicated space by the organization to health-related issues may serve to normalize health as an organizational practice; this should also create new places for engaging in health behaviors and discussion (see May, this volume, for a counterpoint on corporate colonization of the body).

Finally, this focus on space and place also resonates with recent theorizing on communication design. We can draw on the works of Nelson and Stolterman (2012), and others (e.g., Barbour & Gill, 2014; Harrison, 2014; Jackson & Aakhus, 2014; and Morgan & Mouton, this volume), as they focus on situating broad principles to specific sites of action. Analysis of the interaction environment provides mechanisms to modify and transform organizations into places where health messages are part of our expected experiences.

Unexpected Outcomes

It is critical that scholars recognize that social diffusion processes have strong effects on health campaigns, but that social diffusion processes can backfire. Increased numbers of conversations and increased levels of peer influence can work in a negative fashion and may actually dissuade individuals in organizations from acquiring the knowledge, attitudes, or behaviors intended. Understanding more about the nature of work in different industries will help us to improve our understanding of how people engage in information seeking and information processing and will subsequently help us tailor our messages and message dissemination processes to utilize social diffusion in a positive manner.

One way to overcome issues related to the potential negative consequences of peer influence is to identify opinion leaders or key peers and provide them with communication strategies to disseminate accurate information, although this may or may not negate the effects of spontaneous interactions where diffusion of health messages occur. But, the combination of positive peer influence with effective campaign strategies and messages that utilize the interaction environment to its fullest should lead to the most positive outcomes.

DISCUSSION QUESTIONS

1. If your organization had a campaign, what messages would you find most influential, well-designed campaign messages or messages from your colleagues? Why?
2. How would you choose a peer educator in your organization?
3. How does the physical space of your organization facilitate or hinder social diffusion processes?
4. Describe the interaction environment of your organization. How would you adapt a campaign to best utilize that environment?

Suggested Reading

Greenhalgh, T., Robert, G., Macfarlane, F., Bate, P., & Kyriakidou, O. (2004). Diffusion of innovations in service organizations: Systematic review and recommendations. *The Milbank Quarterly, 82*, 581–629.

Harrison, T. R., Morgan, S. E., Chewning, L. V., Williams, E., Barbour, J., Di Corcia, M., & Davis, L. (2011). Revisiting the worksite in worksite health campaigns: Evidence from a multi-site organ donation campaign, *Journal of Communication, 61*(3), 535–555.

Morrill, C., Buller, D. B., Buller, M. K., & Larkey, L. L. (1999). Toward an organizational perspective on identifying and managing formal gatekeepers. *Qualitative Sociology, 22*, 51–72.

References

Barbour, J. B. & Gill, R. (2014). Designing communication for the day-to-day safety oversight of nuclear power plants. *Journal of Applied Communication Research, 42,* 168–189.

Bull, S. S., Levine, D. K., Black, S. R., Schmiege, S. J., & Santelli, J. (2012). Social media-delivered sexual health intervention: A cluster randomized controlled trial. *American Journal of Preventive Medicine, 43,* 467–474.

Buller, D. B., Andersen, P. A., Walkosz, B. J., Scott, M. D., Cutter, G. R., Dignan, M. B., Zarlengo, E. M., Voeks, J. H., & Giese, A. J. (2005). Randomized trial testing a worksite sun protection program in an outdoor recreation area. *Health Education & Behavior, 32,* 514–535.

Buller, D. B., Andersen, P. A., Walkosz, B. J., Scott, M. D., Cutter, G. R., Dignan, M. B., Kane, I. L., & Zhang, X. (2012). Enhancing industry-based dissemination of an occupational sun protection program with theory-based strategies employing personal contact. *American Journal of Health Promotion, 26,* 356–365.

Buller, D. B., Morrill, C., Taren, D., Aickin, M., Sennott-Miller, L., Buller, M. K., Larkey, L., Alatorre, C., & Wentzel, T. M. (1999). Randomized trial testing the effect of peer education at increasing fruit and vegetable intake. *Journal of the National Cancer Institute, 91,* 1497–1500.

Dale, K. & Burrell, G. (2008). *The spaces of organisation and the organisation of space: Power, identity, and materiality at work.* New York: Palgrave Macmillan.

de Souza, R., Dauner, K. N., Goei, R., LaCaille, L., Kotowski, M. R., Schultz, J. F., LaCaille, R., & Nowa, A. L. V. (2014). An evaluation of the peer helper component of Go!: A multimessage, muli-"step" obesity prevention intervention. *American Journal of Health Education, 45,* 12–19.

eVeritas (November 3, 2013). Cyclists 'gear' up to fight cancer. Retrieved from, http://everitas.univmiami.net/2013/11/03/cyclists-gear-up-to-fight-cancer/.

Ferlie E. B. & Shortell, S. M. (2001). Improving the quality of health care in the United Kingdom and the United States: A framework for change. *The Milbank Quarterly, 79,* 281–315.

Greenhalgh, T., Robert, G., Macfarlane, F., Bate, P., & Kyriakidou, O. (2004). Diffusion of innovations in service organizations: Systematic review and recommendations. *The Milbank Quarterly, 82,* 581–629.

Harrison, T. R. (2014). Enhancing communication interventions and evaluations through communication design. *Journal of Applied Communication Research, 42,* 135–149.

Harrison, T. R. (2012). Increasing the likelihood of consent in deceased donations: Point-of-decision campaigns, registries, and the law of large numbers. In G. Randhawa (Ed.), *Organ Donation and Transplantation: Public Policy and Clinical Perspectives* (pp. 97–114). Rijeka, Croatia: Intech. Available from http://www.intechopen.com/books/organ-donation-and-transplantation-public-policy-and-clinical-perspectives/increasing-the-likelihood-of-consent-in-deceased-donations-point-of-decision-campaigns-registries-an.

Harrison, T. R., Morgan, S. E., Chewning, L. V., Williams, E., Barbour, J., DiCorcia, M., & Davis, L. (2011). Revisiting the worksite in worksite health campaigns: Evidence from a multi-site organ donation campaign, *Journal of Communication, 61,* 535–555.

Harrison, T. R., Morgan, S. E., & DiCorcia, M. J. (2008). The impact of organ donation education and communication training for gatekeepers: DMV clerks and organ donor registries. *Progress in Transplantation, 18,* 301–309.

Harrison, T. R., Morgan, S. E., King, A. J., DiCorcia, M. J., Williams, E. A., Ivic, R. K., & Hopeck, P. (2010). Promoting the Michigan Organ Donor Registry: Evaluating the impact of a multi-faceted intervention utilizing media priming and communication design. *Health Communication, 25*, 700–708.

Harrison, T. R., Morgan, S. E., King A. J., & Williams, E. A. (2011). Saving lives branch by branch: The effectiveness of driver licensing bureau campaigns to promote organ donor registry sign-ups to African Americans in Michigan. *Journal of Health Communication, 16*, 805–819.

Harrison, T. R., Morgan, S.E., & Williams, E. A. (2012). A method for assessing the interaction environment of organizations. *Journal of Modern Auditing and Accounting, 8*, 1512–1522.

Hopkins, J. M., Glenn, B. A., Cole, B. L., McCarthy, W., & Yancey, A. (2012). Implementing organizational physical activity and healthy eating strategies on paid time: Process evaluation of the UCLA WORKING pilot study. *Health Education Research, 27*, 385–398.

Hornik, R. & Yanovitzky, I. (2003). Using theory to design evaluations of communication campaigns: The case of the national youth anti-drug media campaign. *Communication Theory, 13*, 204–224.

Jackon, S. & Aakhus, M. (2014). Becoming more reflective about the role of design in communication. *Journal of Applied Communication Research, 42*, 125–134.

King, A. J., Williams, E. A., Harrison, T. R., Morgan, S. E., & Havermahl, T. (2012). The "Tell Us Now" campaign for organ donation: Using message immediacy to increase donor registration rates. *Journal of Applied Communication Research, 40*, 229–246.

Larkey, L. K., Alatorre, C., Buller, D. B., Morrill, C., Buller, M. K., Taren, D., & Sennott-Miller, L. (1999). Communication strategies for dietary change in a worksite peer educator intervention, *Health Education Research, 14*, 777–790.

Morgan, S. E. (2009). The intersection of conversation, cognitions, and campaigns: The social representation of organ donation. *Communication Theory, 19*, 29–48.

Morgan, S. E., Harrison, T. R., Chewning, L. V., DiCorcia, M. J., & Davis, L. A. (2010). The Workplace Partnership for Life: The effectiveness of high- and low-intensity worksite campaigns to promote organ donation. *Communication Monographs, 77*, 341–356.

Morgan, S., Miller, J., & Arasaratnam, L. (2002). Signing cards, saving lives: An evaluation of the worksite organ donation promotion project. *Communication Monographs, 69*, 253–273.

Morgan, S. E., Harrison, T. R., Long, S. D., Afifi, W. A., & Stephenson, M. (2008). In their own words: The reasons why people will (not) donate organs. *Health Communication, 23*(1), 23–33.

Morrill, C., Buller, D. B., Buller, M. K., & Larkey, L. L. (1999). Toward an organizational perspective on identifying and managing formal gatekeepers. *Qualitative Sociology, 22*, 51–72.

Nelson, H. G. & Stolterman, E. (2012). *The design way: Intentional change in an unpredictable world*. Cambridge, MA: MIT Press.

Pratt, C. A., Lemon, S. C., Fernandez, D., Goetzel, R., Beresford, S. A., Vogt, T. M. & Webber, L. S. (2007). Design characteristics of worksite environmental interventions for obesity prevention. *Obesity, 15*, 2171–2180.

Rogers, E. M. (2003). *Diffusion of Innovations*. New York, NY: Free Press.

Smith, A., Matthews, R., & Fiddler, J. (2011). Blood donation and community: Exploring the influence of social capital. *International Journal of Social Inquiry, 4*, 45–63.

Southwell, B. G. & Yzer, M. C. (2009). When (and why) interpersonal talk matters for campaigns. *Communication Theory, 19*, 1–8.

Sque, M., Payne, S., & Vlachonikolis, I. (2000). Cadaveric donotransplantation: Nurses attitudes, knowledge, and beahviour. *Social Science & Medicine, 50*, 541–552.

Valente, T. W. (2012). Network interventions. *Science, 337*, 49–53.

Walkosz, B. J., Buller, D. B., Andersen, P. A., Scott, D. M., Dignan, M. B., Cutter, G. R., Liu, X., & Maloy, J. A. (2014). Dissemination of Go Sun Smart in outdoor recreation: Effects of program exposure on sun protection of guests at high-altitude ski areas. *Journal of Health Communication, 19*, 999–1016.

Weiner, B. J., Lewis, M. A., & Linnan, L. A. (2009). Using organization theory to understand the determinants of effective implementation of worksite health promotion programs. *Health Education Research, 24*, 292–305.

15

SERIOUS GAMES, HEALTH, AND ORGANIZING

Nick Carcioppolo, Jessica Wendorf, and Lien Tran

Organizational communication scholars can utilize serious games as a means to develop and maintain relationships between the organization and the public, foster intra- and interorganizational relationships, and more generally as a novel and predominantly unexplored method of organizing. Serious games represent an appealing medium for organizations seeking to change the ways in which members view health, as they can facilitate health-related outcomes through increased engagement, motivation, attention, and retention of health information (Connolly, Boyle, MacArthur, Hainey, & Boyle, 2012; Corti, 2006; Lee & Peng, 2006; Lieberman, 2006). While games have long been an important part of organizations and a useful tool to achieve health outcomes, there has been little cross-pollination of ideas between these literatures. Considering this, the present chapter will detail the intersections of organizational theory, serious games, and health interventions and suggest areas of focus to incorporate games-based approaches into research on health in organizations.

Over the years, serious games have been conceptualized in a variety of ways, tracing back to Clark Abt (1970) who defined the concept as games that concern "matters of great importance, raising questions not easily solved, and having important possible consequences" (p. 10). More recent definitions describe serious games (sometimes referred to as "games for change," or "game-based learning") as those that leverage entertainment for social and health outcomes, focusing on persuasion, including the formation or change of attitudes, awareness, and behavior (Games for Change, 2014; Hopelab 2014a; Peng, Lee, & Heeter, 2010; Ritterfeld & Weber, 2006; Ritterfeld, Cody, & Vorderer, 2009; Susi, Johannesson, & Backlund, 2007). The following sections detail how different industries have used games to facilitate and maintain relationships, the unique features of games that can achieve organizational goals, the theoretical constructs that can explain how games can affect health-based outcomes, and propose future directions for organizational research.

Serious Games in Organizations

Serious games have been developed and assessed across a wide variety of contexts and fields, including public policy, education, health care, government, the military, and in corporate organizations (Alessi & Trollip, 2001; Michael & Chen, 2005). In 2013, U.S. spending on corporate training exceeded $70 billion, and worldwide spending was estimated at over $130 billion (Berson, 2014). Clearly, not all of that spending was in support of gaming, but games are an important and growing part of organizational spending (Berson, 2014). Games can function as activators of informational processes (e.g., dissemination, acquisition, diffusion, & innovation) within organizations. They can be helpful when content is uninteresting or overly technical and are useful for developing job-specific skills, including skills related to occupational safety and health, communication skills training, and other organization-specific skills (Michael & Chen, 2005). Similar to on-site educational training, games provide individuals with valuable knowledge within organizations. This includes information on their role (professional socialization; see Lammers & Proulx and Myers & Gailliard, this volume), expectations as members of teams, the role of conflict and culture at the individual and organizational level, as well as benefits and consequences to specific behavior both as members of organizations and as individuals with desired health outcomes.

An apt example of a game that has been used extensively within organizations is *BaFá BaFá*. In *BaFá BaFá*, people explore cultural differences and similarities with the aim of reaching shared understandings (Simulation Training Systems, 2006). Having been previously used as a diversity training tool within organizations as they prepare for mergers and other large-scale changes in organizational culture (Shirts, 2009), *BaFá BaFá* has become a standard in business settings that require cultural competence. After a brief introduction, participants are divided into two groups, or cultures, the Alphans and Betans. Individuals are then introduced to their new culture's language, social norms, and expectations. Groups are given time to adapt and practice their new culture, after which visitors are exchanged between groups. Visitors are encouraged to interact with the other culture in an effort to determine the values held by the group (Jarrell, Alpers, Brown, & Wotring, 2008). Once all members have interacted with the other culture, each group discusses the other culture's attitudes, beliefs, values, roles, and cultural characteristics before reuniting as a larger group for discussion. Through this game, participants can gain insight regarding the impact of cultural differences on organizational functions and practices as well as the role of conflict in the presence of competing viewpoints. In short, *BaFá BaFá* demonstrates the ability of games to affect organizational culture.

Games and Health

Game-based health interventions can be traced back as far as the early 1980s when Szer (1983) successfully utilized a video game to deliver a physiotherapeutic intervention for arm injuries. Others have demonstrated that simulation games can be an effective tool to prepare doctors for complicated surgeries (Rosser, Rosser, & Savalgi, 1997). In fact, gaming interventions have been used to influence a litany of health-based outcomes, including physiological, psychological, physical, knowledge-based, skills-based, and pain and disease management outcomes (Kato, Cole, Bradlyn, & Pollock, 2008; Primack et al., 2012).

One noteworthy game-based health intervention is *Re-Mission*, created to influence adherence to cancer treatment among adolescents. *Re-Mission* was designed to elicit empathy through narrative components embedded within the game, and although the analysis of the narrative-based mechanism of effect has not yet been published (Hopelab, 2014b), nonetheless, the game is notable as it is the largest randomized, controlled study of a video game intervention ever conducted (Kato et al., 2008). The study followed 375 cancer patients ages 13–29 over a three-month period of treatment. Participants were randomly assigned to either the control condition, which received PCs pre-loaded with a popular video game, or the experimental condition, which received that same popular video game as well as *Re-Mission* (Kato et al., 2008). Hopelab found that playing *Re-Mission* resulted in lasting effects on outcomes, including a better understanding of cancer and increased willingness to fight it, as well as significant increases in antibiotic adherence, oral chemotherapy adherence, cancer related knowledge, and cancer-specific self-efficacy compared to children who played the control game (Kato el al., 2008).

Modality and Features of Serious Games

Games allow people to experience situations, perspectives, and events that they would otherwise never encounter (Corti, 2006). The unique situations and events encountered while gaming engage processes such as experiential and active learning, problem-based role-playing, and immediate feedback that are qualitatively different from the ways in which people experience typical health intervention materials (Boyle, Connolly, & Hainey, 2011; Peng, 2009). These experiences allow message recipients to learn, practice, and interact with health content in simulated environments that traditional media interventions and training cannot replicate. Indeed, game-based interventions can influence health outcomes through activation of numerous cognitive mechanisms, including enhanced self-monitoring, problem recognition, problem solving, decision-making, collaboration, and negotiation (for a review, see Susi et al., 2007).

In addition to the interactive contexts afforded by games, there are at least five formal features of games relevant to organizational scholars that can help to achieve desired outcomes: (1) competition, (2) goal-setting, (3) the establishment of rules, (4) choice, and (5) novel contexts and settings (see Charsky, 2010 for a review). Not all features are included in any given game; their presence varies depending on the goals of the organization or developer, and the most compelling strategies to reach those goals. These features mirror organizing processes and allow us to conceptualize the use of games as an organizing process itself. To explain, we use two games introduced earlier, *BaFá BaFá* and *Re-Mission*, as examples of how these five features serve as organizing processes.

Competition, be it with other players, a computer, or a timer, can motivate players to achieve learning outcomes in pursuit of winning the game (Alessi & Trollip, 2001). Competition can encourage people to internalize health-related content that they may not have otherwise. For example, in *Re-Mission* players are in direct competition with leukemia, playing the role of a nanobot injected into a patient to fight cancer. This serves as an organizing mechanism whereby in-game learning outcomes can mirror real-world organizational priorities and where a sense of competition motivates people to internalize health information. In *Re-Mission*, patients are motivated to learn about their own cancer treatment through gameplay.

In-game goals can go hand-in-hand with competition. In any game, participants have in-game goals that they are directed to achieve. As an example, the goal of many tabletop games is to achieve more victory points than your competitors in order to win the game. However, serious games often set goals that are beyond a traditional win-lose dichotomy present in many pure entertainment games (Charsky, 2010). For instance, in *BaFá BaFá* players are tasked with intimately learning the qualities of another culture. These goals do not dictate win/lose game scenarios, but instead determine the extent to which one engages, understands, and accepts cultural differences. Goals in serious games are often set to achieve organizational objectives. As an example, cultural differences between health care providers and the communities they serve are often a major barrier to effective care; however, researchers in transcultural nursing care found that *BaFá BaFá* was effective in overcoming this barrier to increase cultural awareness among nurses (Tuck & Harris, 1988; Graham & Richardson, 2008). In essence, setting goals in games can assist organizations in dictating agendas concerning health outcomes.

Game rules, which provide constraints on players' actions, help advance the goals of serious games by replicating the limits of real-world situations (Alessi & Trollip, 2001; Charsky, 2010). Rules can also be educational by demonstrating the amount of control or power that an individual or group can have in a given situation (Hannafin & Peck, 1988). Additionally, rules may be helpful in establishing, demonstrating, and reinforcing organizational norms. To illustrate, the communication of game rules can establish codes of conduct that participants may understand as being emblematic of organizational practices and values, which can help new members or non-members identify with the organization (Giddens, 1991). Rules also recreate hierarchies found within organizations. These constraints provide a framework of behavior for individuals while at the same time possibly challenging held beliefs. This "trade-off" is not dissimilar to the acculturation process employees undergo as new members of organizations. In *BaFá BaFá*, the rules establish cultural competence as a value of the organization, encouraging participants to interact with and understand the viewpoints of others.

Emerging from the rules is choice, which refers to the options and decisions that players can enact (Hannafin & Peck, 1988). In-game choices can motivate players to engage with educational content embedded within the game (Charksy, 2010). Increased motivation from gameplay can lead to more in-depth processing of health-related messages, which could ultimately lead to stronger and more lasting outcomes (Klimmt, 2009). In-game choices can also act as proxies for real health-based decisions that people may make, adding experiential learning to gameplay. In *BaFá BaFá*, although interaction is expected and encouraged through rules, ultimately individual motivations and choices determine the extent to which one personally explores and understands the others' culture. Some games intentionally limit choice to reflect the limited amount of efficacy that some people may face in difficult situations. This game feature can be seen in *Spent*, a game designed to simulate the struggle with homelessness and poverty, where players have severely limited resources to devote to a litany of essential expenses (Urban Ministries of Durham, 2014). From playing *Spent*, organizational members begin to see the choices inherent in organizing and consequences of those choices as they relate to goal hierarchies.

Finally, serious games can place participants into contexts and situations that they would not otherwise experience. In this way, games can function as fantasy-based narratives that have the capacity to affect outcomes in ways similar to entertainment education interventions (Wang & Singhal, 2009). For example, *Re-Mission* immerses players into cancer treatment on a cellular level. This provides young cancer patients with a unique perspective on how specific medicines and treatments fight cancer within their own bodies. This change in roles and contexts could be used in various health and organizational contexts to change perspective, knowledge, learning, and action.

Theoretical Approaches to Serious Gaming

Various theoretical frameworks have been studied to both develop and assess serious games. For instance, some have utilized the theory of reasoned action and theory of planned behavior to develop games that promote healthy eating among young adults (Peng, 2009). Others have used the elaboration likelihood model to explain how games can increase the likelihood that people critically think about underlying health messages (Baranowski, Buday, Thompson, &

Baranowski, 2008). From a meta-theoretical perspective, some understand serious games through the lens of symbolic interaction theory, viewing games as a safe play space where people can experience and interact with their social world (Kato, 2010; Mead, 1982).

However, recent research assesses the effects of serious games interventions from an entertainment education perspective, borrowing constructs from such theories and models as Bandura's (1986) social cognitive theory (SCT), the extended elaboration likelihood model (EELM; Slater & Rouner, 2002), and the entertainment overcoming resistance model (EORM; Moyer-Gusé, 2008; Moyer-Gusé & Nabi, 2010). Further, health organizations could also take a cultural schema theory (Garro, 2000) perspective when conducting game-based research.

Social Cognitive Theory

SCT posits that knowledge and behavior are influenced by observing others' experiences and using those observations to inform future behavior (Bandura, 1986; Bandura, 1998). SCT is perhaps the most common theoretical framework used by researchers to inform the development of serious games interventions, infer how serious games can affect health-based outcomes, and in limited capacities, to assess the mechanism of effect through which games can influence health. SCT is an appropriate framework for the study of serious games because of the ways in which learning occurs in response to gameplay. Games allow people to learn both by observing other players/characters and directly through enactive experience in a safe, simulated environment (Peng, 2008; Lin, 2013), a process analogous to new members' assimilation and socialization into an organization.

Many serious games can facilitate enactive learning among players. Take, for instance, *Humans vs. Mosquitoes*, a game designed to communicate the role mosquitoes and breeding grounds play in exposing humans to vector-borne diseases, including dengue fever and chikungunya (Ewing et al., 2014). This game has been used to facilitate enactive learning in a fun and interactive environment. The game can be played in varying formats for different age groups and situations, including gesture-based, physical play-based, and card-based versions. The different versions of the game highlight the ways in which games can function at multiple levels of an organization to engage community action. *Humans vs. Mosquitoes* works on both a policy level to convey organizational goals and norms to community leaders, and an individual level as an educational tool to engage children with the message and teach them community-based solutions to a significant health threat.

To begin, two to eight players divide equally into two teams: humans and mosquitoes. The humans' goal is to eliminate all mosquitoes by removing all 'egg' tokens from play, while the mosquitoes' goal is to 'bite' the human players to both deplete a human's strength and gain a new egg token. In each round, each human player must choose to either clear a particular breeding ground of

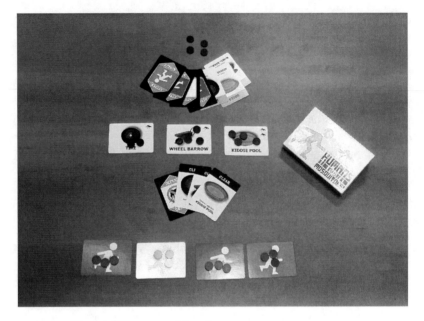

FIGURE 15.1 Photo of *Humans vs. Mosquitoes*.

one egg token or take preventive measures to avoid all attacks by mosquitoes. Each mosquito player must choose one of the following options: attack a specific human player in hopes that they are not protected, or, if the mosquito team has an available egg, breed in a particular location. This interconnected gameplay requires players to cooperate as a team, anticipate others' strategy, and act strategically. The game provides a safe space for individuals to learn about disease vectors in a hypothetical situation, mitigating risk of infection. Through situated learning players are able to apply information on the relationship between breeding grounds and disease to the real world. In this way, the game demonstrates the potential for community-based collective action: individuals who play the game become change agents for a community by influencing others around them (see Taylor & Kent, this volume) with further potential to affect community-level norms and actions. In this way, games can serve as tools to disseminate information and behavior through communities.

Some of the prominent organizing features of serious games showcased in *Humans vs. Mosquitoes* are goal-setting, rules, and choice. To demonstrate, each group has competing goals to eradicate one another in a zero-sum game, which encourages cooperation among teammates, shared decision-making, and the development of a common strategy, as individual actions in the game can affect team outcomes. The rules help players visualize distinct types of breeding grounds, which can be modified to match typical breeding grounds of a particular country or region. These features can help organize communities towards collective action by highlighting a particular health threat and providing the tools necessary to change the environment. Finally, each player can choose between several options on their turn; however, the goals of the game reward cooperative decision-making, as individual decisions affect team-based outcomes.

Some researchers have proposed several indirect effects of serious games derived from SCT, including enhanced attention, motivation to engage in message processing, self-efficacy, behavioral modeling, and behavioral feedback (see Baranowski et al., 2008 for a review). One example of a game that can increase perceptions of self-efficacy can be seen in *Awkward Moment*, a card game designed to address stereotype threat, prejudice, and implicit bias against women in science, technology, engineering, and math (STEM) fields (Flanagan et al., 2014). The game confronts this issue by encouraging associations between women and STEM to reduce stereotypes and show girls that they can pursue these professions. *Awkward Moment*, developed by the Tiltfactor lab at Dartmouth University, is a serious game disguised as a party game for middle-school-aged children. Players take turns being the Decider, who reveals both a Moment Card that describes a "hysterical, embarrassing, or stressful situation" and a Decider Card that provides a guideline for choosing a winning Reaction card (Tiltfactor, 2014a). All non-Decider players must choose which one of the Reaction cards in his or her hand best matches the Moment based on the Decider criteria. The Decider shuffles all the selected cards, reads them aloud, and selects the card he or she thinks is the best response. The player who has the greatest number of best responses at the end of the game wins. Game features such as competition and goals inspire players to identify card pairings that break traditional gender stereotypes regarding STEM participation.

Preliminary findings suggest that gameplay results in increased associations between women and STEM and increased perceived assertiveness to confront social bias (Tiltfactor, 2014b). *Awkward Moment* demonstrates the power of games to increase self-efficacy to overcome perceived cultural barriers and stigmas. This game can function in part by providing vocational anticipatory socialization messages (see Myers & Gailliard, this volume) for adolescent girls to normalize female participation in STEM fields. In short, *Awkward Moment* provides middle-school-aged children, principally girls, with encouragement to pursue STEM education and careers, as well as the potential to form identities associated with those careers (Myers, 2005; Jahn & Myers, 2014). *Awkward Moment* disrupts the established, gendered assumptions associated with health care occupations (see Barbour, Gill, & Dean, this volume).

Models of Entertainment Persuasion

The EELM was developed to explain how persuasion takes place in contexts where the primary goal of a message is not to persuade (Slater & Rouner, 2002). The model specifies six different routes through which receivers can process messages, one of which, hedonic processing, is engaged when individuals consume media for entertainment purposes (Slater, 1997). Given the fact that games are created to entertain and increase enjoyment, it is likely that games, and potentially serious games, are processed hedonically. Hedonic message processing differs from the traditional central and peripheral processing routes specified by the elaboration likelihood model (Petty & Cacioppo, 1986), in that issues involvement, source credibility, and argument quality become less relevant, and the relationship between message exposure and outcomes is influenced primarily by character involvement, or identification, and absorption into a narrative, or transportation (Slater & Rouner, 2002).

The EORM describes how changes in attitudes, beliefs, and behaviors can occur from exposure to an entertainment narrative (Moyer-Gusé, 2008; Moyer-Gusé & Nabi, 2010). The model proposes that engagement with characters and narrative can be useful as a way to overcome cognitive resistance to persuasion. In total, the model posits seven different media exposure variables and seven mediators that can influence persuasive outcomes (Moyer-Gusé, 2008). However, to date, only some of the propositions of the EORM have been formally assessed. Based on initial propositions put forth in the EELM, the EORM posits that transportation and identification are crucial factors that can explain persuasive outcomes in response to entertainment media.

Problematically, conceptual definitions for identification and transportation have been historically confounded. Identification in entertainment contexts is defined as personally experiencing the attitudes, beliefs, and emotions of another (Cohen, 2001; Moyer-Gusé & Nabi, 2010). Transportation refers to the process of becoming lost in a narrative, leading to story-consistent attitudes and beliefs, and increased emotional attachment to characters (Green & Brock, 2000). Recent work has sought to conceptually and operationally distinguish the measures, conceptualizing identification as emotional and cognitive connection with characters, and transportation as a more general sense of cognitive and affective involvement with the plot rather than associations with particular characters (Tal-Or & Cohen, 2010).

Identification is thought to increase persuasive outcomes in two important ways. First, increased identification with characters in narratives is associated with increased perceived vulnerability to harms experienced by that character (Moyer-Gusé & Nabi, 2010). To provide more context, if one feels similar to a character and experiences thoughts and emotions from the perspective of that character, he or she may feel more susceptible to the same health threats encountered by that character. This could be particularly important in the context of serious games to address health outcomes. Additionally, both identification and transportation into a narrative are hypothesized to be associated with decreased counter-arguing (Moyer-Gusé, 2008). Generally, the more one identifies with a character and transports into a narrative, the more likely one should experience story-consistent attitudes and beliefs, as well as diminished counter-arguing against information presented in the narrative (Moyer-Guse, 2008).

Examples that highlight the impact of identification and transportation on outcomes can be seen in *Cops and Rubbers*, a facilitated tabletop game in which players take on the role of sex workers (Tran, 2014), whose health and human rights are often at risk due to policy that allows condoms to be treated as contraband (Shields, 2012). This game was commissioned by Open Society Foundations to provide an experiential learning opportunity that addresses the consequences of the condoms-as-evidence-of-prostitution policy from the perspective of a vulnerable sex worker. To begin, players are each given a persona card which provides background about their in-game character. Each player then works towards two goals: (a) earn money for basic needs (e.g., paying rent,) and (b) avoid sexually transmitted infections. These in-game goals are consistent with most people's values, which allows players to more easily identify with their game character and potentially reduces stigmatization of sex workers. Through the use of narrative elements, players are drawn into their roles. Players are assigned names to go along with their character's identity and backstory, and players are referred to by these names throughout the game, increasing the likelihood that players will transport into the narrative and identify with their characters. In each round of the game, players attempt to 'hide' condoms in order to have safe sex with a client. If the police catch a player in possession of a condom, it may be confiscated. Alternatively, the police may destroy it and threaten to arrest the player unless he or she gives money or sex to the police. Thus, players quickly realize the emotional struggle faced by this population due to the condoms-as-evidence policy.

Cops and Rubbers utilizes multiple, interrelated game features, including goal-setting, rules, choice, and placing players in novel contexts to facilitate outcomes. First, players are presented with competing goals: meet your financial objectives in the game while also avoiding sexually transmitted infections. These goals often place players in situations where they have a difficult choice to make: if the police take their condom, they can either take a client at the risk of their own health, or choose not to make any money that turn, sacrificing financial goals for personal health. The rules of the game were designed purposefully to limit the amount of choice that players have in-game. For instance, there is no option for players to acquire condoms outside of the limited confines of the rules, or to negotiate prices with clients. These restrictive rules allow players to experience situations that actual sex workers may experience themselves, including feeling limited efficacy or control over their choices in difficult situations. These strategies can increase empathy for others who are dealing with hardships that are ordinarily too difficult, complex, or deeply personal to intuitively understand without the role-playing perspectives afforded by serious games.

Cops and Rubbers exemplifies Ganesh and colleagues' (2005) call for increased attention to modes of resistance that transform the dominant narratives and disrupt power relationships to influence large-scale policy changes. In addition to

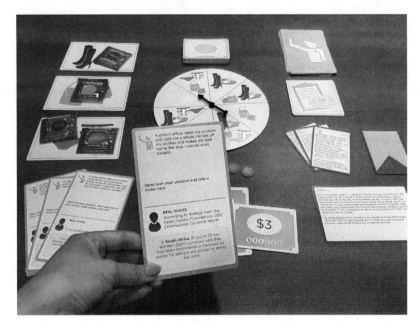

FIGURE 15.2 Photo of *Cops and Rubbers.*

shifting public perceptions on policy change, the game can function to institute organizational change within policing agencies. For instance, in high-reliability organizations like law enforcement, it is not uncommon to see high levels of concertive control, where organizational norms, policies, and values are developed through a negotiated consensus among members (Barker, 1993; Myers & McPhee, 2006). Through the narrative of the game, police officers may attain a more holistic and empathic understanding of the difficulties faced by sex workers that can counter the typical law enforcement narratives of their daily lives, thus leading to institutional changes from within police organizations with policies such as condoms-as-evidence.

At the time of this writing, *Cops and Rubbers* is still being evaluated; however, preliminary evidence suggests that the game results in higher intentions to oppose the condoms-as-evidence policy than an informational brochure on the issue, and no difference in knowledge compared to the brochure, suggesting that people can get similar knowledge about the policy from playing the game as reading educational materials (Tran, Lang, Carcioppolo, & Beyea, 2014).

Cultural Schema Theory, Role-Taking and Role-Playing

According to cultural schema theory, when individuals are engaged in situations within their own culture, they utilize pre-existing knowledge and information, or schemas, in their interactions (Garro, 2000). Cultural schemas, although habituated, are less rigid than stereotypes and often malleable. In the context of serious games, cultural schema may be present at various levels and may represent existing knowledge about an individual's own culture (specific cultural) or general cultural differences (Abbe, Rentsch, & Mot, 2009). Studies have found that individuals process situations based on experiences they have committed to memory (Barsalou, 1999), such as the narratives, rituals, and norms that shape organizational culture (Eisenberg & Riley, 2001). Using these stored memories when engaging in a new activity, individuals are able to run simulation-like moments in their mind and formulate responses to these new situations (Gee, 2009).

In the process of experiencing and interacting within game-based cultural environments, people are engaged in either role-taking or role-playing behavior. Role-playing is the adoption of a character's point of view through the development of empathic feelings (Mead, 1934). Symbol-mediated environments (e.g., simulating a culture or describing a situation) allow individuals to actively engage in role-playing (Peng, Lee, & Heeter, 2010). This is accomplished by creating an environment in which players are able to play roles in which their cultural schema offers very little support in interpreting new experiences (Wendorf, 2014). It is important to differentiate between role-playing and role-taking. Role-taking enables an individual to occupy a familiar position or status, as in the case of a woman taking the role of a mother by care-taking for her child (Coutu, 1951). Role-playing, however, is distinctly different as it involves a purely mental or cognitive process (Mead, 1934). Individuals are said to be role-playing when momentarily suspending previously held ideologies and taking the perspective of another (Coutu, 1951, p. 180). Coutu (1951) states that individuals are able to rehearse the attitudes, perspectives, and perceptions of others through the process of role-playing. This notion of role-taking and role-playing is central to understanding the perspectives of others within organizations, such as the experiences of doctors and nurses, the different perspectives involved in team-based care, as well as the those involved in transdisciplinary research (see Silk & Smith, this volume).

Conclusion and Future Directions

Serious games represent an effective strategy for health organizations to encourage members, communities, and individuals to engage with, process, and internalize health-based messages. From an organizational perspective, serious games integrate well within the autogenetic perspective on organizing, where organization occurs "through the self-organizing capacities of individuals interacting in a social field" (Drazin & Sandelands, 1992; p. 231). As described in this review, the formal features of games allow for a more interactive form of engagement with health messages than traditional health communication intervention materials. As such, these features tend to influence health outcomes through different cognitive mechanisms than traditional health messages, many of which can be described through models of entertainment education.

Still, serious games are more than entertainment education as they represent an interactive, customizable, replicable learning experience, much of which remains under-researched. For years, health organizations—and organizations more broadly—have used games to facilitate understanding of dynamic and multifaceted systems. While there are extant theoretical frameworks that can be used to describe the process through which games exert influence on health outcomes, we know less about specific organizational influences.

One priority of future research should be to identify the organizational communication constructs that can explain how serious games can influence health outcomes. For example, games can be explored in terms of their ability to facilitate perceptions of organizational identity. Many members of health organizations, nonprofit charities in particular, are volunteers who work infrequently and often outside of formal organizational spaces and may not experience the types of organizational identification that other, more traditional workers perceive (Ashcraft & Kedrowicz, 2002). Perhaps serious games can be useful as a tool to facilitate distinct organizational identities among these types of members, which in turn can influence health-related outcomes.

Serious games can also be a useful organizing process to encourage collaboration among members. This can be done through the establishment of in-game goals, which may be useful to elicit collaboration among positions in organizations that are historically contentious, such as doctors and nurses. Games that require collaboration, and competition against a shared opponent, may be able to facilitate more cooperative working environments in real life. Considering this, future research should explore the utility of using a games-based approach to encourage cooperation among team members.

Additionally, games represent a compelling strategy to influence knowledge and compliance with occupational health and safety issues within organizations. As one example, previous research has shown that handwashing compliance is quite poor in health care settings (Pittet et al., 2000). There remains a clear disconnect between the knowledge that health care providers possess regarding the relationship between hand hygiene and disease, and their own hand washing behavior. Perhaps games can serve as a novel training strategy to increase compliance with safety procedures that suffer from low adherence. Seeing the outcomes of poor versus adequate handwashing adherence in a game setting can help reinforce the need for such policies at the organizational level. Future work should explore how incorporating game-based training procedures compares to typical organizational training endeavors.

Games can also provide a safe space in which high-reliability organizations are able to increase knowledge with minimal risk (e.g., developing best practices for infectious outbreaks such as Ebola). Similarly, games can be adapted to specialties (i.e., infectious disease or pediatrics) and modified with relative ease, allowing numerous learning opportunities for health care professionals (Castro-Sanchez, Charani, Moore, Gharbi, & Holmes, 2014). Digital games can also be tailored to individual needs. Tailoring, or the process of customizing a message for an individual, has demonstrated a small but significant effect on intervention outcomes. In their meta-analysis Noar, Benac, and Harris (2007) found that tailoring is more effective when intervention materials are perceived as attractive and visually appealing, suggesting that professionally designed, visually appealing, tailored games may find success. Future work in this area should explore how tailored experiences influence game outcomes.

Lastly, games offer novel methods of organizing that can demonstrate organizational norms, rules, and values. As Allport (1962) suggests, rules and other-directed behaviors guide actions and consequences, generating the social structure of the organization. Therefore, in-game rules can help organizations instill norms and social structure in their members, and also easily demonstrate those norms, values, and collective structure to those in the community. Although some theories of entertainment education describe how entertainment media can influence behavioral outcomes through normative mechanisms (Moyer-Gusé, 2008), little research has been conducted to explore this phenomenon, particularly within organizational situations.

DISCUSSION QUESTIONS

1. How can serious games function to encourage collaboration among organizational members?
2. Describe the ways in which the formal features of games can be useful as methods of organizing.
3. What is the difference between role-taking and role-playing? How can the adoption of new roles in the context of a game affect organizational culture?
4. Why may serious games be particularly useful as a training or intervention tool among high-reliability organizations?
5. What theoretical components can explain how serious games can impact health outcomes?

Suggested Reading

Moyer-Gusé, E. (2008). Toward a theory of entertainment persuasion: Explaining the persuasive effects of entertainment-education messages. *Communication Theory*, 18, 407–425.

Peng, W. (2009). Design and evaluation of a computer game to promote a healthy diet for young adults. *Health Communication*, 24, 115–127.

Ritterfeld, U., Cody, M., & Vorderer, P. (Eds.). (2009). *Serious games: Mechanisms and effects*. New York: Routledge.

References

Abbe, A., Rentsch, J., & Mot, I (2009). *Cultural schema: Mental models guiding behavior in a foreign culture.* U.S. Army Research Institute for the Behavioral and Social Sciences. Retrieved from http://www.deomi.org/eoeeoresources/documents/Cultural_Schema-Abbe.pdf.

Abt, C. C. (1970). *Serious games.* New York: Viking Press.

Alessi, S. M. & Trollip, S. R. (2001). *Multimedia for learning: Methods and development* (3rd ed.). Boston, MA: Allyn and Bacon.

Allport, F. H. (1962). A Structuronomic conception of behavior: Individual and collective. *Journal of Abnormal and Social Psychology, 64,* 3–30.

Ashcraft, K. L. & Kedrowicz, A. (2002). Self-direction or social support? Nonprofit empowerment and the tacit employment contract of organizational communication studies. *Communication Monographs, 69,* 88–110.

Bandura, A. (1986). *Social foundations of thought and action: A social cognitive theory.* Upper Saddle River, NJ: Prentice Hall.

Bandura, A. (1998). Health promotion from the perspective of social cognitive theory. *Psychology and Health, 13,* 623–649.

Baranowski, T., Buday, R., Thompson, D. I., & Baranowski, J. (2008). Playing for real: Video games and stories for health-related behavior change. *American Journal of Preventive Medicine, 34,* 74-82.e10.

Barsalou, L. W. (1999). Perceptual symbol systems. *Behavioral and Brain Sciences, 22,* 577–660.

Berson, J. (2014, February 4th). Spending on corporate training soars: Employee capabilities now a priority. *Forbes.* Retrieved from http://www.forbes.com/sites/joshbersin/2014/02/04/the-recovery-arrives-corporate-training-spend-skyrockets/.

Boyd, C. (2006, July 6th). *Darfur activism meets video games.* BBC. Retrieved from: http://news.bbc.co.uk/2/hi/technology/5153694.stm.

Boyle, E. A., Connolly, T. M., & Hainey, T. (2011). The role of psychology in understanding the impact of computer games. *Entertainment Computing, 2,* 69–74.

Castro-Sánchez, E., Charani, E., Moore, L., Gharbi, M., & Holmes, A. (2014). "On call: antibiotics": Development and evaluation of a serious antimicrobial prescribing game for hospital care. In *Games for health* (pp. 1–7). Wiesbaden, Germany: Springer Fachmedien Wiesbaden.

Charsky, D. (2010). From edutainment to serious games: A change in the use of game characteristics. *Games and Culture, 5,* 177–198.

Cohen, J. (2001). Defining identification: A theoretical look at the identification of audiences with media characters. *Mass Communication & Society, 4,* 245–264.

Connolly, T. M., Boyle, E. A., MacArthur, E., Hainey, T., & Boyle, J. M. (2012). A systematic literature review of empirical evidence on computer games and serious games. *Computers & Education, 59,* 661–686.

Corti, K. (2006). *Games-based Learning: A serious business application.* PIXELearning Limited. Retrieved from https://www.cs.auckland.ac.nz/courses/compsci777s2c/lectures/Ian/serious%20games%20business%20applications.pdf.

Coutu, W. (1951). Role-playing vs. role-taking: An appeal for clarification. *American Sociological Review, 16,* 180–187.

Drazin, R. & Sandelands, L. (1992). Autogenesis: A perspective on the process of organizing. *Organization Science, 3,* 230–249.

Eisenberg, E. M. & Riley, P. (2001). Organizational culture. In F. M. Jablin & L. L. Putnam (Eds.), *The new handbook of organizational communication: Advances in theory, research, and methods* (pp. 291–322). Thousand Oaks, CA: Sage.

Ewing, C., Tran, L., Dutta, M. F., Norskov, B., Labay, E. Colantonio, S. . . . Shrestha, K. (2014). *Humans vs. Mosquitoes*. Retrieved from http://humansvsmosquitoes.com/.

Flanagan, M., McClave, A., Ramos, V., Seidman, M., Downs, Z., & Punjasthikul, S. (2014). *Awkward Moment*. Retrieved from http://www.tiltfactor.org/game/awkward-moment/.

Games for Change (2014). *About games for change*. Retrieved from http://www.gamesfor-change.org/about/.

Ganesh S., Zoller, H. M., & Cheney, G. (2005). Transforming resistance: Critical organizational communication meets globalization from below. *Communication Monographs, 72*, 161–169.

Garro, L. (2000). Remembering what one knows and the construction of the past: A comparison of cultural consensus theory and cultural schema theory. *Ethos, 28*, 275–319.

Gee, J. P. (2009). Deep learning properties of good game: How far can they go? In U. Ritterfeld, M. Cody, and P. Vorderer (Ed.), *Serious games: Mechanisms and effects* (pp. 67–82). New York: Routledge.

Giddens, A. (1991). *Modernity and self-identity: Self and society in the late modern age*. Stanford, CA: Stanford University Press.

Graham, I. & Richardson, E. (2008). Experiential gaming to facilitate cultural awareness: Its implication for developing emotional caring in nursing. *Learning in Health and Social Care, 7*, 37–45.

Green, M. C. & Brock, T. C. (2000). The role of transportation in the persuasiveness of public narratives. *Journal of Personality and Social Psychology, 79*, 701–721.

Hannafin, M. J. & Peck, K. (1988). The design, development and evaluation of instructional software. New York: MacMillan.

Hopelab (2014a). About us. Retrieved from: http://www.hopelab.org/about-us/.

Hopelab (2014b). Our research: Narrative and empathy in remission. Retrieved from http://www.hopelab.org/our-research/narrative-empathy-remission/.

Jahn, J. L. S. & Myers, K. K. (2014). Vocational anticipatory socialization of adolescents: Messages, sources and frameworks that influence interest in STEM careers. *Journal of Applied Communication Research, 42*, 85–106.

Jarrell, K., Alpers, R., Brown, G., & Wotring, R. (2008). Using BaFá BaFá in evaluating cultural competence of nursing students. Teaching and Learning in Nursing, 3, 141–142. Doi: 10.1016/j.teln.2008.08.001.

Kato, P. M. (2010). Video games in health care: Closing the gap. *Review of General Psychology, 14*, 113–121.

Kato, P. M., Cole, S. W., Bradlyn, A. S., & Pollock, B. H. (2008). A video game improves behavioral outcomes in adolescents and young adults with cancer: A randomized trial. *Pediatrics, 122*, e305–e317.

Klimmt, C. (2009). Serious games and social change: Why they (should) work. U. Ritterfeld, M. Cody, & P. Vorderer (Eds.) *Serious games: Mechanisms and effects* (pp. 248–270). New York: Routledge.

Lee, K. M. & Peng, W. (2006). A brief biography of computer game studies. In P. Vorderer & J. Bryant (Eds.), *Playing computer games: Motives, responses, and consequences* (pp. 325–345). Mahwah, NJ: Erlbaum.

Lieberman, D. (2006). What can we learn from playing interactive games? In P. Vorderer & J. Bryant (Eds.), *Playing computer games: Motives, responses, and consequences* (pp. 379–398). Mahwah, NJ: Erlbaum.

Lin, J.-H. (2013). Identification matters: A moderated mediation model of media interactivity, character identification, and video game violence on aggression. *Journal of Communication, 63*, 682–702.

Mead, G. H. (1934). *Mind, self, and society*. Chicago, IL: University of Chicago Press.

Mead, G. (1982). *The individual and the social self: Unpublished essays by G. H. Mead*. Chicago, IL: University of Chicago Press.

Michael, D. R. & Chen, S. L. (2005). *Serious games: Games that educate, train, and inform*. Boston, MA: Course Technology.

Moyer-Gusé, E. (2008). Toward a theory of entertainment persuasion: Explaining the persuasive effects of entertainment-education messages. *Communication Theory, 18*, 407–425.

Moyer-Gusé, E. & Nabi, R. L. (2010). Explaining the effects of narrative in an entertainment television program: Overcoming resistance to persuasion. *Human Communication Research, 36*, 26–52.

Myers, K. K. (2005). A burning desire. *Management Communication Quarterly, 18*, 344–384.

Myers, K. K. & McPhee, R. D. (2006). Influences on member assimilation in workgroups in high-reliability organizations: A multilevel analysis. *Human Communication Research, 32*, 440–468.

Noar, S. M., Benac, C. N., & Harris, M. S. (2007). Does tailoring matter? Meta-analytic review of tailored print health behavior change interventions. *Psychological Bulletin, 133*, 673–693.

Peng, W. (2008). The mediational role of identification in the relationship between experience mode and self-efficacy: Enactive role-playing versus passive observation. *Cyberpsychology & Behavior, 11*, 649–652.

Peng, W. (2009). Design and evaluation of a computer game to promote a healthy diet for young adults. *Health Communication, 24*, 115–127.

Peng, W., Lee, M., & Heeter, C. (2010). The effects of a serious game on role-taking and willingness to help. *Journal of Communication, 60*, 723–742.

Petty, R. E. & Cacioppo, J. T. (1986). The elaboration likelihood model of persuasion. *Advances in Experimental Social Psychology, 19*, 123–205.

Pittet, D., Hugonnet, S., Harbarth, S., Mourouga, P., Sauvan, V., Touveneau, S., & Perneger, T. V. (2000). Effectiveness of a hospital-wide programme to improve compliance with hand hygiene. *The Lancet, 356*, 1307–1312.

Primack, B. A., Carroll, M. V., McNamara, M., Klem, M. L., King, B., Rich, M., . . . Nayak, S. (2012). Role of video games in improving health-related outcomes: A systematic review. *American Journal of Preventive Medicine, 42*, 630–638.

Ritterfeld, U., Cody, M., & Vorderer, P. (2009). Introduction. In U. Ritterfeld, M. Cody, & P. Vorderer (Eds.) *Serious games: Mechanisms and effects* (pp. 3–9). New York: Routledge.

Ritterfeld, U. & Weber, R. (2006). Video games for entertainment and education. In P. Vorderer & J. Bryant (Eds.), *Playing video games: Motives, responses, and consequences* (pp. 399–413). Mahwah, NJ: Erlbaum.

Rosser, J. C., Rosser, L. E., & Savalgi, R. S. (1997). Skill acquisition and assessment for laparoscopic surgery. *Archives of Surgery, 132*, 200–204.

Shields, A. (2012). *Criminalizing Condoms: How policing practices put sex workers and HIV services at risk in Kenya, Namibia, Russia, South Africa, the United States, and Zimbabwe*. Open Society Foundations.

Shirts, G. (2009). *Train the trainer: When used for diversity* [Powerpoint slides]. Retrieved from http://indstate.edu/diversity/docs/Bafa-Diversity-10-01-09.pdf.

Simulation Training Systems (2006). *BaFá BaFá*. Retrieved from http://stsintl.com/schools-charities/bafa.html.

Slater, M. D. (1997). Persuasion processes across receiver goals and message genres. *Communication Theory, 7*(2), 125–148. Doi: 10.1111/j.1468-2885.2002.tb00265.x.

Slater, M. D. & Rouner, D. (2002). Entertainment education and elaboration likelihood: Understanding the processing of narrative persuasion. *Communication Theory, 12,* 173–191.

Susi, S., Johannesson, M., & Backlund, P. (2007). *Serious games: An overview.* Technical Report HS- IKI -TR-07-001, School of Humanities and Informatics, University of Skövde, Sweden.

Szer, J. (1983). Video games as physiotherapy. *Medical Journal of Australia, 1,* 401–402.

Tal-Or, N. & Cohen, J. (2010). Understanding audience involvement: Conceptualizing and manipulating identification and transportation. *Poetics, 38,* 402–418.

Tiltfactor (2014a). *Tiltfactor Laboratory announces two new party games: Buffalo and Awkward Moment.* Retrieved from http://www.tiltfactor.org/tiltfactor-laboratory-announces-two-new-party-games-buffalo-and-awkward-moment/.

Tiltfactor (2014b). *Research projects.* Retrieved from http://www.tiltfactor.org/research/.

Tran, L. (2014). *Cops & Rubbers.* Retrieved from http://lienbtran.com/games/cops-rubbers/.

Tran, L., Lang, K., Carcioppolo, N., & Beyea, D. (2014, June). *Role-taking as an advocacy strategy for policy reform: A comparative analysis of presentation modes in evoking empathy and willingness to act.* Paper presented at the Games, Learning & Society Conference, Madison, WI.

Tuck, I. & Harris, L. (1988). Teaching students transcultural concepts. *Nurse Educator, 13,* 36–39.

Urban Ministries of Durham (2014). McKinney launches mobile version of *Spent.* Retrieved from http://umdurham.org/assets/files/PR_UMD_SPENT%20tablet_final.pdf.

Wang, H. & Singhal, A. (2009). Entertainment education through digital games. In U. Ritterfeld, M. Cody, & P. Vorderer (Eds.) *Serious games: Mechanisms and effects* (pp. 271–292). New York: Routledge.

Wendorf, J. (2014, November). *"Jugando a lo seguro" (playing it safe): An exploration of experiential game play for dengue awareness in Colombia.* Presented 100th Annual National Communication Association Conference. Chicago, IL.

Zagal, J. P., Nussbaum, M., Rosas, R. (2000). A model to support the design of multi-player games. *Presence, 9,* 448–462.

16

CONSTRUCTING ORGANIZATIONAL KNOWLEDGE

Theorizing Processes and Practices Conducive to Health

Heather E. Canary

For the past several decades, organizational theorists, researchers, and practitioners have investigated the phenomenon of *organizational knowledge* (Canary & McPhee, 2011). These investigations represent a number of disciplines, including management, information technology, communication, and many others. This chapter presents an overview of communication-centered approaches to organizational knowledge, although much of the literature reviewed comes from other disciplines. The focus throughout the chapter is on how processes and practices of organizational knowledge construction have varying potentialities for health and well-being.

Organizational knowing processes and practices impact a number of constituencies, including members of organizational sub-systems (e.g., Majchrzak, Faraj, Kane, & Azad, 2013; McWilliam et al., 2009; Sørensen & Holman, 2014) and external stakeholders such as patients (e.g., Stock, McFadden, & Gowen III, 2010), community members (e.g., Boyko, Lavis, Abelson, Dobbins, & Carter, 2012), and members of affiliated organizations (e.g., Gabbay et al., 2003; Sylla, Robinson, Raney, & Seck, 2012). The chapter begins with an overview of theoretical approaches to organizational knowledge. A majority of the chapter focuses on connections between knowing processes and health-related outcomes and how organizational knowledge theory and research translate to practice. The chapter concludes with a section that addresses future directions for communication approaches to organizational knowledge processes related to health and several questions to stimulate discussion of key concepts covered in the chapter.

Theoretical Approaches to Organizational Knowledge

Because of the variety of perspectives reflected in organizational knowledge work, several definitions exist for the term. For the purposes of this essay, I adopt a practice-based view of organizational knowledge put forth by McPhee, Corman, and Dooley (1999): "the symbolic and/or practical routines, resources, and affordances drawn on by organization members and social units as they maintain the institutional organization and/or coordinate their action and interaction" (p. 4). This definition highlights the collective feature of organizational knowledge that differentiates it from stocks of individual knowledge. That is, organizational knowledge specifically relates to those rules and resources that enable coordination among organizational members and that maintain the organization. So individual-level knowledge, such as how to treat a particular illness, becomes organizational knowledge when it is used within an organizational group to coordinate action in patient treatment. This definition also reflects a social-practice view of knowledge that has emerged as a dominant perspective on organizational knowledge in the twenty-first century. A practice view focuses research interests on what *happens* to construct knowledge, or on *how* people deem particular information sets as relevant or valued *as* knowledge, or on the *influence* of organizational structures, power, and procedures on knowledge construction and sharing. The emphasis in this perspective, then, is less on the *what* of knowledge and more on the *how* of knowledge in organizational settings.

Knowledge and Knowing

Although a practice view of organizational knowledge focuses on process, there has remained interest in different types of knowledge that are used to coordinate action in organizations. Scholars offer several typologies of organizational knowledge to account for different ways knowledge manifests to coordinate organizational action. One widely recognized distinction is between *explicit* knowledge and *tacit* knowledge, first posed by Polanyi (1967). Explicit knowledge is that which can be articulated, codified, and easily transferred or shared between organizational members. Standard operating procedures, codes of conduct, and other such organizational documents are examples of collections of explicit knowledge that help maintain the organization and coordinate action. Tacit knowledge, on the other hand, involves the more nuanced, practice-based knowledge that comes from embodied experiences and that may be more difficult to articulate. For example, experienced triage nurses in emergency departments might know by sight if an incoming patient is experiencing an "emergency" medical situation or a more routine medical problem, but such tacit knowledge is difficult to articulate. Rather, more explicit information such as vital signs and checklists become the explicit knowledge to coordinate patient care (see Reimer, Russell, & Roland, this volume, for further discussion of explicit and implicit knowledge in health care team's decision-making processes). Recent approaches to organizational knowledge recognize the importance of *both* dimensions and hold that organizational attempts to "make explicit that which is implicit" miss the point that Polanyi was making originally, which is that both types of knowledge co-exist and are necessary (McPhee, Canary, & Iverson, 2011). Indeed, many scholars have asserted that organizational knowledge is multi-dimensional, including experiential knowledge, abstract information, and culturally-bound understandings (see Canary, 2011, for overview of typologies). The importance of such typologies lies in their contribution to investigating how different processes might be involved, or needed, for capturing the richness of organizational knowledge to lead to positive outcomes.

The emphasis in most communication research of organizational knowledge has been less on knowledge as a possession than on knowing as a process. Empirical questions concern ways organizational members communicatively construct and share various types of knowledge in the ongoing accomplishment of organizational activities (e.g., Kuhn & Porter, 2011; Murphy & Eisenberg, 2011). This is particularly the case when examining organizational knowledge processes related to outcomes concerning health and well-being of various constituencies (Boyko et al., 2012; Leiter, Day, Harvie, & Shaughnessy, 2007; Stock et al., 2010). Prior empirical research has demonstrated that organizational structures, cultures, and more specifically policies, procedures, and practices, either support or stifle organizational knowledge construction processes (Leiter et al., 2007; Stock et al., 2010; McWilliam et al., 2009). This occurs within single location organizations as well as in complex, multi-location organizations (Sobo, Bowman, Aarons, Asch, & Gifford, 2008). Several theoretical approaches or frameworks have emerged in this work to explain knowledge processes and health-related outcomes. The discussion that follows elaborates on two practice-based constructs and two broader theories that have gained currency in recent empirical investigations of organizational knowledge and health-related outcomes.

Practice-Based Constructs

In health professions, the phenomenon of knowledge transfer and exchange (KTE) has become an important research focus (e.g., Boyko et al., 2012; Contandriopoulos, Lemire, Denis, & Tremblay, 2010; Dobbins et al., 2009; Mitton, Adair, McKenzie, Patten, & Perry, 2007). Early approaches to knowledge sharing in health professions focused on knowledge *transfer* between researchers and health practitioners. This approach focused on ways researchers could "push" information concerning their research results to relevant providers who were then expected to translate those results to clinical practice. Such an approach reflected a cognitive approach to knowledge that privileged expert-generated, explicit information as the most important component for clinical knowledge. That one-way, cognitive approach has been recently critiqued and replaced with the current approach, knowledge transfer and exchange (KTE; Boyko et al., Contadriopoulos et al., Mitton et al.).

KTE involves both "push" and "pull" processes, recognizing the social, situated nature of knowledge. There may be important information that should be "pushed" to relevant practitioners, but productive knowledge construction also includes the ability of practitioners to "pull" information they need to incorporate into clinical practice and the ability of relevant parties to negotiate *what* and *how* knowledge is to be used. In this way, KTE reflects a social practice perspective on organizational knowledge. Boyko et al. (2012) provide a broad definition of KTE: "a dynamic and iterative process that includes the synthesis, dissemination, exchange and ethically sound application of knowledge to improve health status, provide more effective health services and products, and strengthen the healthcare system" (p. 1938). Key features of constructive KTE processes include appropriate meeting environments (sufficient time, appropriate rules of engagement, adequate resources, etc.), the appropriate mix of participants (representing multiple interests and including people who are motivated to engage in the process), and the appropriate use of research evidence (providing information for balanced and inclusive discussion) (Boyko et al., 2012).

Some KTE research has investigated the role of "knowledge brokerage" in the KTE process (e.g., Burgess & Currie, 2013; Currie & White, 2012; Dobbins et al., 2009a; Dobbins et al., 2009b). This role, which may be filled by a person or by a group of people, "uses his/her in-between vantage position to support innovation through connecting, recombining and transferring to new contexts otherwise disconnected pools of ideas" (Burgess & Currie, p. S132). Because knowledge processes are influenced by, and dependent upon, organizational cultures, procedures, resources, etc., a knowledge broker who is familiar with all relevant cultures and contexts may facilitate more effective knowledge construction between groups (Burgess & Currie, 2013; Dobbins et al., 2009a). Knowledge brokers might facilitate knowledge construction between people situated in different organizations, such as between university-based researchers and hospital-based practitioners (Dobbins et al., 2009a, b). However, knowledge brokers might also facilitate knowledge construction between people in different professions or functions within the same organization, such as between nurses, doctors, and administrators (Burgess & Currie, 2013; Currie & White, 2012). Indeed, Currie and White argue that knowledge brokering may be a collective endeavor, dispersed across an organization that values knowledge sharing and the co-construction of practical knowledge such that the focus should be more on characteristics of knowledge brokering processes rather than on characteristics of a particular knowledge broker(s).

Some investigators of knowledge brokering processes have asserted that such efforts also might increase capacities to make decisions that are both based on relevant research and that are appropriate for the given organizational context (Contandriopoulos et al., 2010; Crisp, Swerissen, & Duckett, 2000; Dobbins et al., 2009a; Dobbins et al., 2009b). However, research of knowledge brokering situations has not demonstrated that there are better outcomes in terms of satisfaction with the process or actionable outcomes than in KTE processes that do not involve knowledge brokers (Dobbins et al., 2009b). For example, Currie and White (2012) found that their case study of dispersed knowledge brokering in a health care organization was not sustained long term after budget cuts eliminated key roles that engendered a knowledge-sharing organizational culture. As with the broader KTE construct, lessons learned from knowledge brokering research should not be construed as constituting a "one-size-fits-all" approach to effective knowledge processes in health care contexts (Burgess & Currie, 2013). Furthermore, Currie and White argue that conclusions drawn concerning knowledge brokering processes in health care contexts may be generalizable to other organizational contexts that have similar professional boundaries and bureaucratic structure. Such contexts, they assert, constitute important directions for future research that will elaborate and enrich understandings of the role of knowledge brokering in organizational outcomes. Theoretical approaches to knowledge construction, discussed below, provide further insights into outcomes of such practice-based constructs.

Theoretical Approaches

Institutional theory, with roots in sociology, has been used to explain organizational knowledge processes in health care organizations (e.g., Currie & Suhomlinova, 2006; Yang, Fang, & Huang, 2007). Institutional theory focuses on structural influences, both inside and outside organizations, on organizational knowledge processes. Lammers and Lambert (this volume) provide an excellent overview of using institutional theory to explain health care organizational processes so I focus my attention specifically on using the theory to explain organizational knowledge processes. Institutional theory asserts that norms, rules, and regulations of particular professions (such as academics or medical doctors) and of particular industries (such as health care or air transportation) create particular pressures that become institutional structures for practice. By extension, scholars adopting institutional theory assert that these institutional structures influence what counts as knowledge, who is recognized as sources of such knowledge, and what procedures are accepted for creating and disseminating requisite knowledge (Currie & Suhomlinova, 2006).

This theory is useful for contextualizing KTE and knowledge brokering processes discussed above by theoretically explaining latent influences on manifest processes. Currie and Suhomlinova (2006) observed in their study that in spite of government-level emphases on interprofessional knowledge sharing to improve health outcomes, institutional pressures of the medical profession, research institutions, and organizational functional divisions constituted stronger influences on knowledge sharing than policy mandates. Accordingly, knowledge sharing was thwarted in ways that involved parties had not recognized or questioned.

Importantly, this theory is not only applicable to health care organizations. As the discussion below concerning health-related outcomes will make clear, knowledge construction processes in a variety of organizational contexts influence the health and well-being of stakeholders. Accordingly, institutional theory may be productively applied across organizational contexts to explain knowledge processes and how they associate with various health-related outcomes.

Another theory rooted in sociology, structuration theory (Giddens, 1984), also has guided recent efforts to explain connections between organizational knowledge processes and outcomes. Briefly, this theory rejects divides between structure and agency and between macro-features and micro-features as explanatory mechanisms for social action and outcomes. Rather, the theory asserts that institutional structure is produced, reproduced, and even transformed *in* action and that it is only in action that we can identify structural features being drawn on to enable and constrain ongoing actions and interactions. This is the concept of *duality of structure*. Giddens also proposes that people act knowledgably, even if that knowledge is unarticulated and rooted in routine practices. The theory describes three levels of knowledgeability—unconscious knowledgeability (below the surface of recognition, such as instinctive responses to put your hand out to break a fall), practical consciousness (experiential, routine knowledge, such as how to participate in a weekly staff meeting), and discursive consciousness (articulated and perhaps codified, such as the steps involved in sterilizing equipment). Most organizational knowledge research focuses on the second and third levels of knowledge because those are the levels of knowledge most commonly used to maintain the organization and coordinate actions/interactions among members.

One structuration-based line of research concerns developing evidence-based practices in health services (McWilliam, Kothari, Kloseck, Ward-Griffin, & Forbes, 2008; McWilliam et al., 2009). The framework, participatory action knowledge translation (PAKT), emphasizes the social and interactive nature of knowledge in health care contexts and accounts for the influence of social structures such as professional hierarchies and organizational bureaucracies. Drawing on the importance of individual-level agency and experience of involved people, meso-level structures of health care teams, and macro-level structures of involved organizations and professions, interventions are designed and implemented to facilitate five knowledge processes: (a) consider the evidence and opportunities; (b) reflect on barriers and facilitators; (c) brainstorm and prioritize strategies; (d) implement and evaluate change; and (e) instituionalize and diffuse change (McWilliam et al., 2008, p. 238). These elements of the PAKT process are rooted in the structuration theory concept of duality of structure, emphasizing the importance of reflective action and interaction that both draws on and transforms structural rules and resources for the purposes of translating relevant research-based information into appropriate practice-based knowledge.

Another structuration theory-based approach to organizational knowledge is represented in policy communication work conducted by my colleauges and me, in which we developed and applied structurating activity theory (SAT; Canary, 2010a; 2010b; Canary & Cantú, 2012; Canary & McPhee, 2009). SAT builds upon the structuration theory concept of duality of structure by incorporating meso-level constructs from cultural historical activity theory (Engeström, 1987). This work demonstrates how different elements of activity systems, which are collectivities of people, practices, and objects, influence ongoing accomplishment of activity and in the process structure future activity. These projects examined various aspects of organizational knowledge development in the context of disability policy dissemination, interpretation, and implementation.

As with other approaches discussed above, SAT work has focused on cross-system knowledge processes to explain how members of intersecting activity systems (such as different professions, organizational functions, and lay communities) communicatively construct requisite knowledge. This work elaborates on five communicative processes that were shaped by system-level elements and that structured future interactions and actions about disability policy in the focal organization: (a) identifying priorities; (b) expressing lack of knowledge; (c) explanations and clarifications; (d) posing potential consequences; and (e) expressing difference. These knowledge construction processes emerged in three frames of knowledge develoment: (a) orientation; (b) amplification; and (c) implementation (Canary, 2010a). Consistent with other policy research and with other knowledge research discussed above, these frames were not linear "stages" but rather represented different ways of talking about and working with policy that influenced policy knowledge and practices. Ultimately, these communication processes and knowledge frames influenced how policy was implemented, which in turn impacted the educational programs of children with disabilities. This approach to organizational knowledge will be discussed later in the chapter as well, in the section concerning translating theory to practice.

Knowledge Processes and Health-Related Outcomes

Processes through which organizational members and stakeholders develop requisite knowledge for effective functioning relate to health issues in a number of ways. Sometimes organizational knowledge processes relate to the health and well-being of organizational members, either directly through organization-sponsored information dissemination about health and well-being issues, or indirectly through interactional and socio-emotional processes such as conflict and feelings of efficacy at work. Steve May (this volume) provides an intriguing perspective on ways that employee assistance programs (EAPs), an increasingly popular element in health offerings for employees, constitute a way of constructing knowledge about health and well-being. Other times, knowledge processes relate to the health and well-being of people outside of the organization, such as by reducing health risks, implementing preventative health measures, and providing high quality care to patients. Both types of connections are discussed below.

Internal Stakeholder Well-Being

Burnout constitutes one dimension of organizational member well-being that has been linked to organizational knowledge processes. Typically, studies of employee burnout have focused on associations with stress, conflict, and other phenomena one might characterize as negative (see Wright & Nicotera, this volume, for overview). The research attention is warranted, considering the strong empirical support for negative job experiences and employee burnout, particularly in the helping professions such as health care.

It is less intuitive to investigate how organizational processes perceived as rather benign, such as knowledge transfer, might associate to negative outcomes such as burnout. Leiter et al. (2007) developed and tested a model of individual knowledge transfer (KT) activities, an organizational environment that values and supports knowledge transfer, and three dimensions of the work burnout–engagement continuum. Results revealed that organizational KT positively influenced personal KT, which in turn positively influenced reports of work efficacy. Additionally, manageable workload and organizational KT negatively correlated with burnout indicators of exhaustion and cynicism. These findings, while cross-sectional and preliminary, point to the important role that knowledge processes have for employee well-being dimensions, such as workplace efficacy, exhaustion, and cynicism. Sørensen & Holman (2004) conducted a study of occupational health interventions in six knowledge work organizations. Key concerns about workplace well-being among knowledge workers were:

> the difficulties of crafting solutions to ill-defined problems; knowing when a solution was acceptable; the complexity associated with administering, planning and coordinating several projects; and working on tasks that require uninterrupted problem-solving time but which also require knowledge-sharing and coordination with others.
>
> *(p. 80)*

Each organization implemented organization-specific interventions to address these problems, and two organizations did not actually implement any interventions. At the post-intervention evaluation, the two organizations that had implemented the most widespread changes in terms of work and relationship processes showed improvements on all eight indicators: job autonomy, workload, work tempo, manager relationship quality, leader skill, leader support, coworker support, and burnout. The medium-implementation and non-implementation organizations had either minimal changes or lower scores on those indicators. Although all participants in this study were engaged in the business of creating, harnessing, and/or disseminating knowledge as their jobs, communication-centered implementations such as increased feedback from supervisors and coworkers, improved meeting procedures, and the implementation of interaction rules were associated with indicators of workplace well-being.

Employee safety represents another health-related outcome empirically linked to organizational knowledge processes. Two contexts are highlighted in empirical investigations of this association. First, recent studies of high-reliability organizations (HROs) focus on the importance of productive organizational knowledge processes for keeping members of such organizations out of danger. These organizations involve high-risk, life-and-death work activities, such as fire and police departments, hospital emergency departments, military units, and other such organizational contexts where member knowledge is vital to successfully performing in high-danger situations (Myers, 2011; Weick & Roberts, 1993). In these organizations, organizational knowledge is valuable not because it leads to profit or successful project completion. Rather, it is valuable because it increases the reliability with which practices are enacted and lives are protected, both for organizational members and for those whom they serve (such as citizens at risk or patients).

One conclusion from studies of knowledge construction in HROs is that reliable, safe work activities are not solely the result of formal, codified knowledge sharing procedures. Myers (2011) describes the importance of group-level, informal knowledge construction for creating reliable organizational members. For example, she points out through a synthesis of prior empirical investigations that most organizational newcomers in HROs participate in formal training and orientation sessions when they first join a workplace. These are contexts for sharing explicit, codified knowledge and practices that, of course, are important for coordinating action and maintaining the organization. However, Myers notes that retrospective accounts by seasoned organizational members note that the "real" knowledge comes from long-term members sharing stories, from newcomers being corrected by old timers, and from work team members sharing work experiences together in real-time (see Myers and Gailliard, this volume for further discussion of socialization and assimilation into health care organizations). Weick and Roberts (1993) coined the phrase "collective mind" in their study of aircraft carrier work teams. Findings indicated that it was through ongoing coordinated action and the construction of embodied, encultured, and embedded knowledge that carrier crews developed a group-level, "collective" way of thinking that facilitated reliable and safe work procedures.

A second context for empirically examining the knowledge–safety link is in various occupational health and safety models and interventions. For example, Guzman, Yassi, Baril, and Loisel (2008) proposed that many occupational injuries and disabilities could be prevented by incorporating effective knowledge construction processes. Although the authors label such processes "knowledge transfer," the specific procedures they recommend (e.g., seeking input from all relevant stakeholders, conducting needs assessments with multiple methods, and disseminating information through multiple channels) reflect the KTE construct discussed above. These authors assert that high occupational injury and disability rates across contexts are closely tied to a lack of understanding of knowledge construction processes. Consistent with the idea of KTE, Kramer and colleagues (2010) employed the construct of knowledge brokering when they conducted a study using members of intermediary organizations as knowledge brokers between research organizations and work organizations in four industries. The goal was to examine the process of knowledge construction and perceptions of the process by members of the three types of organizations. Results indicated that the knowledge brokerage model was effective for making adjustments to interventions that would account for research-based knowledge as well as context-based knowledge of the workplaces. However, results were not reported regarding long-term outcomes such as reductions in musculoskeletal disorders, which were the focus of three of the four interventions.

These studies concerning worker exhaustion, burnout, and safety point to important consequences organizational knowledge processes have for members of a variety of organizations. The few studies focusing on both process and outcome indicate that there is a clear need for further theoretically-based work in this area. I will return to this issue in the final section of the chapter.

External Stakeholder Well-Being

The lion's share of research about health-related outcomes of organizational knowledge processes has focused on external stakeholders such as patients and community members. This emphasis is understandable in a contemporary organizational climate that extols quality customer service across professional sectors, including health care. Two predominant outcomes in this line of research are: (1) patient care and safety, and (2) knowledge outcomes for policy-related stakeholders that have longer-term health implications.

Many researchers have focused on how knowledge construction within health care organizations associates to patient care outcomes, including patient safety and medical errors (e.g., Murphy & Eisenberg, 2011; Sobo, Bowman, Aarons, Asch, & Gifford, 2008; Stock, McFadden, & Gowen III, 2010). However, little of this research uses objective measures of such outcomes. For example, Stock et al. (2010) measured patient safety by asking hospital employee participants to report on their perceptions of reductions in the frequency, severity, and impact of medical errors. Other studies have relied on similar self-reports from health care provider participants about improvements in patient care processes and connections between organizational knowledge processes and patient care and safety.

For instance, Murphy and Eisenberg (2011) discuss three frames of knowledge used by health care teams: knowledge as routinized, knowledge as emergent, and knowledge as political. Their qualitative study provides examples of how health care providers identified ways in which the nature of knowledge used, and the processes by which that knowledge was constructed, impacted patient care. Sobo and colleagues (2008) studied an intervention to improve HIV testing rates with organizational knowledge processes in Veteran's Administration hospitals but, like other studies, focused more on the *process* than on the outcome.

These studies, in combination with research discussed earlier in the chapter, indicate that there is widespread recognition in the organizational research community that process matters for health-related outcomes. However, so much emphasis has been placed on process that less rigor has been enacted to measure and describe outcomes related to those processes. Stock et al. (2010) noted the important role that organizational culture played in making connections between patient safety perceptions and knowledge acquisition, dissemination, and responsiveness. Although patient safety was measured by assessing hospital employee perceptions, their results come close to identifying predictive connections between cultural elements such as an emphasis on participation and openness ("group culture" elements) along with a focus on accomplishment and productivity ("rational culture" elements), organizational knowledge processes, and patient outcomes. Cumulatively, we know from this line of research that knowledge sharing cannot be taken for granted as occurring, that organizational cultures may facilitate or hinder requisite knowledge construction, that context needs to be considered to know what knowledge processes are constructive, and that constructive knowledge processes are perceived as leading to positive outcomes for patient care and safety.

Many studies have focused on how organizational knowledge processes relate to broader policy agendas and to policy-related stakeholders. Much of this research has employed the constructs of knowledge transfer and exchange (KTE) and knowledge brokering discussed earlier in the chapter. In fact, so much research has focused on these two concepts that several years ago a systematic review of literature identified research themes that could be used to guide further research (Mitton, Adair, McKenzie, Patten, & Perry, 2007). Not surprisingly, these themes comport with important issues discussed throughout this chapter, such as individual-level, organizational-level, communication-based, and timing-based barriers and facilitators to knowledge transfer and exchange processes. At the time Mitton et al. conducted their review of KTE articles, the focus on such research was not on tying process to concrete outcomes, such as specific ways knowledge processes resulted in policy or practice changes. However, research since that time has addressed this shortcoming (e.g., Dobbins et al., 2009a, b). For instance, Dobbins and colleagues compared three KTE strategies and found little impact on public health policy outcomes, although one difference emerged when taking the organizational research culture into account. The main take-away from this long line of research is that there is not one right way to impact policy or broader public health programs, although more recent KTE research points to general communication strategies that foster cross-system knowledge construction that may lead to policy outcomes that will impact the public health at large.

The importance of context for identifying appropriate organizational knowledge processes is also evident in more recent international public health work. For example, Sylla, Robinson, Raney, and Seck (2012) concluded that the form and function of communication strategies differed for various parties involved in providing health care in Senegal. They noted:

> [...] the crucial role that hierarchy and social organization play in the flow of communication and in knowledge exchange. Depending on where a given provider or manager is in the organizational, social, or community structure, he or she may be a central lynchpin in information sharing, may have access to information, or conversely may have little access to information.
>
> *(p. 61)*

Results from prior research concerning connections between organizational knowledge processes and health-related outcomes indicate future directions for translating theory and research into practice.

Translating Theory Into Practice

Empirical research quite clearly points to the inadequacy of relying solely on formal knowledge sharing processes for developing knowledge that relates to positive health outcomes. People are not simply information processing systems. We are social beings, and knowledge is social. Different processes work in varying ways across contexts. The most productive approaches to organizational knowing allow for flexibility in application across social systems. However, such conclusions from prior empirical work do not indicate that theory is irrelevant for practice. On the contrary, researchers and practitioners can apply theory to practice while also tailoring specific processes and procedures to particular organizational contexts. Theories used in prior work, such as institutional theory, structuration theory, and systems theory, are abstract enough to provide explanatory constructs that can be applied in a variety of organizational situations. Silk and Smith (this volume) describe an exemplar case study of a transdisciplinary research team developed to take a new approach to breast cancer. Their case study discussion is an excellent example of applying theories of *learning organizations* and the *communicative constitution of organizations* to the practice of team science oriented to improve health outcomes.

Structurating activity theory (SAT) is one theory that can be used to guide formative organizational knowledge research and the operationalization of constructs into organizational practices. Previous SAT-based work used the theory to examine policy knowledge processes across organizational systems and also between professional and family systems. Focal outcomes in those studies were different ways policy was implemented for educating children with disabilities. This work can easily be applied to other organizational contexts and to investigating connections between organizational knowledge processes and other health-related outcomes for various stakeholders, including patients, patient families, and organizational members. SAT constructs of mediating system elements (subject, rules, community, division of labor, and mediating resources) are abstract enough to apply across contexts. Researchers can use these system-level concepts, as well as the broader concepts of social structure and structuration, to theoretically explain how various organizational knowledge processes, such as development of health risk knowledge, result in particular health-related outcomes, such as changes in cancer screening behaviors.

A current project is using SAT to translate this type of research to an interaction tool that practitioners can use to improve their interactions with people at increased risk for cancer, a cross-system knowledge process with implications for how members of various social systems approach cancer screening. Our pilot study of conversations between trained genetic counselors and people at increased risk for colorectal cancer due to their family history resulted in a new coding system, the Resource-Based Interaction Coding System (R-BICS; Canary, Cummings, Bullis, & Kinney, 2013). Findings revealed ways in which elements of family, primary health care, cancer prevention and treatment, and health insurance systems emerged in intervention conversations and were associated with colonoscopy completion in unexpected ways. Although not a focus of the intervention design, results indicate greater prevalence of family stories, roles, rules, and relationship references among participants who completed colonoscopies after the intervention than for those who did not. One surprising finding of this pilot work is an apparent contradiction between participants' articulated positions that their healthy living and eating practices constitute sufficient preventative behaviors and counselors' positions that genetics play a large role in risk for CRC that healthy living alone cannot avert. Future work in progress will continue to reveal ways in which elements of our various social systems influence knowledge construction and how those processes influence how we talk about health and risk, make decisions for, and take actions that impact our health.

Conclusions and Future Directions

Several conclusions may be drawn from the issues reviewed in this chapter. I first discuss problematic knowledge processes that might be avoided when translating theory to practice. Second, I suggest future directions for research and theory of organizational knowledge processes as they relate to health outcomes. Finally, I highlight the most important issues from the chapter concerning the connections between theory and practice for organizational knowing and health.

Prior research has clearly pointed to problems that arise when knowledge is viewed as an object that should be uni-directionally passed from experts or upper management to others who are then expected to "use" that objective knowledge for some practical purpose. Such an over-simplified approach to knowledge-sharing results in a *loss* of knowledge across organizational systems, which may then result in poor outcomes for internal and/or external stakeholders. Furthermore, an objective, one-way approach to organizational knowledge processes truncates the rich, social process of knowledge *construction* that has been linked to positive outcomes such as workplace efficacy, satisfaction with organizational processes, and improved patient care. By extension, the research reviewed in this chapter clearly indicates that there is no one-size-fits-all approach to organizational knowledge processes that result in positive health and well-being outcomes. Context matters. Study after study indicates that researchers, administrators, and practitioners need to take time to establish relationships that foster knowledge co-construction and to identify potential barriers to putting knowledge into practice.

Just as important as taking context into consideration is the importance of translating theory into practice so that involved parties know *how* and *why* particular knowledge processes unfold and what explains their connections to outcomes for stakeholders. That is how knowledge processes can increase capacity for organizational members to use lessons learned from one knowledge process and successfully transfer relevant elements to other contexts. Using theoretical mechanisms such as organizational structures, organizational culture, agency and knowledgeability, and system mediating elements are all ways that theory can be translated into positive outcomes in terms of health and well-being for internal and external stakeholders without erasing the importance of organizational context and situational variables.

Future research can build upon what we know about constructive organizational knowledge processes in health care and other organizational contexts to more rigorously investigate connections to various health and well-being outcomes. The research that has so carefully examined aspects of process has been less focused on systematically measuring health-related outcomes of those processes. Participant self-reports or narratives about perceived outcomes have often been used as the measure of organizational knowledge outcomes. Future research needs to move beyond participant perceptions, particularly when impacted stakeholders may not be represented in those perceptions. Communication scholars are well-situated to take on such future work that will approach organizational knowledge as a situated, social process and that will rigorously examine health-related outcomes of such processes.

DISCUSSION QUESTIONS

1. How might a communication researcher engage the concepts of knowledge translation and exchange (KTE) and knowledge brokering to conduct research of health-related outcomes in a variety of organizational contexts?
2. This chapter presents structuration and institutional theories as representative of theoretical approaches to explaining knowledge construction processes in health-related contexts. What other theories might productively be applied to such processes and contexts?
3. What are communication-centered studies one might conduct to better understand connections between organizational knowledge processes and outcomes for employee health and well-being? What theoretical frameworks would productively guide such investigations?
4. If prior research indicates that organizational knowledge processes must be context-specific to be effective, how do we build a body of theoretical knowledge about associations between organizational knowledge processes and health-related outcomes?

Suggested Reading

Boyko, J. A., Lavis, J. N., Abelson, J., Dobbins, M., & Carter, N. (2012). Deliberative dialogues as a mechanism for knowledge translation and exchange in health systems decision-making. *Social Science & Medicine, 75*, 1938–1945.

Sørensen, O. H. & Holman, D. (2014). A participative intervention to imrove employee well-being in knowledge work jobs: A mixed-methods evaluation study. *Work & Stress, 28*, 67–86.

References

Boyko, J. A., Lavis, J. N., Abelson, J., Dobbins, M., & Carter, N. (2012). Deliberative dialogues as a mechanism for knowledge translation and exchange in health systems decision-making. *Social Science & Medicine, 75*, 1938–1945.

Burgess, N. & Currie, G. (2013). The knowledge brokering role of the hybrid middle level manager: The case of healthcare. *British Journal of Management, 24*, S132–S142.

Canary, H. E. (2010a). Constructing policy knowledge: Contradictions, communication, and knowledge frames. *Communication Monographs, 77*, 181–206.

Canary, H. E. (2010b). Structurating activity theory: An integrative approach to policy knowledge. *Communication Theory, 20*, 21–49.

Canary, H. E. (2011). Knowledge types in cross-system policy knowledge construction. In H. E. Canary & R. D. McPhee, *Communication and organizational knowledge: Contemporary issues for theory and practice* (pp. 244–263). New York, NY: Routledge.

Canary, H. E. & Cantu, E. (2012). Making decisions about children's disabilities: Mediation and structuration in cross-system meetings. *Western Journal of Communication, 76*, 270–297.

Canary, H. E., Cummings, J., Bullis, C., & Kinney, A. Y. (2013, November). Counselor-client conversations in a colorectal cancer screening intervention: An analysis of intersecting activity systems. Paper presented at the annual convention of the National Communication Association, Washington, DC.

Canary, H. E. & McPhee, R. D. (2009). The mediation of policy knowledge: An interpretive analysis of intersecting activity systems. *Management Communication Quarterly, 23*, 147–187.

Canary, H. E. & McPhee, R. D. (2011). Introduction: Toward a communicative perspective on organizational knowledge. In H. E. Canary & R. D. McPhee, *Communication and organizational knoweldge: Contemporary issues for theory and practice* (pp. 1–14). New York, NY: Routledge.

Contandriopoulos, D., Lemire, M., Denis, J.-L., & Tremblay, E. (2010). Knowledge exchange processes in organizations and policy arenas: A narrative systematic review of literature. *The Milbank Quarterly, 88*, 444–483.

Crisp, B. R., Swerissen, H., & Duckett, S. J. (2000). Four approaches to capacity building in health: Consequences for measurement and accountability. *Health Promotion International, 15*, 99–107.

Currie, G. & Suhomlinova, O. (2006). The impact of institutional forces upon knowledge sharing in the UK NHS: The triumph of professional power and the inconsistency of policy. *Public Administration, 84*, 1–30.

Currie, G. & White, L. (2012). Inter-professional barriers and knowledge brokering in an organizational context: The case of healthcare. *Organization Studies, 33*, 1333–1361. Doi: 10.1177/0170840612457617.

Dobbins, M., Hanna, S. E., Ciliska, D., Manske, S., Cameron, R., Mercer, S. L., . . . Robeson, P. (2009a). A randomized controlled trial evaluating the impact of knowledge translation and exchange strategies. *Implementation Science, 4*, 61–76.

Dobbins, M., Robeson, P., Ciliska, D., Hanna, S., Cameron, R., O'Mara, L., . . . Mercer, S. (2009b). A description of a knowledge broker role implemented as part of a randomized controlled trial evaluating three knowledge translation strategies. *Implementation Science, 4*, 23–31.

Engeström, Y. (1987). *Learning by expanding: An activity-theoretical approach to developmental research.* Helsinki, Finland: Orienta-Konsultit Oy.

Gabbay, J., le May, A., Jefferson, H., Webb, D., Lovelock, R., Powell, J., & Lathlean, J. (2003). A case study of knowledge management in mult-agency consumer-informed 'communities of practice': Implications for evidence-based policy development in health and social services. *Health: An Interdisciplinary Journal for the Social Study of Heatlh, Illness, and Medicine, 7*, 283–310.

Giddens, A. (1984). *The constitution of society.* Berkeley, CA: University of California Press.

Guzman, J., Yasi, A., Baril, R., & Loisel, P. (2008). Decreasing occupational injury and disability: The convergence of systems theory, knowledge transfer and action research. *Work, 30*, 229–239.

Kramer, D. M., Wells, R. P., Bigelow, P. L., Carlan, N. A., Cole, D. C., & Hepburn, C. G. (2010). Dancing the two-step: Collaborating with intermediary organizations as research partners to help implement workplace health and safety interventions. *Work, 36*, 321–332.

Kuhn, T. & Porter, A. J. (2011). Heterogeneity in knowledge and knowing: A social practice perspective. In H. E. Canary & R. D. McPhee, *Communication and organizational knowledge: Contemporary issues for theory and practice* (pp. 17–34). New York, NY: Routledge.

Leiter, M. P., Day, A. L., Harvie, P., & Shaughnessy, K. (2007). Personal and organizational knowledge transfer: Implications for worklife engagement. *Human Relations, 60,* 259–283.

Majchrzak, A., Faraj, S., Kane, G. C., & Azad, B. (2013). The contradictory influence of social media affordances on online communal knowledge sharing. *Journal of Computer-Mediated Communication, 19,* 38–55.

McPhee, R. D., Canary, H. E., & Iverson, J. O. (2011). Conclusion: Moving forward with communicative perspectives on organizational knowledge. In H. E. Canary & R. D. McPhee, *Communication and organizational knowledge: Contemporary issues for theory and practice* (pp. 304–313). New York, NY: Routledge.

McPhee, R. D., Corman, S. R., & Dooley, K. (1999, May). Theoretical and methodological axioms for the study of organizational knowledge and communication. *Paper presented at the 49th Annual Conference of the International Communication Association, San Francisco, CA.*

McWilliam, C. L., Kothari, A., Kloseck, M., Ward-Griffin, C., & Forbes, D. (2008). Organizational learning for evidence-based practice: A 'PAKT' for success. *Journal of Change Management, 8,* 233–247.

McWilliam, C. L., Kothari, A., Ward-Griffin, C., Forbes, D., Leipert, B., & SW-CCAC. (2009). Evolving the theory and praxis of knowledge translation through social interaction: A social phenomenological study. *Implementation Science, 4*(26).

Mitton, C., Adair, C. E., McKenzie, E., Patten, S. B., & Perry, B. W. (2007). Knowledge transfer and exchange: Review and synthesis of the literature. *The Milbank Quarterly, 85,* 729–768.

Murphy, A. G. & Eisenberg, E. M. (2011). Coaching to the craft: Understanding knowledge in health care organizations. In H. E. Canary & R. D. McPhee, *Communication and organizational knowledge: Contemporary issues for theory and practice* (pp. 264–284). New York, NY: Routledge.

Myers, K. K. (2011). Socializing organizational knowledge: Informal socialization through workgroup interaction. In H. E. McPhee, *Communication and organizational knowledge: Contemporary issues for theory and practice* (pp. 285–303). New York, NY: Routledge.

Polanyi, M. (1967). *The tacit dimension.* Garden City, NY: Anchor Books.

Sobo, E. J., Bowman, C., Aarons, G. A., Asch, S., & Gifford, A. L. (2008). Enhancing organizational change and improvement prospects: Lessons from an HIV testing intervention for veterans. *Human Organization, 67,* 443–453.

Sørensen, O. H. & Holman, D. (2014). A participative intervention to imrove employee well-being in knowledge work jobs: A mixed-methods evaluation study. *Work & Stress, 28,* 67–86.

Stock, G. N., McFadden, K. L., & Gowen III, C. R. (2010). Organizational culture, knowledge management, and patient safety in U.S. hospitals. *The Quality Management Journal, 17,* 7–26.

Sylla, A., Robinson, E. T., Raney, L., & Seck, K. (2012). Qualitative study of health information needs, flow, and use in Senegal. *Journal of Health Communication, 17,* 46–63.

Weick, K. & Roberts, K. (1993). Collective mind in organizations: Heedful interrelating on flight decks. *Administrative Science Quarterly, 38,* 357–381.

Yang, C., Fang, S., & Huang, W. (2007). Isomorphic pressures, institutional strategies, and knowledge creation in the health care sector. *Health Care Management Review, 32,* 263–270.

17

INSTITUTIONAL THEORY AND THE COMMUNICATION OF HEALTH CARE ORGANIZATIONS

John C. Lammers and Natalie J. Lambert

Institutional theory is concerned with the origins, endurance, and changes in rules and practices shared across organizational fields. The perspective has flourished in management and sociological studies—including studies of health organizations—over the last 30 years because it offers scholars a way of explaining phenomena at a macro level as well as at a micro level (Scott, Ruef, Mendel & Caronna, 2000; Shortell, Gillies, & Devers, 1995). Moreover, the institutional perspective emphasizes the shared cognitive strategies, value orientations, and beliefs that undergird common practices of organizations (Greenwood, Oliver, Sahlin, & Suddaby, 2008). For many years, institutionalists theorized and researched at a structural level of analysis, pointing out consistencies in organizational strategies and structures. Today, however, institutionalists have begun to attend to the communicative processes by which these strategies arise, are maintained, and changed. The approach has recently been adopted in studies of organizational communication (Barbour & Lammers, 2007; Barbour, 2010; Lammers & Barbour, 2006; Lammers & Barbour, 2009; Lammers & Garcia, 2013). Thus it is appropriate that studies of health communication take up this perspective, which, while consistent with intra-organizational communication studies, embraces inter- and cross-organizational communicative behavior as well.

In its communicative sense, institutional theory concerns the endurance, reach, and incumbency of messages (Lammers, 2011; Lammers & Jackson, 2014). Endurance refers to the establishment or sustained repetition of messages and ideas. Reach refers to the size and number of audiences influenced by a message. Encumbency refers to the tendency of some messages to require particular responses or behaviors from recipients. Institutions are therefore characterized by enduring patterns of communication that reach large audiences and have behavioral consequences. Researchers have recently employed a wide range of communication concepts to understand institutional influences, including framing (Cornelissen, Holt, & Zundel, 2011), rhetoric (Green, Babb, & Alpaslan, 2008), discourse (Phillips, Lawrence, & Hardy, 2004), messages (Lammers, 2011), and logics (Thornton, Ocasio, & Lounsbury, 2012; see also Lammers & Proulx, this volume). Indeed, a recently published essay on institutions, communication, and cognition urges that communication be placed front and center in institutional studies (Cornelissen, Durand, Fiss, Lammers, & Vaara, 2015).

Institutional theory is especially relevant to health communication because of the profound extra-organizational forces present in modern systems of care. These forces include government funding, regulations, and policies; private insurers' and health plans' contracts and reimbursement rules; professional roles, associations, and accrediting organizations; and the mass media, including new social media. Each of these phenomena exists independently of particular health care providers or organizations, and penetrates the affairs of organizations including the interactions between individual providers and patients. For example, the kind of health insurance coverage that an individual has is a strong predictor of timely or delayed care seeking. Institutional analysis would identify regularities in the strategies organizations such as hospitals employ to govern interaction with employees, patients, reimbursers, and the broader community. Thus, using an institutional approach, we might develop a greater understanding of local phenomena, identify sources of regularity and difference in practices, and ultimately participate in the improvement of care by identifying practice patterns that are or are not consistent with widely shared values.

This chapter focuses on the intersection of three strands of research and theory: health communication, organizational communication, and institutional analysis. After a brief review of the institutional approach, we review institutional research that pertains specifically to health care, mapping the literature onto the major concerns of health communication scholars, including interpersonal health communication research (patient–provider communication, including social support and family health communication); organizational health communication (communication about professional roles and service delivery arrangements); and mass-mediated health communication (health campaigns, social marketing, health effects of the media, and eHealth). Institutional insights are not typically made in these areas of health communication. However, in our last section we argue that the institutional perspective encourages fresh attention to the patient as a consumer who is awash in information and responsible for more choices than in the past; that providers face a new environment in which their expertise is constrained by the growth of clinical and administrative communication technologies and wide-spread regulations; and that the focus of mass mediated health messages has shifted to include new audiences of public policy decision-makers.

The Approach of Institutional Theory

The institutional approach to organizational analysis has deep roots in the socio-logical tradition (Weber, 1968; Selznick, 1949; Meyer & Rowan, 1977; DiMaggio & Powell, 1983; see Greenwood et al., 2008 and Lammers & Garcia, 2013 for summaries). Here we emphasize its general elements most useful at the intersections of institutions, health communication, and organizations: endurance, fields, and legitimacy. First, institutional analysis is concerned with social conduct which has "the greatest time-space extension within [societal] totalities" (Giddens, 1984, p. 17). Put more plainly, it concerns long-established, widely spread ways of getting work done. It is appropriate to refer to individual hospitals as institutions because of their *endurance* as social forms within communities (health communication scholars refer to hospitals as institutions, drawing on the gravitas of the term). It is also appropriate to refer to private health insurance (which affects many hospitals) as an institution. Note that the Affordable Care Act left private employer-sponsored insurance largely intact so that the institution of workplace coverage continues to characterize the way that most Americans pay for health care. It is also appropriate to refer to the long-established National Health Service in Britain and Medicare in Canada as institutions—enduring ways of delivering health care in those countries.

Second, institutional analysis is concerned with how this endurance character-izes not only individual organizations such as the local hospital, but also how it characterizes whole *fields* of organizations, "recognized area(s) of institutional life: key suppliers, resource and product consumers, regulatory agencies, and other organizations that produce similar services or products" (DiMaggio & Powell, 1983, p. 148). For example, grass-roots-based community clinics exist in many American towns and cities, and each has a unique character, staffed in part by local volunteers and supplied in part by local charitable organizations. But these clinics also survive in the same institutional environment as other public and private health organizations, subject to the same rules, regulations, and policies as others, so the institutionalists' attention is drawn to field-wide forces of consist-ency (termed *isomorphism*—see below).

Third, institutionalists commonly draw attention to *legitimacy* as the sym-bolic glue that holds institutional fields together (Ruef & Scott, 1998; Reay & Hinings, 2005). Organizational legitimacy is "a status conferred by social actors" that a particular organization "is one whose values and actions are congruent with that social actor's values and expectations for action. The social actor accepts or endorses the organization's means and ends as valid, reasonable, and rational" (Deephouse, 1996, p. 1025). For example, Scott, Ruef, & Mendel (1996) studied technical and managerial sources of legitimacy in a regional population of hospi-tals. They found that hospitals whose managerial structures achieved a high degree of legitimacy by shaping their structures to prevailing norms. Institutionalists, in other words, direct our attention to sources of legitimacy that characterize com-munication in health organizations.

Thus the foundations of institutional theory include the insights that organizations endure in fields of similar organizations where perceptions of organizational conduct as legitimate help assure the survival of particular forms. Organizational change efforts therefore must take field-level effects and forces into account, as the symbolic representations of legitimacy constrain and enable change. In looking at communication in health care organizations, we can see the persistence of forms that may be of dubious functionality but survive because of established norms of legitimacy. Daily struggles about the status or identity of health occupations and professions, or about the behavior of organizations such as nonprofit hospitals or federally qualified community health centers, or even the promulgation of the Affordable Care Act, all occur in an institutional context of established ways of doing work that are perceived as legitimate across organizational settings. Before applying the approach to health communication we turn to the most common conceptual tools institutionalists employ.

The Conceptual Tools of Institutional Theory

Institutionalists have been concerned about health care for many years (Alexander & D'Aunno, 1990; Lammers & Krikorian, 1997), but only recently have confronted communication as a body of scholarship. In this section we review four conceptual tools used in institutional analysis: isomorphism, logics, discourse analysis, and messages.

Isomorphism in Institutional Fields

A commonly observed phenomenon in institutional studies is isomorphism (DiMaggio & Powell, 1983). The tendency for organizations within fields to adopt similar forms via mimetic (i.e., competitive), normative, and coercive forces has been well-established (Deephouse, 1996). Zorn, Flanagin & Shoham (2011) noted institutional pressures on nonprofit organizations' adoption of communication technologies over and above functional requirements. More specifically in health communication, Berteotti & Seibold (1994) observed isomorphic forces at work in the establishment of a hospice team's members. The hospice team they studied "experienced coercive isomorphic processes as it tried to implement a team approach to health care within the context and [the] constraints of hierarchically structured organizations" (p. 127). They also observed that the team's members "had to struggle to avoid modeling [the team] on non-hospice organizations," and "that normative pressures played a role as the members tried to create organizational norms to define the conditions" (p. 127) of their tasks. Thus their study revealed the *reach* of institutional norms into the actions enacted by team members. Similarly, Lewis (2007) employed the concepts of institutional isomorphic forces in her predictive model of organizational stakeholder change communication.

Institutional Logics

Thornton and Ocasio (2008) defined institutional logics as "the socially con-structed, historical patterns of material practices, assumptions, values, beliefs, and rules by which individuals produce and reproduce their material subsistence, organize time and space, and provide meaning to their social reality" (p. 804). The goal of work using logics is, according to Thornton and Ocasio (2008), to connect micro interaction with macro structures (see the chapter by Lammers & Proulx, this volume, and below on the connection to institutional messages). Much management research and theorizing has focused on logics, and a good deal of it has to do with health care organizations (Currie & Guah, 2007; Goodrick & Reay, 2011; Kitchner 2002; Scott, 2004).

The logic approach sees organizations as the units of analysis and field-level phenomena as explanatory variables. For example, Kantola and Jarvinen (2012) examined the institutional logics of late-adopters of the treatment classification system known as Diagnosis Related Groups (DRGs) in Finland, which lagged the U.S. by nearly 20 years (see Geist & Hardesty, 1992). They found that the timing of adoption depended upon the prevailing logic employed by health ser-vices managers; that is, whether they saw their hospitals as independent of or connected to other municipal functions. In another example, through an exami-nation of the American Hospital Association's periodical *Modern Hospital* and other publications between 1920 and 1930, Arndt and Bigelow (2006) showed how the logic of efficiency became institutionalized in American hospitals. While norms of efficiency influenced practices at individual hospitals, the logics per-spective helps identify the field-wide forces at work in the spread and establish-ment of standardization and business practices from beyond health care (similarly, see Kennedy & Fiss, 2009 for an application of logics to the adoption of Total Quality Management in U.S. hospitals). Nigam and Ocasio (2010) showed how the Clinton health system reform effort had the somewhat ironic effect of cement-ing the logic of managed care both as a set of practices and a vocabulary for how the health care system should be maintained. The institutional logic of managed care subsequently superseded both the older logic of physician authority and the managed competition logic of the Clinton reform effort for nearly 20 years.

Discourse and Rhetoric

Institutionalists have employed rhetorical and discourse analysis in their studies (Sillince & Barker, 2012; Green, Babb, & Alpaslan, 2008). Rhetorical scholars have also applied their skills to communication and institutional issues in health care organizations. For example, Keränen (2007) examined the "interlocking institutional, technical, and vernacular deathbed rhetoric" (p. 179) surrounding implementation of do-not-resuscitate orders in a hospital. While Keränen did not explicitly couch her work in institutional theory, she did link the behavior of hospital staff to established and enduring rules. Geist and Hardesty (1992) identified the rhetorical standpoints of health care workers when the DRG system was implemented in two hospitals. They found that practitioners took up various persuasive positions as DRGs came to be the established way that procedures were to be classified. Some advocated for the system as a source of efficiency, others strategized ways to make the system work to obtain better care, still others worked as referees between the advocates and strategists, and a last group (bystanders) remained unengaged. While their purpose was to show how the order of the hospital was negotiated by the rival rhetorical standpoints, they also showed how the externally imposed DRG system was rhetorically engaged.

Institutional Messages

In an effort to extend institutional theory toward communication studies and organizational communication in particular, Lammers (2011) explored the colloquial and technical meanings of the term *institutional message*. The notion of institutional message, a "collation of thoughts that take on lives independent of senders and recipients" (p. 154), captures the sustaining effect of communication in established arrangements. Thus Lammers (2011) argued that institutional messages endure, reach wide audiences, call for a specific response, and have a rational purpose. Moreover, he argued that institutional logics are in practice actually carried in institutional messages. This work has begun to develop in studies of health care organizations (Smets & Jarzabkowski, 2013; Gray, Purdy, & Ansari, 2015; White, 2013). White, Thompson, and Griffith (2011) studied the prevailing institutional message of American hospitals, arguing that it needs to change in view of a reformed health care environment. Kulkarni (2014) examined the messages of three institutional orders (the state, profession, and corporation) to understand the process of change surrounding the implementation of electronic health records. In summary, the idea of the institutional message as a force (Lammers & Jackson, 2014) on organizations suggests that scholars seek those regular and established communicative arrangements that are similar across organizations. With foundational elements and conceptual tools in mind, we now turn to opportunities to improve communication research in health organizations from the vantage point of institutionalism.

Improving Health Communication Research With Institutional Theory

In this section we review samples of recent health communication research in three areas and offer institutional insights into that research. Health communication research may very broadly be divided into studies that spring from interpersonal communication (e.g., patient–provider and social support communication); organizational communication (including interprofessional communication and policy communication); and mass communication (persuasion, health campaigns, and electronically mediated health messages). Because these areas are so broad, our discussion of each area is limited to illustrate institutional themes. In particular, our focus on the mass communication area is limited to eHealth.

Patient–Provider Communication

Patient–provider communication research clearly demonstrates that both patients and doctors have firmly established expectations about their interactions with one another. Patients' satisfaction with a physician is correlated with their perceptions of the doctor's credibility, nonverbal behavior, and the waiting times patients experience before seeing the doctor (Moore et al., 2009). Simultaneously, doctors have expectations regarding how their interactions with patients should occur. Beisecker's (1989) study of communication between physicians and patients discovered that doctors' preferred communication routines are severely disrupted when a patient advocate is present. Doctors in that study chose to speak almost exclusively with patients, even when addressed most frequently by the patient advocate. Doctors exerted control during these conversations to attempt to return the communication to the 'normal' doctor–patient routine.

Examining patient–provider communication expectations from an institutional perspective helps to illuminate where communication expectations originate. Traditional doctor–patient interaction has become institutionalized (i.e., enduring, widespread, incumbent, and functional), so that professional expectations are the most influential predictors of doctor and patient satisfaction. This theoretical perspective compliments research findings that patients' locus of control can be influenced through positive interactions with physicians who assign patients concrete tasks towards improving their health (Arntson et al., 1989).

Institutional theory can also be used to understand the changing landscape of patient–provider communication. Not only do patients have preconceived expectations about providers' behaviors, they also alter their own communication strategies with providers. O'Hair (1989) found that although physicians try to maintain control of communication interactions with their patients, patients frequently attempt (and sometimes succeed) to exert communicative control over their doctors. Patients and doctors in his study attempted to exert control equally as often, but overall doctors retained more control of the communication interactions. Patients are clearly trying to take more control over their interactions with doctors than they have in the past (Street et al., 2003), and this behavior is better understood through an institutional perspective. The days of unassisted physicians providing care are long past, and with the current managed care arrangements, patients are more aware of health costs, alternative treatments, and how to navigate the health care system. Patients also arm themselves with health information from various online sources, so it is unsurprising that patients have more questions and concerns to voice to their health care providers. These changing communication patterns are one symptom of a large shift in how patients are responding to the institutional changes in medical care. There is much work left to understand how managed care has affected patients, providers, and other stakeholders.

Organizational Communication Research in Health Care Settings

Research concerning health organizations demonstrates that institutional structures have great influence on communication flow. Both institutional messages and interpersonal support messages adhere to institutional structures in a hospital setting. Communication training of subordinate employees such as pharmacists (Denvir & Brewer, 2015) and nurses (Kalbfleisch & Bach, 1998) is thought to be necessary to improve situations where hierarchical power relations exist. While emphasizing individual physicians' attitudes or subordinates' poor communication skills, these arguments tend to overlook the institutionalized hierarchical structures that constitute domination.

Kalbfleisch and Bach (1998), for example, researched how mentoring and job expectations increase job reward value. Their study demonstrated how interpersonal and institutional messages are intertwined, moving along predefined hierarchical pathways. "Job expectation" from an institutional perspective is education that teaches subordinates how to navigate and sometimes resist the power relations in the institutional environment of a hospital.

Such power relations can protect subordinates as well, as demonstrated by Noland and Carl (2006). In that study medical residents rationalized malpractice lawsuits as unavoidable risks, but were not worried about being affected because their supervising physicians were held liable during lawsuits, not the residents who made the mistakes. Therefore, while the institutional hierarchy of a teaching hospital put residents under administrative and physician power, they gained protection by being lower in the hierarchy.

We believe that there are some misunderstood ideas around health occupations and the responsibility of subordinates to improve communication with superiors. The fact that communication is dependent upon existing institutional and hierarchical channels is taken for granted in much patient–provider communication research. Both institutional messages and interpersonal support messages use the same channels (see Figure 17.1). Subordinate employees like nurses receive the most messages, both supportive and institutional. Because of their positions in the institutional hierarchy, nurses and other subordinates are dependent on their superiors for institutional knowledge. Administrators are in the best position to support, resist, or change institutional messages.

eHealth

The health and communication technology literature is increasingly focusing on health organizations' use of social media and new technologies in an attempt to

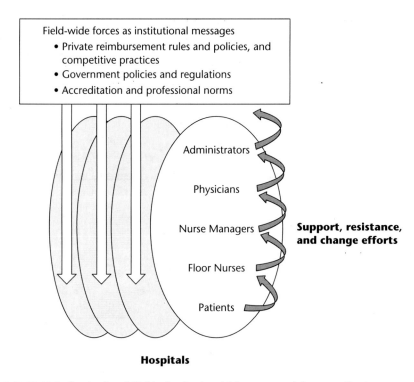

Field-wide forces as institutional messages
- Private reimbursement rules and policies, and competitive practices
- Government policies and regulations
- Accreditation and professional norms

Administrators

Physicians

Nurse Managers

Support, resistance, and change efforts

Floor Nurses

Patients

Hospitals

FIGURE 17.1 Institutional Fields, Institutional Messages, and Support, Resistance, and Change Efforts in Hospital Communication.

improve clinical outcomes and increase health provider efficiency (Hawn, 2009). An institutional view of these new behaviors can help to explain how some of these attempts are successful, while others are not. McCarroll et al. (2014) described how a hospital launched a social networking site to increase patient health knowledge, and found that the vast majority of users were young females. This demographic (young, trend-hungry, and in possession of disposable income) is a desirable target for many businesses. The "customers" of hospitals, by contrast, can be of any age, but are frequently middle-age and senior patients—who are not being reached by the case study's social media website. An institutional perspective suggests that hospitals and other health care organizations are engaging in behavior that is isomorphic (DiMaggio & Powell, 1983) with commercial business organizations. The customers and goals of these organizations are unlike each other, so a hospital using Facebook to educate its patients risks missing its broader population of stakeholders. An institutional perspective could help health organizations make better use of social media by suggesting that, as health care institutions mimic other types of organizations by utilizing social networking sites, they remember their unique patient needs and choose media outlets that effectively permeate their local community.

Other experiments with new health technologies include telemedicine and physicians' use of email to communicate with patients. Online message boards and blogs can greatly benefit both patients and doctors. Scheerhorn et al. (1995) studied a message board created for hemophiliacs and their caregivers that was very successful in creating an online community for information-sharing, cost saving, and interpersonal support. Online communities have completely changed the way that many people with rare or isolating illnesses are able to get information and support. Many blogs are run by individuals who suffer from the illness of discussion, and this marks an important shift from traditional methods of receiving health information from health care institutions. Physicians have also begun going online to disseminate health information. There are numerous websites (such as WebMD) and blogs (such as Autism Buddy) where doctors log in to answer questions posted by individuals before they have approached their own doctors for care.

Walden (2013) found that naturopathic physicians who use holistic methods in the prevention and treatment of illness are using blogs to build credibility for their approach to the practice of medicine. Naturopathic doctors are not fully accepted by the mainstream medical profession, nor are their methods understood by all patients. Walden (2013) found that these doctors utilize online blogs for three primary purposes: (a) introducing the public to naturopathic medicine, (b) advancing science and research, and (c) answering questions and addressing criticisms. This is not just a study of the new media communication strategies of a minority profession; this case study represents the development of a profession that has been rejected in many ways by prevailing medical institutions. New technology can serve to connect patients and legitimize doctors. These behaviors represent adaptations that fill gaps that the current medical system has not addressed. As such, the use of this technology represents what Lawrence, Suddaby, and Leca (2011) refer to as institutional work: "the practices of individual and collective actors aimed at creating, maintaining, and disrupting institutions" (p. 52).

In addition to social media, email is used by some (but not many) doctors to communicate with their patients. Patt, Houston, Jenckes, Sands and Ford (2003) studied physicians who communicate with their patients via email every day. Doctors most satisfied with communicating with patients via email found that doing so was time saving and helped them to deliver better care, whereas doctors unsatisfied with email communication found that patient-requested email communication was time-consuming and put them as risk for liability. Overall, 25% of doctors surveyed would not recommend that their colleagues email their patients, while over 80% of patients would like to communicate via email with their doctor.

It is clear those changes in technologies and their use by patients put pressure on traditional health organizations to adopt new communication practices. Health organizations' forays into social media, blogs, and other new media forms of communication indicate that an institutional change has begun. Tolbert and

Zucker's (1996) model of the institutionalization process is useful for understanding how these changes are being initiated, and how adopted behaviors may affect health institutions over time. By examining the macro institutional effects of new technologies we can move from examining separate case studies to a larger understanding of patterns effecting health care organizations and institutions.

The foregoing discussion shows that expanding health communication research to include institutional insights offers opportunities to increase our explanatory power. In the section below we discuss the implications of an institutional view in future communication research on health organizations.

Organized Health Communication and Institutional Stability or Institutional Change

The question we now turn to is how organized health communication is subject to forces of institutional stability or institutional change. Several possibilities have already been discussed: within organizations, particular actors, such as nurses, physicians, or even patients may resist institutional messages, disrupting the stability that the acceptance of such messages might bring, or offer supportive or adaptive communication strategies that reinforce institutional stability. Here we suggest that in the field of health communication we may identify both forces of stability and forces of change in institutional structures (summarized in Table 17.1). Once again we organize our work around the areas of patient–provider, organizational, and mass health communication research, and emphasize the features of institutional messages, endurance, reach, incumbency, and clarity.

Patient–Provider Communication

Patient–provider communication has traditionally attended to the behaviors of providers and patients and the adaptive or maladaptive interactions between them. The institutional context in which this has taken place is however one characterized by a corps of medical and health management professionals who have been highly socialized to particular enduring roles and sets of beliefs (Groopman, 2007; Freidson, 2001; see also Lammers & Proulx, and Meyer & Gaillard, this volume). Moreover, for most medical encounters studied by health communication scholars, patient provider interactions have taken place in the rule-bound context of either a private or public health insurance system. By the time that the International Communication Association founded the Therapeutic Communication Interest Group in 1975 (later named the Health Communication Division), Medicare and Medicaid had been established for 10 years, lending considerable reach to the institutional messages of entitlement and access. Between 1960 and 1975, the share of health spending paid out of pocket had dropped from 55 percent of total health spending to less than 30 percent, and continued to drop to less than 20 percent in the early 2000s (CMS, 2014). In other words, private and public payers

TABLE 17.1 Implications of an Institutional Perspective for Health Communication Research

Subfield of Health Communication	Source of Institutional Stability	Source of Institutional Change	Implication for Health Communication Research
Patient–provider	Throughout the 20th century, professions and patients with health insurance	Since the 1960s and the rise of broad access to care; markets and policy changes	Attend to the patient's experience as a quasi-consumer; instead of focusing on doctor–patient communication, critical work on the patient as a consumer/citizen responsible for navigating a bureaucracy; and to the provider as a worker facing new arrangements, technologies, etc.; lists of patients
Communication in and around health organizations	Since 1965, Medicare, Medicaid, and traditional insurance	Since the 1980s, managed care; health reform; sale and new management of medical practices	Attend to influence of new technologies like EHRs; new reimbursement arrangements (Geist and Hardesty, 1992); competition among providers; contracts between providers and health plans
Mass-mediated health persuasion	Throughout the post-war period, federally funded public health initiatives	Since the 1990s, reduced government funding; rising private interests	Attend to different audiences, such as schools and lawmakers, rather than general public, go after the audience that the private interests are pursuing

were silent, invisible partners in widespread, enduring, well-defined, and rule-guided patient provider communication. The political agreements that provided for Medicare and the economic agreements that provide for employer-sponsored private insurance lent substantial stability to the system.

Since the early 2000s, however, the numbers of uninsured people in the United States have grown, physicians and hospitals have struggled with reimbursement rates, and employers, unwilling to shoulder the burden of increasing costs alone, have begun to push costs back upon employees. This is not only a financial matter, because, in efforts to control costs, some plans and self-insured employers have begun to require patients to disclose health information, such as smoking or dietary habits (Flaherty, 2013). The stability of the patient–provider relationship is not influenced only by requirements on patients. Recently enacted laws also limit what physicians can talk about with their patients. For example, in Florida, physicians may not legally inquire about whether there are firearms in a patient's home, and four states (Pennsylvania, Ohio, Colorado, and Texas) have passed legislation relating to disclosure of information about exposure to chemicals used in the process of hydraulic fracturing ("fracking") (Weinberger et al., 2012). In addition, "many contracts between health insurers and providers contain 'gag clauses' that bar both parties from disclosing claims data or prices paid for care" (Dentzer, 2013).

Finally, a number of elements of the Affordable Care Act also spell changes in the provider–patient relationship. First, while requiring citizens to purchase health insurance, the Act left intact the established system of private health insurance. We can expect that the accompanying broad access to care will force hospitals and clinics to rationalize the provider role, making physicians busier and more regimented, and bringing increasing numbers of physicians' assistants and nurse practitioners into the work force, challenging providers to standardize and routinize their interactions. At the same time, under pressure to shop for insurance, patients are likely to behave more like consumers than in the past (Lammers & Geist, 1997). All of the aforementioned factors we suggest lend themselves to interruption rather than endurance, fragmented reach, confusing and contradictory rules, and a lack of clarity. Therefore instead of focusing on a traditional doctor–patient relationship, we should anticipate critical work on the patient as a consumer-citizen responsible for navigating a bureaucracy and on the provider as a bureaucratic worker. For example, health communication scholars might include patients' consumer behaviors and providers' institutional constraints in their studies of patient provider communication.

Communication in and Around Health Organizations

Some of the forces that will alter patient provider communication affect organizational communication in health settings (Lammers, Lindholm, & Hazeu, 2004). In the mid-1960s the establishment of Medicare and Medicaid, based on the principles of traditional indemnity insurance, had the overall effect of increasing the size of the health care industry and its component organizations. In general this could be recognized as a force of stability in the traditional structure of hospitals and insurance companies. Hospitals everywhere came to resemble each other under a regime of similar rules and requirements.

Since the 1980s, however, the prevailing logic of health organizations has been managed care (Lammers, Barbour, & Duggan, 2003), as a means to control the rising costs that consistently outstrip inflation. Practices such as prospective payment and capitation, along with Health Maintenance Organizations and Preferred Provider Organizations, drove health organizations toward a corporate model of organization. Physicians found it lucrative to sell their practices to investor-owned companies, but thereby became employees. Hospitals found it necessary to create or join health care systems and in some cases to purchase or affiliate with health insurance organizations to assure a flow of 'covered lives.' These moves have made the field of health care turbulent.

The Affordable Care Act has if anything propelled health organizations toward an integrated corporate design, the largest cost component of which is employment. Thus the Act encourages and rewards the use of medical technologies, especially the electronic health record; it refines the idea of the Accountable Care Organization, which makes a single organization responsible for a population of patients in a community so that each member of the community has a "medical home" and is entitled to a defined list of "essential health benefits." With respect to the traditional community hospital, the Affordable Care Act must be seen as a force of instability (that is, a lack of endurance, fragmented reach, lack of clarity, and weakly enforced—*unencumbent*—rules) until the U.S. sees its population more fully and directly covered. During this time, employment and bureaucratic roles will be seen to grow rapidly.

Mass-Mediated Health Communication

Prior to the era of technologically assisted social networking, and throughout the latter half of the 20th century, federally funded public health initiatives drove outreach efforts to persuade mass audiences to adopt healthful or risk-preventative behaviors. This fairly steady flow of funds may be seen as a source of institutional stability. However, the public health infrastructure has not been widely recognized by the population it serves, but rather fragmented with overlapping jurisdictions (that is, audiences), and characterized by fairly weak rules and modest clarity.

This situation actually deteriorated over the last fifty years. According to Kinner and Pellegrini (2009) "as a percentage of all US health expenditures, federal public health spending was lower in 2008 than it was in 1966" (p. 1781). While a modest increase in public health expenditures was recognized in the post-September 11, 2001 period, "annualized growth in discretionary outlays at the CDC ultimately declined" as a percentage of gross domestic product, "as did federal grants to state and local governments for disease prevention–related activities" (p. 1787). The West African Ebola crisis of 2014 brought the role of state and municipal public health agencies and the Centers for the Disease Control and Prevention back into the public's and policy makers' attention. Fears of the spread of Ebola, and the tactical and technical challenges associate with limiting its spread may be seen as sources of institutional instability.

As we discussed above however, in the current age of social networking assisted by a global data network (Lammers & Jackson, 2014), health communication is taking on new forms and following an almost infinite number of channels. While the reach of public health messages has increased, their endurance and clarity seem doubtful, and the extent to which public health messages actually require actions of recipients seems contended. In general, we view this as a source of instability.

Summary and Conclusion

In this chapter we have offered a review of an institutional approach to health communication. We have identified the elements of the institutional perspective— endurance, field-level effects, and legitimacy—and conceptual tools—isomorphism, logics, rhetorical analyses, and messages—that apply to health communication phenomena. We have argued that attending to the endurance, reach, encumbency, and clarity of messages will help communication researchers identify sources of stability and change in health organizations. In reviewing the institutional stability of the settings in which health communication occurs, it seems appropriate to observe that the field is now in a time of institutional instability in the U.S. More Americans have access to care today than five years ago, but consumerism is likely to drive them to challenge the authority of providers. New organizational arrangements are developing that challenge traditional physicians' offices and hospitals. The global data network reduces barriers to information, but has not replaced the traditional systems by which health information is considered legitimate. Finally, the public health infrastructure, which has operated on a cooperative and loosely federated basis for years, is facing new challenges with the advent of globally portable highly infectious diseases. All of these shifts make for an exciting time to be studying health communication, and raise the salience and importance of its institutional context.

DISCUSSION QUESTIONS

1. Thinking about your own experience with a particular hospital, why do you think it is appropriate to refer to it as an *institution*? How does that square with the definitions offered here?
2. What do you think is the *institutional message* of the Patient Protection and Affordable Care Act? Can you apply the ideas of endurance, reach, incumbency, or clarity to it? Why or why not?
3. How would you characterize the *logic* of the U.S. health care system? Is it fair to say there are competing logics? What are they?
4. Thinking about the logics you identified in question 3, how would you say they are communicated? Can you identify specific communication channels or rhetorical strategies by which the logic(s) is (or are) sustained?

Author note

The authors gratefully acknowledge Ariel Alexander, Kylee Lukacena, and Christofer Skurka for bibliographic assistance.

Suggested Reading

Lammers, J. C. & Barbour, J. B. (2009). Exploring the institutional context of physicians' work: Professional and organizational differences in physician satisfaction. In D. Goldsmith & D. Brashers (Eds.), *Managing health and illness: Communication, relationships, and identity* (pp. 91–112). Mahwah, NJ: Erlbaum.

Lammers, J. C., Lindholm, K., & Hazeu, H. (2004). Re-organized medical practice: An institutional perspective on neonatal care. In E. Ray (Ed.). *Health communication in practice: A case study approach* (pp. 297–310). Mahwah, NJ: Lawrence Erlbaum Associates.

References

Alexander, J. A. & D'Aunno, T. A. (1990). Transformation of institutional environments: Perspectives on the corporatization of U.S. health care. In S. S. Mick (Ed.), *Innovations in health care delivery: Insights for organization theory* (pp. 53–85). San Francisco, CA: Jossey-Bass.

Arndt, M. & Bigelow, B. (2006). Toward the creation of an institutional logic for the management of hospitals: Efficiency in the early nineteen hundreds. *Medical Care Research and Review, 63,* 369–394.

Arntson, P., Makoul, G., Pendleton, D., & Schofield, T. (1989). Patients' perceptions of medical encounters in Great Britain: Variations with health loci of control and sociodemographic factors. *Health Communication, 1*(2), 75–95. Doi:10.1207/s15327027hc0102_1.

Barbour, J. B. (2010). On the institutional moorings of talk in health care organizations. *Management Communication Quarterly, 24,* 449–456.

Barbour, J. B. & Lammers, J. C. (2007). Health care institutions, communication, and physicians' experience of managed care: A multilevel analysis. *Management Communication Quarterly, 21,* 201–231.

Beisecker, A. E. (1989). The influence of a companion on the doctor-elderly patient interaction. *Health Communication, 1,* 55–70.

Berteotti, C. R. & Seibold, D. R. (1994). Coordination and role-definition problems in health-care teams: A hospice case study. In L. R. Frey (Ed.), *Group communication in context: Studies of natural groups* (pp. 107–131). Hillsdale, NJ: Lawrence Erlbaum.

CMS (2014). National Health Expenditures by Type of Service and Source Of Funds: Calendar Years 1960 to 2013. Centers for Medicare & Medicaid Services, Office of the Actuary, National Health Statistics Group. Retrieved from http://www.cms.gov/Research-Statistics-Data-and-Systems/Statistics-Trends-and-Reports/NationalHealthExpendData/NationalHealthAccountsHistorical.html.

Cornelissen J. P., Holt, R., & Zundel, M. (2011). The role of analogy and metaphor in the framing and legitimization of strategic change. *Organization Studies, 32,* 1701–1716.

Cornelissen, J. P., Durand, R., Fiss, P., Lammers, J. C., & Vaara, E. (2015). Putting communication front and center in institutional theory and analysis. *Academy of Management Review, 4,* 10–27

Currie, W. & Guah, M. (2007). Conflicting institutional logics: A national programme for IT in the organisational field of healthcare. *Journal of Information Technology, 22,* 235–247.

Deephouse, D. (1996). Does isomorphism legitimate? *Academy of Management Journal, 39,* 1024–1039.

Dentzer, S. (2013). Five takeaways from the National Transparency Summit: An issue whose time has come. *Culture of Health Blog.* Retrieved from http://www.rwjf.org/en/blogs/culture-of-health/2013/12/five_takeaways_from.html.

Denvir, P. & Brewer, J. (2015). "How dare you question what I use to treat this patient?": Student pharmacists' reflections on the challenges of communicating recommendations to physicians in interdisciplinary health care settings. *Health Communication, 30*(5), 504–512. Doi:10.1080/10410236.2013.868858.

DiMaggio, P. J. & Powell, W. W. (1983). The iron cage revisited: Institutional isomorphism and collective rationality in organization fields. *American Sociological Review, 48*, 147–160.

Flaherty, C. (2013, July 22). Weigh In or Pay. *The Chronicle of Higher Education.* Retrieved from https://www.insidehighered.com/news/2013/07/22/penn-state-faculty-object-details-new-preventive-health-care-plan.

Freidson, E. (2001). *Professionalism: The third logic.* Chicago, IL: The University of Chicago Press.

Geist, P. & Hardesty, M. (1992). *Negotiating the crisis: DRGs and the transition of hospitals.* Hillsdale, NJ: Lawrence Erlbaum.

Giddens, A. (1984). *The constitution of society: Outline of the theory of structuration.* Cambridge, UK: Polity.

Goodrick, E. & Reay, T. (2010). Florence Nightingale endures: Legitimizing a new professional role identity. *Journal of Management Studies, 47*, 55–84.

Goodrick, E. & Reay, T. (2011). Constellations of Institutional Logics: Changes in the professional work of pharmacists. *Work and Occupations, 38*, 372–416.

Gray, B., Purdy, J., & Ansari, S. (2015). From interactions to institutions: Microprocesses of framing and mechanisms for the structuring of institutional fields. *Academy of Management Review, 40*(1), 115–143. Doi:10.5465/amr.2013.0299.

Green, S., Jr., Babb, M., & Alpaslan, C. M. (2008). Institutional field dynamics and the competition between institutional logics: The role of rhetoric in the evolving control of the modern corporation. *Management Communication Quarterly, 22*, 40–73.

Greenwood, R., Oliver, C., Sahlin, K., & Suddaby, R. (2008). Introduction. In R. Greenwood, C. Oliver, K. Sahlin, & R. Suddaby (Eds.), *The SAGE handbook of organizational institutionalism* (pp. 1–46). Thousand Oaks, CA: Sage.

Groopman, J. (2007). *How doctors think.* New York: Houghton Mifflin.

Hawn, C. (2009). Take two aspirin and tweet me in the morning: How Twitter, Facebook, and other social media are reshaping health care. *Health Affairs, 28*, 361–368.

Kalbfleisch, P. J. & Bach, B. W. (1998). The language of mentoring in a health care environment. *Health Communication, 10*(4), 373–392. Doi:10.1207/s15327027hc1004_5.

Kantola, H. & Jarvinen, J. (2012). Analysing the Institutional Logic of Late DRG Adopters. *Financial Accountability & Management, 28*(3), 269–285.

Kennedy, M. T. & Fiss, P. C. (2009). Institutionalization, framing, and diffusion: The logic of TQM adoption and implementation decisions among U.S. hospitals. *Academy of Management Journal, 52*, 897–918.

Keränen, L. (2007). "Cause someday we all die": Rhetoric, agency, and the case of the "patient" preferences worksheet. *Quarterly Journal of Speech, 93*, 179–210.

Kinner, K. & Pellegrini, C. (2009). Expenditures for public health: Assessing historical and prospective trends. *American Journal of Public Health, 99*, 1780–1791.

Kitchener, M. (2002). Mobilizing the Logic of Managerialism in Professional Fields: The Case of Academic Health Centers Mergers. *Organization Studies, 23*, 391–420.

Kulkarni, V. (2014). *Discourse of institutional change.* (Unpublished doctoral dissertation). New Brunswick, NJ: University of New Jersey.

Lammers, J. C. (2011). How institutions communicate: Institutional messages, institutional logics, and organizational communication. *Management Commmunication Quarterly, 25,* 154–182.

Lammers, J. C. & Barbour, J. B. (2006). An institutional theory of organizational communication. *Communication Theory, 16,* 356–377.

Lammers, J. C. & Barbour, J. B. (2009). Exploring the institutional context of physicians' work: Professional and organizational differences in physician satisfaction. In D. Goldsmith & D. Brashers (Eds.), *Managing health and illness: Communication, relationships, and identity* (pp. 91–112). Mahwah, NJ: Erlbaum.

Lammers, J. C., Barbour, J., & Duggan, A. (2003). Organizational forms of the provision of health care: An institutional perspective. In T. Thompson, A. Dorsey, K. Miller, & R. Parrot (Eds.). *Handbook of health communication* (pp. 319–345). Mahwah, NJ: Lawrence Erlbaum Associates.

Lammers, J. C. & Garcia, M. A. (2013). Institutional theory and organizational communication. In L. Putnam & D. Mumby (Eds.), *The handbook of organizational communication* (pp. 195–216). Newbury Park, CA: Sage.

Lammers, J. C. & Geist, P. (1997). The transformation of caring in the light and shadow of managed care. *Health Communication, 9,* 45–60.

Lammers, J. C., Lindholm, K., & Hazeu, H. (2004). Re-organized medical practice: An institutional perspective on neonatal care. In E. Ray (Ed.), *Health communication in practice: A case study approach* (pp. 297–310). Mahwah, NJ: Lawrence Erlbaum Associates.

Lammers. J. C. & Jackson, S. A. (2014). The institutionality of a mediatized organizational environment. In J. Pallas & L. Strannegård (Eds.), *Organizations and the media: Organizing in a mediatized world* (pp. 33–47). New York, NY: Routledge.

Lammers, J. C. & Krikorian, D. (1997). Theoretical extension and operationalization of the bona fide group construct with an application to surgical teams. *The Journal of Applied Communication Research, 25,* 17–38.

Lawrence, T. B., Suddaby, R., & Leca, B. (2011). Institutional work: Refocusing institutional studies of organization. *Journal of Management Inquiry, 20,* 52–58.

Lewis, L. K. (2007). An organizational stakeholder model of change implementation communication. *Communication Theory, 17,* 176–204.

McCarroll, M. L., Armbruster, S. D., Chung, J. E., McKenzie, A. & von Gruenigen, V. E. (2014). Health care and social media platforms in hospitals. *Health Communication, 29,* 947–952.

Meyer, J. W. & Rowan, B. (1977). Institutionalized organizations: Formal structure as myth and ceremony. *American Journal of Sociology, 83,* 340–363.

Moore, S. D., Wright, K. B., & Bernard, D. R. (2009). Influences on health delivery system satisfaction: A partial test of the ecological model. *Health Communication, 24*(4), 285–294. Doi: 10.1080/10410230902889225.

Nigam, A. & Ocasio, W. (2010). Event attention, environmental sensemaking, and change in institutional logics: An inductive analysis of the effects of public attention to Clinton's health care reform initiative. *Organization Science, 21,* 823–841.

Noland, C. & Carl, W. J. (2006). "It's not our ass": Medical resident sense-making regarding lawsuits." *Health Communication, 20,* 81–91. Doi: 10.1207/s15327027hc 2001_8.

O'Hair, D. (1989). Dimension of relational communication and control during physician-patient interactions. *Health Communication, 1,* 97–115.

Patt, M. R., Houston, T. K., Jenckes, M. W., Sands, D. Z., & Ford, D. E. (2003). Doctors who are using e-mail with their patients: a qualitative exploration. *Journal of Medical Internet Research, 5*(2). Doi: 10.2196/jmir.5.2.e9.

Phillips, N., Lawrence, T., & Hardy, C. (2004). Discourses and institutions. *Academy of Management Review, 29,* 635–652.

Reay, T. & Hinings, C.R. (2005). The recomposition of an organizational field: Health care in Alberta. *Organization Studies, 26,* 351–384.

Ruef, M. & Scott, W. R. (1998). A multidimensional model of organizational legitimacy: Hospital survival in changing institutional environments. *Administrative Science Quarterly, 43,* 877–904.

Scheerhorn, D., Warisse, J., & McNeilis, K. S. (1995). Computer-based telecommunication among an illness-related community: Design, delivery, early use and the functions of Highnet. *Health Communication, 7,* 301–325.

Scott, W. R. (2004). Competing logics in health care: Professional, state, and managerial. In F. Dobbin (Ed.), *The sociology of the economy* (pp. 267–287). New York, NY: Russell Sage Foundation.

Scott, W. R., Ruef, M., Mendel, P. J., & Caronna, C. A. (2000). *Institutional change and healthcare organizations: From professional dominance to managed care.* Chicago, IL: University of Chicago Press.

Selznick, P. (1949). *TVA and the grass roots: A study in the sociology of formal organization.* Berkeley, CA: University of California Press.

Shortell, S. M., Gillies, R. R., & Devers, K. J. (1995). Reinventing the American hospital. *The Milbank Quarterly, 73,* 131–160.

Sillince, J. A. A. & Barker, J. R. (2012). A tropological theory of institutionalization. *Organization Studies, 33,* 7–38.

Smets, M. & Jarzabkowski, P. (2013). Reconstructing institutional complexity in practice: A relational model of institutional work and complexity. *Human Relations, 66,* 1279–1309.

Street, R. L., Jr., Krupat, E., Bell, R., Kravitz, R. L., & Haidet, P. (2003). Beliefs about control in the physician-patient relationship: Effect on communication in medical encounters. *Journal of General Internal Medicine, 18,* 609–616.

Thornton, P. H. & Ocasio, W. (2008). Institutional logics. In R. Greenwood, C. Oliver, K. Sahlin & R. Suddaby (Eds.), *Handbook of organizational institutionalism* (pp. 99–129). London: Sage.

Thornton P. H., Ocasio W., & Lounsbury, M. (2012). *The institutional logics perspective: A new approach to culture, structure, and process.* New York: Oxford University Press.

Tolbert, P. S. & Zucker, L. G. (1996). The institutionalization of institutional theory [Electronic version]. In S. Clegg, C. Hardy and W. Nord (Eds.), *Handbook of Organization Studies* (pp. 175–190). London: Sage. Retrieved from http://digitalcommons.ilr.cornell.edu/articles.

Walden, J. (2013). A medical profession in transition: Exploring naturopathic physician blogging behaviors. *Health Communication, 28,* 237–247.

Weber, M. (1968). *Economy and society* (G. Roth & C. Wittich, Trans.). Berkeley, CA: University of California Press. (Original work published 1906–1924).

Weinberger, S. E., Lawrence, H. C., Henley, D. E., Alden, E. R., & Hoyt, D. B. (2012). Legislative interference with the patient–physician relationship. *New England Journal of Medicine, 367,* 1557–1559.

White, K. R. (2013). When institutions collide: The competing forces of hospitals sponsored by the Roman Catholic Church. *Religions, 4*, 14–29.

White, K. R., Thompson, S., & Griffith, J. R. (2011). Transforming the dominant logic of hospitals. *Advances in Health Care Management, 11*, 133–145.

Zorn, T. E., Flanagin, A. J., & Shoham, M. (2011). Institutional and non-institutional influences on information and communication technology adoption and use among nonprofit organizations. *Human Communication Research, 37*, 1–33.

PART III

Collaboration, Design, and Interorganizational Efforts to Improve Health

18

ORGANIZING TRANSDISCIPLINARY RESEARCH

A Breast Cancer and the Environment Collaborative Model

Kami Silk and Sandi Smith

Organizing health research so that it is collaborative and integrative of multiple disciplines is increasingly common, especially within the context of federally funded research projects. The complex nature of health issues requires that a range of perspectives, knowledge bases, and approaches is used to fully understand, address, and impact health issues. Interdisciplinary and multidisciplinary research are familiar terms for describing the research process where individuals from more than one discipline are working together on a research problem; however, transdisciplinary research is less familiar (Mitchell, 2005). A transdisciplinary model integrates cross-disciplinary perspectives with the aim of synthesizing them to create a new approach of team science for addressing a research problem (Kreps & Maibach, 2008). It requires collaboration, information exchange, resource sharing, and integration of disciplines (Rosenfield, 1992). The organizing strategies used to create a transdisciplinary model are fundamental, yet complex, as the integration of multiple research agendas into a cohesive structure that facilitates and forges novel and rigorous research is not a simple task. In many ways, a transdisciplinary approach has yet to be proven as superior to a more traditional research model (Stokols, Misra, Moser, Hall, & Taylor, 2008), particularly if the key metrics for determining the model's effectiveness are the quality and quantity of the research outputs created by the team. While it is unclear at present whether organizing health research into a transdisciplinary model results in synergistic research outcomes, it is undoubtedly the case that in order to solve complex health issues, research that is not unilateral in its focus and that is informed by multiple perspectives and disciplines is necessary.

This chapter takes an organizing perspective to present the transdisciplinary research model, using the Breast Cancer and Environment Research Center/

Program (BCERC/P) as a primary exemplar. Integrating a team of researchers from multiple disciplines so they form a cohesive strategy to address a complex health problem such as breast cancer is an evolving process that merits considerable attention, especially as transdisciplinary research models have not been evaluated systematically for their effectiveness (Stokols, 2006). We will first examine the transdisciplinary model and will explicate how the BCERC/P was structured and functioned as a system striving to collectively reveal new knowledge related to the influence of environmental factors in breast cancer and strategies for prevention (Interagency Breast Cancer and Environmental Research Coordinating Committee, 2013). Next we will frame the BCERC/P as a learning community (Senge, 1990) comprised of a range of stakeholders in need of developing a unified approach to solving the problem of breast cancer. Then we will elaborate on the four flows of the learning organization to discuss relevant factors that helped constitute the BCERC/P (McPhee & Zaug, 2000). Finally, we will discuss potential pitfalls and lessons learned from organizing within the BCERC/P transdisciplinary model.

The Transdisciplinary Research Model

Transdisciplinary research is defined as "research efforts conducted by investigators from different disciplines working jointly to create new conceptual, theoretical, methodological, and translational innovations that integrate and moves beyond discipline-specific approaches to address a common problem" (Harvard School of Public Health, 2014, p.1). A transdisciplinary model "transcends individual departments or specialized knowledge bases because they intend to solve . . . research questions that are, by definition, beyond the purview of the individual disciplines" (Gebbie, Rosenstock, & Hernandez, 2003, pp. 117–118). Canary (this volume) discusses the construction of interorganizational knowledge and participatory action knowledge translation showing that organizational knowledge can transcend specialized knowledge bases. One key component of the transdisciplinary research model is its focus on translating research findings, including both in the health science and practice arenas as well as in the communication/prevention forum. In other words, it is not enough for the transdisciplinary team to engage in scientific endeavors; there is a great onus on the transdisciplinary team to also ensure the state of the science is communicated beyond academic journals so that interventions and public communication efforts are informed by the most recent scientific findings. This additional responsibility of translating research findings is novel for many researchers; thus, including communication scientists to lead translational efforts is helpful in developing theoretically informed, evidence-based message content and dissemination strategies.

Transdisciplinary teams are organized to be inclusive of not only researchers from different disciplines, but also members of the lay public, particularly advocates focused on a specific health issue. Transdisciplinary teams often are comprised of members from across many institutions and communities to create a team inclusive of the necessary areas of expertise to accomplish research goals. Contextual factors that influence transdisciplinary research collaborations include intrapersonal (e.g., attitude, leadership style), interpersonal (e.g., familiarity, social cohesiveness, diversity), organizational (e.g., incentives, participatory goal setting, meetings, climate of sharing), technologic (e.g., infrastructure and member readiness), societal and political (e.g., cooperative research policies, ethical reviews, intellectual property), and the physical environment (e.g., spatial proximity of workspaces, meeting areas, environmental resources) (Stokols et al., 2008). All of these contextual factors are important considerations for often-dispersed transdisciplinary teams to collaborate effectively. Multiple leaders, clear coordination, and communication processes need to be built in to the team structure (Gray, 2008). In other words, a clear system for organizing and doing work that considers the aforementioned contextual factors is necessary for the transdisciplinary team to be successful in effectively investigating the research problem.

One helpful way to frame the transdisciplinary research team from a communication orientation is as a learning organization that needs to integrate the expertise of its members to facilitate systems thinking (Senge, 1990). Learning organizations are holistic and integrative in their approach to identifying and addressing the evolving needs and challenges presented to them, which mirrors the assumptions of the transdisciplinary model. Before delving into a discussion of learning organizations, the background, structure, and goals of the BCERC/P are explained to provide a foundation for considering it further as an exemplar of the transdisciplinary model and as a learning organization.

Organizing the BCERC/P

The BCERC/P provides an excellent exemplar of the transdisciplinary research model with its inclusion of a range of researchers and advocates and its organizational structure. The National Institute of Environmental Health Sciences (NIEHS) and the National Cancer Institute (NCI) co-funded the BCERC for seven years, and the BCERP was subsequently funded for an additional five years to continue the programs of research fostered in the BCERC. The overarching research problem of the BCERC/P is to investigate and communicate about the impact of environmental exposures on breast cancer risk and it meets the mandate of identifying innovative models to more comprehensively study environmental and genomic factors related to breast cancer (Breast Cancer and Environmental Research Act, 2008). The specific goals of the BCERC/P are to investigate mammary gland development in animal models when environmental exposures are introduced, study the timing of pubertal events with a focus on environmental factors that may affect maturation, and develop public health messages for women and girls based on the scientific findings (bcerc.org/ about.htm). To accomplish its goals the BCERC/P is organized as a transdisciplinary model with three cores, including epidemiology, biology, and community outreach and translation (COTC) (Osuch, Silk, Price, Barlow, Miller, Hernick, & Fonta, 2012). Each of the three cores includes representatives from the other two cores, so that every core has the benefit of the knowledge base and input from all of the cores. Researchers from multiple universities and advocates from across the United States work within and across the three cores so that no core is geographically bound in its representation (Silk, Neuberger, Nazione, & Osuch, 2011).

The epidemiology core has implemented longitudinal studies with cohorts of young girls where they gather data regarding the girls' weight, height, BMI, pubertal development, and diet as well as certain chemical exposures as determined from blood draws. In more recent years, the epidemiology core has continued to gather data on the girls' development. Additionally, a "windows of susceptibility" foci was added to further examine the concept that during certain periods of time females are more susceptible to exposures; molecular mechanisms and gene-environment interactions are the focus of the windows of susceptibility line of research. The biology core has worked with animal models (both rat and mouse) to examine how certain diets and chemical exposures affect normal tissue and/or tumor development. The COTC, primarily comprised of breast cancer advocates and a few social scientists, has developed educational materials focused on breast cancer risk reduction and has used a range of strategies to disseminate the state of the scientific evidence associated with BCERC/P. Overall, the three cores are aligned to address different facets of the breast cancer problem so that a more comprehensive picture of the role of environmental exposures in breast cancer can be understood and communicated to the public.

Learning Organizations

Senge (1990) defined *learning organizations* as those " . . . where people continually expand their capacity to create the results they truly desire, where new and expansive patterns of thinking are nurtured, where collective aspiration is set free, and where people are continually learning to see the whole together" (p.3). Although seemingly idealistic, the nature of the transdisciplinary model embodies this definition with its collective of researchers and lay persons striving to create synergistic strategies to address complex health problems. Transdisciplinary team members are collaborating to form a novel vision and approach, and therefore are required to not only consider multiple perspectives, but to extend their own perspective as they collectively tackle the research problem. According to Senge (1990), for learning organizations to thrive and grow, the convergence of five disciplines is necessary, including: personal mastery (continual high achievement in building ongoing expertise), mental models (assumptions and understanding of the world), building a shared vision (a genuinely shared vision to bring to fruition), team learning, and systems thinking. Within the transdisciplinary research model of the BCERC/P, we illustrate how these five disciplines interact to impact the effectiveness of the model.

Personal Mastery

The transdisciplinary model requires that experts from a range of fields work together. Their *personal mastery* in their respective scientific fields and personal experience is fundamental to ensure the success of the model because experts have the greatest opportunity to address and potentially solve the research problem. The expertise of lay individuals is not an oxymoron, because lay individuals not only offer valuable, often survivor-focused, perspectives, but also because those in advocacy roles often are experts in the issues they support. It is important to note that personal mastery also pertains to self-awareness and how to engage effectively within the team. Thus, personal mastery across all stakeholders might be a strength of transdisciplinary teams as they views their roles as pioneers with the model, each one offering a variable and valuable perspective. In the BCERC/P, epidemiologists, biologists, and social scientists who are experts in their respective disciplines, along with breast cancer advocates who are pivotal players in breast cancer advocacy, formed the team. Across 11 years of collaboration with each other, it is fair to say that some BCERC/P partners garnered more personal mastery than others. For example, some scientists were able to connect and value the contributions of breast cancer advocates, while others perceived their role as less essential to BCERC/P functioning. Similarly, many breast cancer advocates fully engaged with the BCERC/P and were able to facilitate collaborative outreach activities with the scientists.

Mental Models

The transdisciplinary model challenges researchers to move beyond their *mental models* of how research should be conducted (Senge, 2006), and it asks researchers to broaden their perspectives about participatory research models (Hall, Feng, Moser, Stokols, & Taylor, 2008). Every collaborator in the BCERC/P comes to the project with a certain understanding and training related to their specific disciplines and fields of experience. Assumptions about what is a rigorous research model and what are the important questions to answer are variable, but the transdisciplinary model should provide the infrastructure and connectivity so that a collective appreciation for the range of research possibilities can evolve. For example, BCERC/P biologists use animal models for their research to understand underlying mechanisms for breast tissue development, while the epidemiologists work with pre-adolescent and adolescent girls to track their chemical exposures. By broadening their perspectives beyond their own disciplines, the biologists have been able to take findings from the epidemiologists to inform one avenue of research related to perfluorooctanoic acid (PFOA). Based on this PFOA research from both biologists and epidemiologists, breast cancer advocates have disseminated risk reduction information to mothers and their daughters, primary audiences for the BCERC/P, and social scientists have tested knowledge gain from messages derived through collaboration with the biologists on the team (Smith, Hitt, Russell, Nazione, Silk, & Atkin, 2013).

Shared Vision

An overarching *shared vision* is essential for the transdisciplinary model so that all of the different stakeholders can organize their approaches around helping that vision come to fruition. However, a shared vision can be a challenge as researchers move forward with answering specific research questions pertaining to their own disciplines. While all BCERC/P stakeholders would agree that the goal of the program is to investigate and communicate about environmental exposures to breast cancer, each stakeholder might also identify different goals related to what exposures are most relevant to breast cancer and what information is the most critical to share with the lay public. In other words, at the macro level, a shared vision has been accomplished for the BCERC/P, but because the scope of the projects under the larger umbrella vision is so great, there is some flexibility in how stakeholders might communicate about this shared vision.

Team Learning

Creating opportunities for *team learning* is inherent to the transdisciplinary model. Efforts to learn from the collective are highly valued in the transdisciplinary model so that stakeholders learn to think together as a team. Annual integration meetings, annual conferences, monthly conference calls, webinars, and other face-to-face as well as technology-enabled interactions provide mechanisms and opportunities for team learning in the BCERC/P. Team learning, however, is not simply one-way knowledge sharing from researchers to researchers or researchers to lay individuals; it also includes team learning from lay individuals to researchers, particularly because advocates help to inform research processes. For more than a decade, BCERC/P collaborators have learned from each other and tried to use their collective knowledge to identify potential areas for novel research, understand research findings, and identify key messages to communicate with lay audiences.

Systems Thinking

Systems thinking is fundamental to the transdisciplinary model because the model views the problem at hand as complex and interrelated, thereby requiring a diverse team of individuals to more comprehensively begin to address the problem. Senge's five disciplines converge to create a synergistic approach that influences team members so that ideally they view the health problem more wholly rather than from the limited lens of their own discipline or singular experience. Within the BCERC/P, it is unclear how much researchers maintained a systems perspective as they focused on their own laboratories and cohorts of participants. It is the case, however, that the structure of the BCERC/P helped to facilitate systems thinking as researchers shared emerging findings and approaches at regular junctures, which then allowed researchers to more fully consider their own research findings and approaches. Overall, there is the potential for creativity, productivity, and synergy within the transdisciplinary model due to its unique structure of teams and collaborations that are inclusive of a range of stakeholders (Senge, 2006).

In sum, the learning organization framework provides a prescriptive model that the BCERC/P embodies in its most pure form. With its organizing and organizational structure, the BCERC/P strives to create an environment for synergy so that the greatest potential for addressing the fight against breast cancer can be realized. To state that the BCERC/P has reached its highest potential as a learning organization would be inaccurate; however, as an early pioneer for transdisciplinary approaches, the BCERC/P does function as an evolving learning organization. While the five disciplines provide a lens to help elucidate how the BCERC/P can be instantiated as a learning organization, a consideration of the Four Flows Approach provides further insight into the communication processes that helped constitute the BCERC/P as a learning organization (McPhee & Zaug, 2000).

The Four Flows of the Learning Organization

Communication is a key element that undergirds learning organizations because it provides the means by which the five disciplines can thrive and converge. The Communicative Constitution of Organizations (CCO) approach centralizes communication as the organizing force that helps create and maintain organizations (Cooren, Kuhn, Cornelissen, & Clark, 2011; Schoeneborn, Blaschke, Cooren, McPhee, Seidl, & Taylor, 2014). In their communication-centered CCO approach with the Four Flows Model, McPhee and Zaug (2000) identify four specific flows of communication that need to occur during the organizing process. An examination and application of the these four flows to the BCERC/P transdisciplinary research model provides insight into how communication processes shaped the organizing of the BCERC/P into a transdisciplinary learning organization.

Membership Negotiation

The first flow of the Four Flows Model, membership negotiation, pertains to all of the communication that occurs between and among organizational members, enabling them to cross and maintain boundaries that help to distinguish organizational members from others. Membership negotiation can include communication about boundary transitions, socialization of members into the BCERC/P, and the creation of a shared understanding of basic breast cancer and environmental exposure knowledge. BCERC/P researchers and advocates are connected under the umbrella of the BCERC/P because they have an intimate knowledge of the BCERC/P, its members, and its goals. And they gain legitimacy from their membership as they strive to publish research, present ideas and findings, reach out to communities with prevention ideas, and represent the BCERC/P across many other contexts. One of the early challenges was for the COTC to gain an equivalent level of legitimacy as a critical core of the BCERC/P. As a novel transdisciplinary approach, many scientists did not value the role of the COTC and did not understand why advocates should have "voice" across a range of matters, including the research agenda of the BCERC/P. While this legitimacy issue remains a challenge from many COTC members' perspectives, the BCERC/P has progressed significantly as many researchers expanded their perspectives and now genuinely embrace advocates as equal partners in the project.

Self-Structuring

The self-structuring flow refers to communication that provides norms, standards, and rules for getting work done. This type of communication also includes feedback in the system, organizational policies, and other types of documents necessary for work to be done. In the BCERC/P model, there is quite a bit of self-structuring flow that relies heavily on codifying ways in which researchers should collaborate so as to facilitate and maintain the complex organizational structure. For example, committee structures are heavily utilized within each of the three cores and across the BCERC/P more broadly. A new committee is created each year with full representation from different areas of the BCERC/P to organize the annual conference and integration meeting, a working group serves in an advisory capacity to provide input for NCI and NIEHS about the progress of the BCERC/P, and a publications committee exists to provide authorship and manuscript development guidelines. Self-structuring flow is also evident with the creation of the project website and with the norms for collaboration that developed over the last decade.

Activity Coordination

Another flow, activity structuring, includes the ongoing interaction required for collaboration so that work can get accomplished. It is not enough to create the structures that provide the form, procedures, and standards for getting work done; more communication is necessary to allow for the coordination and collaboration among individuals. This flow illustrates the interdependence of organizational members as they navigate work tasks and challenges. Within the BCERC/P, activity coordination occurred as researchers, advocates, NCI and NIEHS officers, and lay audiences engaged in dialogue with each other to determine new research questions, annual meeting agendas, strategies for communicating the science effectively with lay audiences, and other collaborative endeavors. Activity coordination occurs through regular conference calls, individual phone calls, sometimes daily email interaction, and face-to-face communication. The BCERC/P has a reasonably clear structure as explained previously, but the structure has not been enough to be able to coordinate all activities. The BCERC/P has enabled long-term relationships between BCERC/P researchers and advocates that have served to decrease uncertainty, reduce barriers, and foster trust among BCERC/P members, which ultimately has facilitated communication and collaboration over the duration of the learning organization.

Institutional Positioning

The fourth and final flow, institutional positioning, occurs at a macro level as organizational members interact within a larger environment of external stakeholders to establish and maintain organizational identity. This flow acknowledges the landscape in which organizations exist, the necessary relationships that have to be forged and maintained, and the communication that needs to occur between organizational members and outside entities. The BCERC/P is positioned as a pioneer for transdisciplinary research. Within the research context of National Institutes of Health (NIH) funding of large-scale R01 and Center grants, the BCERC/P is situated as a successful example of transdisciplinary partnerships as illustrated by tens of millions of dollars already invested in the research and new NIH calls to further fund the program. The communication of BCERC/P stakeholders with NCI and NIEHS has positioned the BCERC/P as an integrated body of experts to be called upon when expertise related to breast cancer and environmental exposures is necessary. Within the breast cancer advocacy community, the BCERC/P is considered a model for how to engage with scientists on issues of relevance to specific groups, and being aligned or associated with the BCERC/P provides additional credibility to advocacy efforts. Within academic communities, affiliation with the BCERC/P adds status to one's research credentials based on the high quality of the science being conducted, the millions of dollars in funding it has garnered to date, the longitudinal nature of the funding, the visibility of the project, and the level of productivity associated with the project with presentations and publications as key metrics. The BCERC/P is well positioned as an expert voice on breast cancer and the environment. With continued funding, its visibility and credibility in the breast cancer research context will continue to increase, which will position BCERC/P as the authoritative voice for questions related to breast cancer and the environment.

Overall, the BCERC/P as a novel transdisciplinary model can be framed as a learning organization that is constituted through the Four Flows Model. Personal mastery, mental models, a shared vision, team learning, and the systems thinking required to evolve as a learning organization occur via communication. The specific types of communication identified in the Four Flows Model (membership negotiation, self-structuring, activity coordination, and institutional positioning) are specifically what fosters the evolution of the learning organization. Understanding the BCERC/P through these theoretical lenses provides insight into the organizing of the BCERC/P. It also creates a context for a critique of the BCERC/P so that others seeking to engage in transdisciplinary research can learn from it.

Lessons Learned from BCERC/P Challenges

The transdisciplinary model is not a panacea for solving research problems, but it does provide an opportunity to consider a problem through a novel perspective, as many stakeholders examine the research problem both individually and collectively as a standard practice within the model. An initial consideration of the model may create the perception that transdisciplinary research creates a more comprehensive approach to a research problem, and therefore, a "better" approach than more traditional models. It is not the goal of this chapter to make such a claim as no true evaluation of the transdisciplinary model has provided evidence that organizing research in this way yields truly superior results over more individualized approaches to research (Stokols et al., 2008). However, it is the case that the transdisciplinary model creates a forum for a range of stakeholders focused on the same research problem so they have the opportunity to maximize the knowledge network of the team, have more timely access to recent research findings, and generate new research questions and approaches that may not have been asked without the synergy of the team. Keeping in mind the transdisciplinary model is an evolving research approach that has legitimate status among research models (Emmons, Viswanath, & Colditz, 2008), the challenges associated with the BCERC/P transdisciplinary model will now be addressed. Many of the lessons to be learned from the experiences of the BCERC/P team stem from the complexity of engaging in transdisciplinary research, large number of stakeholders, ingrained ways of pursuing research, and a lack of support for translational activities.

One of the initial challenges faced by the BCERC/P was the lack of collaboration between researchers in developing a unified transdisciplinary center proposal; instead, the projects were developed individually without an integrated vision. For a learning organization, a shared vision is a fundamental feature, yet without experience working together previously on collaborative research, the BCERC/P was constrained initially (Stokols et al., 2008). To better facilitate a shared vision and potential for integration, transdisciplinary projects should have a more organic approach with researchers and advocates required to demonstrate some reasonable track record of collaboration even if only on a small-scale. It is essential that all stakeholders involved in the transdisciplinary research model embrace the full vision that all team members are necessary and valuable for bringing the goals of the project to fruition.

Senge (1990) introduces the idea that organizations can have learning disabilities such that people identify with their position and sometimes are unable to work within, and accept, the larger whole. In the BCERC/P, the roles of participants were often a singularly key identity for members of the project. Every participant was clearly labeled as a biologist, epidemiologist, advocate, member of the COTC, and so forth, inadvertently reinforcing individual level goal achievement rather than a collective BCERC/P focus. BCERC/P biologists and epidemiologists did not truly understand or appreciate the role of the COTC and the role its members had in translation and dissemination efforts, creating a perceived lower status of COTC members. Particularly during the early years of the project before any novel science from the team could be reported, advocates' roles seemed limited to recruitment of young girls for epidemiology studies. While establishing and maintaining young girl cohorts indeed was pivotal for the success of the BCERC/P, the scope of activities for the COTC was much larger than that: a primary aim of the COTC was to translate the state of the science on breast cancer and the environment for lay audiences so that lay audience members could make informed decisions about engaging in risk reduction practices.

In addition to advocates, the COTC included several communication scientists (including the authors of this chapter) who engaged in formative research with lay audiences (Silk et al., 2006), conducted newspaper and website analyses of breast cancer coverage (Atkin, Smith, McFeters, & Ferguson, 2008; Whitten, Munday, LaPlante, & Smith, 2008), and implemented a wide range of experiments to test the effectiveness of breast cancer messages (Smith, Atkin, Munday, Skubisz, Stohl, 2009; Smith et al., 2009; Smith et al., 2010; Smith et al., 2013) based on the formative research conducted by Marshall, Smith, and McKeon (1995) on source, channel, and message preferences for receiving breast cancer information. However, similar to the advocates, our role in the project was unclear to the biologists and epidemiologists. In retrospect, because most of the researchers across the country had not collaborated previously, the expertise of COTC members was not necessarily understood or respected. With the development of trust between BCERC/P stakeholders over time and an understanding of the advocacy and communication science expertise that existed in the COTC, biologists and epidemiologists began to appreciate the personal mastery of the COTC. As Stokols et al. (2008) explains trust is difficult to establish and maintain when team members do not share a social or physical space, social norms, or values. However, trust can be created by early face-to-face contact and socialization, and facilitated and maintained by sustained task and social communication. In other words, as communication about and engagement in successfully completed common tasks and social issues increased, so did trust between the members of each of the cores of the BCERP/C.

Geography certainly was a challenge as the BCERC/P is spread across different universities throughout the United States. Technology was, of course, a facilitator of communication and collaboration, and team members seemed to have access to reliable technology (i.e., computer, internet access, cell/telephone) to engage with BCERC/P members. Although we live in a technology-laden world, there still are benefits to working side-by-side with collaborators as they attempt to solve complex research problems. Geography became a barrier for the annual conference and integration meetings because funding for advocates was scarce at times, limiting the participation of advocates at the two annual meetings, which then revealed an inequitable distribution of resources and thus, decision power in the BCERC/P. Travel scholarships from NIH and other organizations to support advocate attendance ameliorated some of this challenge. However, the lack of budget for advocate travel as well as a minimal budget to fund COTC activities contributed to a perceived, and perhaps very real, imbalance that sent the message that the COTC activities were merely supplemental rather than critical to the BCERC/P's success. A systems approach to the BCERC/P would strive to integrate the COTC fully so that real attention is given to the budget requirements for COTC translation and dissemination efforts. Stokols et al. (2008) would recommend financial, training, education, and recognition incentives for all BCERC/P members, including advocates. Future transdisciplinary grant submissions should commit appropriate budget support for not only advocate time, travel, and outreach activities, but also for communication science activities to meet translational goals.

Perhaps one of the largest hurdles that still pervades the BCERC/P is conflict about information sharing. Biologists, epidemiologists, and advocates do not agree on what and when to share about BCERC/P findings with lay audiences. This conflict is not surprising as it stems from fundamental differences in scientific and advocate world views. Specifically, BCERC/P scientists were much more hesitant to share findings from the BCERC/P and often felt that it was too early to make risk reduction recommendations based on what they perceived as limited or preliminary findings; generally, they wanted more investigation before sharing information and they wanted to make sure it was published prior to any other type of formal release of findings. Advocates, on the other hand, sought to invoke the precautionary principle because they perceived enough evidence existed to warrant the creation of public health messages to warn of potential dangers. This fundamental difference in world view is part of the challenge of navigating a transdisciplinary model with all of its different stakeholders. Identifying when and what to share with lay audiences is not something that is easily codified; thus, good communication involving self-structuring and activity coordination is necessary to negotiate what information is shared. The BCERC/P did go through an elongated process to create toolkits for health practitioners, health educators, and lay audiences (these toolkits are available on the bcerc.org website). While the toolkits have generally been used by the BCERC/P for outreach purposes, BCERC/P advocates do not perceive the toolkits to be comprehensive of potential risks and recommendations. Future transdisciplinary teams might try to create some guidelines or a strategic communication plan for translating research findings.

Another challenge is lack of clarity about decision-making processes. Research decisions ultimately seemed to be in the hands of the principal investigator (PI) of each center. However, there were many other decisions that each core and BCERC/P committees made. For example, in the first few months of the BCERC, drafts of various potential logos were created for the project. While the assignment to create one was put into the hands of the COTC, it was unclear who ultimately decided which logo should be selected. Further evidence of a clear approach to decision-making was the conference calls for different core meetings. Sometimes a democratic vote would be used and for other decisions the chair of the core or an NIH officer used a leader mandate approach to decide. This ambiguity about individuals' decision-making power undermined some of the synergy of the group because all stakeholders need to have a clear understanding for how decisions will be made, even if the decision-making mode varies for different types of issues. Future transdisciplinary teams should strive to clarify modes of decision-making to reduce uncertainty and help facilitate activity coordination.

The challenges faced by the BCERC/P mirror the kinds of challenges identified in research that has begun to elucidate the transdisciplinary model and articulate the factors that impact its effectiveness (Emmons et al., 2008; Gray, 2008; Hall, Stokols et al. 2008; Morgan, Kobus, Gerlach et al., 2003; Stokols, 2006; and Stokols et al., 2008). From the start, the organizing of the BCERC/P was hindered by the lack of previous collaboration between the BCERC/P stakeholders. The BCERC/P was the first time for most of the researchers to ever have engaged with breast cancer advocates and communication scientists, and it took considerable time for relationships to develop. As Canary, this volume, notes "researchers, administrators, and practitioners need to take time to establish relationships that foster knowledge co-construction and to identify potential barriers to putting knowledge into practice." The pioneering spirit of the BCERC/P team helped to solidify some excellent partnerships as the team collectively dealt with barriers and challenges. The continued funding of the BCERC/P has helped secure the continuity of the project for 11 years thus far; new RFPs have been released which will also fund some further iteration of the project. In its current configuration, the BCERP now has greater readiness and potential for effectiveness because of its history of trust, collaboration, and research outputs.

Conclusion

Overall, the effectiveness of the transdisciplinary model is still relatively unknown. Initial evaluation of the model has begun to develop metrics for assessment and readiness to collaborate (Hall, Stokols et al., 2008), and factors that facilitate and constrain team research (Stokols et al., 2008). The assessment metrics include measures of concepts that increase transdisciplinary team effectiveness such as: identification of common goals and outcomes, an equitable division of power, leaders who develop a strong shared vision and encourage cooperation, a previous history of collaboration, and organizational support (Stokols et al., 2008). Readiness to collaborate can be assessed through intrapersonal factors such as personal support for interdisciplinary research, interpersonal factors such as the common history of previous work and the breadth of stakeholders in the project, and contextual-environmental factors such as the physical or virtual proximity of the team members and institutional support for cross-disciplinary research (Hall, Stokols et al., 2008; Stokols et al., 2008). Conceptually, the transdisciplinary model provides an important framework that acknowledges that more than one discipline is needed to solve a health problem. The fact that funding agencies are promoting the model and requiring researchers to collaborate on these complex issues indicates that the model is more than the current vogue and will continue to be used as an organizing research strategy. However, "before a team science initiative is launched, efforts should be made to ensure that, at a minimum, project-specific requirements for collaborative success are present at the outset" (Stokols et al., 2008, p. 112). This recommendation from Stokols remains salient for the BCERC/P because more extensive early planning and collaboration would likely have mitigated many of the challenges faced by team members. Future transdisciplinary teams should aim to assess the effectiveness of the model because it requires further evaluation using recently developed metrics noted here to determine its success compared to more traditional research models.

DISCUSSION QUESTIONS

1. Describe the transdisciplinary approach to organizing and research. Provide evidence for your assessment of whether this is a beneficial approach or not.
2. Identify one research area that should be investigated by a transdisciplinary team and explain why this is the best approach to the proposed research.
3. Show how the five components of a learning organization can be applied to your area of transdisciplinary research.
4. Identify aspects of each of the four flows of communication that occur in your proposed transdisciplinary research.
5. Create a scheme to assess your transdisciplinary model and proposed research.

Suggested Reading

Osuch, J., Silk, K., Price, C., Barlow, J. Miller, K. Hernick, A., & Fonfa, A. (2012). An historical perspective on breast cancer activism in the United States: From education and support to partnership in scientific research. *Journal of Women's Health, 21*, 355–362.

Stokols, D., Misra, S., Moser, R. P., Hall, K. L., & Taylor, B. K. (2008). The ecology of team science: Understanding contextual influences on Transdisciplinary collaboration. *Journal of American Journal of Preventive Medicine, 35*, 96–115.

References

Atkin, C. K., Smith, S. W., Ferguson, V. & McFeters, C., (2008). A comprehensive analysis of breast cancer news coverage in leading media outlets. *Journal of Health Communication, 13*, 3–17

Breast Cancer and Environmental Research Act (2008). Public law 110–354. Retrieved from http://www.gpo.gov/fdsys/pkg/PLAW-110publ354/pdf/PLAW-110publ354.pdf.

Breast Cancer and Environment Research Program (2014). Retrieved from http://www.bcerc.org/about.htm.

Cooren, F., Kuhn, T. R., Cornelissen, J. P., & Clark, T. (2011). Communication, organizing and organization: An overview and introduction to the special issue. *Organization Studies, 32*, 1–22.

Emmons, K. M., Viswanath, K., & Colditz, G. A. (2008). The role of transdisciplinary collaboration in translating and disseminating health research, lessons learned, and exemplars of success. *The American Journal of Preventative Medicine, 35*, S204–S210.

Gebbie, K., Rosenstock, L., & Hernandez, L. M. (Eds.). (2003). *Who will keep the public healthy: Educating health professionals for the 21st century.* Institute of Medicine. Washington, DC: The National Academies Press.

Gray, B. (2008). Enhancing transdisciplinary research through collaborative leadership. *American Journal of Preventive Medicine, 35*, 124–132.

Hall, K. L., Feng, A. X., Moser, R. P., Stokols, D., & Taylor, B. K. (2008). Moving the science of team science forward: Collaboration and creativity. *American Journal of Preventive Medicine, 35*(2S), 243–249.

Hall, K. L., Stokols, D., Moser, R. P., Taylor, B. K, Thornquist, M., Nebeling, L. C., & Ehret, C. C., et al. (2008). The collaboration readiness of transdisciplinary research teams and centers: Findings from the National Cancer Institute's TREC year-one evaluation study. *Journal of American Journal of Preventive Medicine, 35*, 161–172.

Harvard School of Public Health (2014). Harvard transdisciplinary research center in energetic and cancer center. Retrieved from http://www.hsph.harvard.edu/trec/about-us/definitions/.

Interagency Breast Cancer and Environmental Research Coordinating Committee (IBCERCC) (2013). Breast cancer and the environment: Prioritizing prevention. Retrieved from http://www.niehs.nih.gov/about/boards/ibcercc/.

Kreps, G. L. & Maibach, E. W. (2008). Transdisciplinary science: The nexus between communication and public health. *Journal of Communication, 58*, 732–748.

McPhee, R. D. & Zaug, P. (2000). The communicative constitution of organizations: A framework for explanation. *The Electronic Journal of Communication, 10*, 1–16.

Marshall, A. M., Smith, S. W., & McKeon, J. K. (1995). Persuading low-income women to engage in mammography screening: Source, message, and channel preferences. *Health Communication, 7*, 283–299.

Mitchell, P. H. (2005). What's in a name? Multidisciplinary, interdisciplinary, and transdisciplinary. *Journal of Professional Nursing, 21*(6), 332–334.

Morgan, G., Kobus, K., Gerlach, K. K., et al. (2003). Facilitating transdisciplinary research: The experience of the transdisciplinary tobacco use research centers. *Nicotine & Tobacco Research, 5*, S11–S19.

Osuch, J., Silk, K., Price, C., Barlow, J. Miller, K. Hernick, A., Fonfa, A. (2012). An historical perspective on breast cancer activism in the United States: From education and support to partnership in scientific research. *Journal of Women's Health, 21*, 355–362.

Rosenfield, P. L. (1992). The potential of transdisciplinary research for sustaining and extending linkages between the health and social sciences. *Social Science and Medicine, 35*, 1343–57.

Schoeneborn, D., Blaschke, S., Cooren, F., McPhee, R. D., Seidl, D., & Taylor, J. R. (2014). The three schools of CCO thinking: Interactive dialogue and systematic comparison. *Management Communication Quarterly, 28*, 285–316.

Senge, P. M. (1990). *The fifth discipline: The art and practice of the learning organization*. New York, NY: Doubleday/Currency.

Senge, P. (2006). *The fifth discipline: The art and practice of the learning organization* (2nd ed.). New York, NY: Currency/Doubleday.

Silk, K. J., Bigsby, E., Volkman, J., Kingsley, C., Atkin, C. K., Ferrara, M., & Goins, L. A. (2006). Formative research on adolescent and adult risk perceptions for breast cancer. *Social Science and Medicine, 63*, 3124–3136.

Silk, K. J., Neuberger, L., Nazione, S., & Osuch, J. (2011). The Breast Cancer and Environment Research Centers (BCERC): A transdisciplinary model. In M. Brann (Ed.), *Contemporary case studies in health communication: Theoretical and applied approaches* (pp. 258–268). Dubuque, IA: Kendall Hunt.

Smith, S. W., Atkin, C. K., Munday, S., Skubisz, C., & Stohl, C. (2009). The impact of personal and/or close relationship experience on memorable messages about breast cancer and the perceived speech acts of the sender. *Journal of Cancer Education, 24*, 129–134.

Smith, S. W., Clark-Hitt, R., Nazione, S., Russell, J., Silk, K., & Atkin, C. K. (2013). The effects of motivation, ability, and heuristic cues on systematic processing of information about breast cancer environmental factors. *Journal of Health Communication, 7*, 845–865.

Smith, S. W., Hamel, L. M., Kotowski, M. R., Nazione, S., LaPlante, C., Atkin, C. K., Stohl, C., & Skubisz, C. (2010). Action tendency emotions associated with memorable breast cancer messages and prevention and detection behaviors. *Health Communication, 25*, 737–746.

Smith, S. W., Munday, S., LaPlante, C., Kotowski, M. R. Atkin, C. K., Skubisz, C., & Stohl, C. (2009). Topics and sources of memorable breast cancer messages: Their impact on prevention and detection behaviors. *Journal of Health Communication, 14*, 293–307.

Stokols, D. (2006). Toward a science of transdisciplinary action research. *American Journal of Community Psychology, 38*, 63–77.

Stokols, D., Misra, S., Moser, R. P., Hall, K. L., & Taylor, B. K. (2008). The ecology of team science: Understanding contextual influences on Transdisciplinary collaboration. *Journal of American Journal of Preventive Medicine, 35*, 96–115.

Whitten, P., Munday, S., LaPlante, C., & Smith, S. W. (2008). Communication assessment of the most frequented breast cancer websites: Evaluation of design and theoretical criteria. *Journal of Computer-Mediated Communication, 13*, 880–911.

19

GETTING BY WITH A LITTLE HELP FROM MY FRIENDS

Nonprofits' Use of Third Parties to Promote Public Health

Thomas Hugh Feeley and Aisha K. O'Mally

Nonprofit organizations number over 1.6 million in the United States alone and distinguish themselves from for-profit or enterprise organizations along several characteristics (Grobman, 2008). The primary distinguishing feature of a nonprofit organization is how it distributes profits when they exist in a given fiscal year. All surplus revenues in nonprofits are required to be used for the direct benefit of the organization (and are not used as dividends for its shareholders). However, many nonprofits, by their nature, do not deal in profits and are primarily dedicated to promotion of the public good in form of delivery of needed social services, including services related to public health. For example, the Bill and Melinda Gates Foundation (www.gatesfoundation.org) represents the largest nonprofit (NPO) with a 38 billion dollar endowment. As stated clearly on Gates Foundation website, the foundation is dedicated to global health and development. Gidiron, Kramer, and Salamon (1992) further define nonprofits by four other criteria—nonprofits are (a) private; (b) self-governing; (c) voluntary; and (d) for public benefit.

There are many sources of funding to support NPOs' efforts, including endowments (private funding) and public funding (local, state, federal). Some authors suggest the source(s) of funding indicate the NPO's likeliness to engage in collaborative arrangements with for-profit organizations or with private groups toward realization of agency goals (Jang & Feiock, 2007). The forms and consequences of collaborative arrangements with third parties form the basis of this chapter. It is often the case that NPOs whose mandate is the promotion of public health must rely on help from the private sector to help realize their goals.

A realization in recent years for many NPOs is an increased pressure to deliver critical health and social services with shrinking private and public resources at their disposal. Thus, NPOs are challenged to diversify their revenue sources and identify inventive methods to deliver much-needed social services—services that include protecting the environment, feeding the young, and educating the poor (Xue-ying & Wen-wen, 2008). Thus, the incentive for NPOs to partner with third parties to promote public support for a given cause (e.g., breast cancer) is great, although it is understood these collaborative agreements are undertaken with some level of cost and possible risk. After all, these collaborative arrangements do not materialize out of nowhere and it is incumbent on the NPO to clearly communicate their mission and value to the external partner before collaboration occurs (see Silk & Smith, this volume, for a discussion on research collaborations and the similar processes at play).

Before detailing one illustration of a collaborative arrangement between NPOs and partnering organizations to promote a health cause, the current chapter will detail the objectives of the NPOs, forms these collaborations may take, and review the motivations for organizations to undertake such arrangements. Also, a discussion of the communication strategies and challenges will be outlined in relation to the form of relationship detailed in Figure 19.1. Figure 19.1 illustrates the critical elements in NPO–third party relationships, with the most important element represented by the promotion of the health cause. It is the nature and emergency of the health problem that shapes and binds NPOs and third-party partners (Path A).

Figure 19.1 provides a model of the key constituencies in the nonprofit–private section collaborative relationship. Also included in this model is the relations among players denoted by one- or two-way arrows with the arrows representing communication. For example, nonprofits' communicate directly to their target audience and also communicate indirectly to the target group through organizations and groups. Thus, NPOs communicate directly to both their target audience and use media to promote a given cause. At the same time communication is two-way between NPOs and their private partners in cause promotion.

Nonprofit and Enterprise Collaborative Agreements

Before discussing the forms of collaborations/partnerships, it is imperative to address the major objectives of NPOs. Few scholars address the impact of collaboration in relation to nonprofit objectives. Lefroy and Tsarenko (2012) define and measure nonprofit goal achievement as being "the attainment of both organizational and social objectives" (p. 1644). Organizational objectives include payroll for employees, office supplies, travel expenses, or any supplies needed for campaigns. In short, organizational objectives are any costs associated with day-to-day running of the business. Social objectives are directly related to the NPO's primary issue or cause and include any cost related to spreading awareness

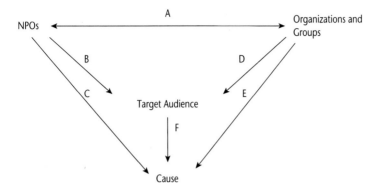

FIGURE 19.1 Collaborative Arrangement Between Nonprofits (NPOs) and Organizations.

or even education to the general public about an issue or cause (Lefroy & Tsarenko, 2012).

A pioneering NPO–corporation agreement is reviewed by Andreasen (1995) and details the decision by American Express in 1982 to donate 5 cents to arts organizations in the San Francisco Bay area for each transaction in the bay area. American Express also donated $2 for every new credit card member from the area and these efforts yielded a $108,000 windfall for the arts. Closer to the spirit of the current chapter, *Glamour* magazine, Hanes Hosiery and the National Cancer Institute (NCI; among other cancer-related organizations involved) partnered to educate young adult women about breast cancer awareness and prevention in the early 1990s. The collaboration among these entities, commonly referred to as *joint-issue promotion*, used magazine articles, in-store promotions and inserts into Hanes Hosiery to promote understanding of breast cancer. It is clear why NCI would be eager to enter into this arrangement with the enterprising organizations. Why would *Glamour* and Hanes enter into such an agreement? The answer to this question will be taken up shortly after a brief description of the forms of collaborations between NPOs and for-profits is provided.

Forms of Collaboration

There are many forms of collaborative agreements among NPOs and enterprises in support of health causes. Organizations should not restrict themselves to precedent, but should be open to inventive ways to ally with organizations. There are many factors that can dictate the form of a given arrangement, with the health problem itself as one primary factor that shapes the collaboration, and the aim of the campaign a second factor. For example, it is one aim to *promote breast cancer awareness* and another aim to *increase screening rates* in a given target population. While the health problem is the same in this example, the audience and effective methods would vary greatly when comparing these two aims. Indeed, the difference in health problems and campaign aims is likely to lead to different collaborative arrangements. Several authors (e.g., Andreason, 1996; Berger, Cunningham, & Drumwright, 2004) detail the forms of these collaborations and for the present purposes six forms will be described in relation to health promotion.

Philanthropy

Companies and groups donate time, cash, products and expertise directly to NPOs on regular basis (i.e Path E in Figure 19.1). These donations or direct giving efforts are not necessarily tied to consumer purchases or behavior. A company may choose to donate a certain amount of money and/or staff time to an NPO or perhaps commit a percentage of profits from sales to the nonprofit. For example, Starbucks offers a hundred or so youth leadership grants yearly to support community efforts globally to engage teens and young adults to give back to their neighbors (Starbucks, 2014).

Volunteer Programs

An inventive method for organizations and independent groups to assist needy causes and the NPOs whose charge it is to promote health is through volunteer work. Organizations can allow employees to either use company time or dock company time toward volunteer work for NPOs. There is also evidence philanthropic volunteer programs help to attract and retain employees through improved work skills and increased job satisfaction (Coy, 1996).

Sponsorship of Cause

A third method of collaboration is for organizations to sponsor causes through underwriting events or campaigns. How sponsorship of causes works is the organization first donates the money or resources (e.g., space, manpower) to make the event possible. The marketing of the sponsorship is thought to increase goodwill perceived by consumers on the part of the organization. This association of the company with the cause is the expected return on investment (in addition to helping the cause directly). It is important to note any contributions to the cause from the public are an addition to the sponsorship commitment – the two are not directly linked.

Cause-Related Marketing

Cause-related marketing (CRM) attracts much attention in the academic literature (Varadarajan & Menon, 1988). The company's philanthropy is a marketing technique. In CRM, the consumer's behavior comes first and then the company makes a donation in relation to the consumer behavior. The earlier example of American Express exemplifies this form of collaboration. American Express may agree to donate 1% of all purchases the first week of December in certain regions to a given cause or NPO representing the cause. Much has been written on the benefits to organizations who participate in CRM in relation to a cause. CRM is a marketing activity that promotes company image by doing well and is independent from other marketing activities, such as sales promotion (Varadarajan & Menon, 1988).

An example is in order to differentiate CRM from philanthropy for a given campaign. Smith Groceries could run a campaign where 1% of all produce sales go to the local food bank and this would be CRM. Smith Groceries could alternatively (or in addition) donate $1 for every transaction in June to the local food bank and this form of donation or support would be philanthropy in the form of joint issue promotion, a form of collaboration taken up next.

Joint Issue Promotion

Joint issue promotion involves collaborations wherein NPOs and organizations fuse together in support of a cause that is ostensibly related to the enterprise, as is the case with Smith Groceries supporting the local food bank. The concept of joint issue marketing is to attract more attention to the cause and set up positive image for the cause and for the organizations involved. Certainly the form of donation or support to a NPO can be non-monetary, such as donation of services, the provision of free flu shots, or no-cost food trucks.

Corporation Charity Fund

A final form of collaboration is a corporation charity fund where donations are solicited to the organization in the name of a given cause. This is particularly common to multinational groups who wish to set up a lasting image with their business environment or constituency. The organization may also conduct fundraising efforts or events that funnel profits or donations directly to the fund.

Before detailing communication efforts related to the collaborative relationship depicted in Figure 19.1, it is necessary to consider the motivation for NPOs and enterprises to work together toward a given cause. The motivations for an NPO to collaborate are certainly more apparent than the motivations for the enterprise, as NPO's motivation to collaborate relates directly to the aims of the organization. It is still important to review these motivations and those of third-party groups as they relate to communication processes that impinge on the development and maintenance of these important joint efforts.

Motivation for Collaboration

Earlier we asked why Hanes or *Glamour* would partner with NCI, and certainly NPOs are keen to know the motivations of for-profit companies if they seek to foster these arrangements. The motivations to corporations and even small companies can be monetary or non-monetary in nature. Very often the distinction between financial/profit gains and intangible benefits is blurred. One interesting and positive effect that can ensue from NPO–enterprise collaboration is the perception of a relationship between the organization and the cause (Path E in Figure 19.1). The result of this perception of corporate responsibility (see May, this volume, for discussion of corporate social responsibility) can be greater customer loyalty and increased sales (Lichtenstein, Drumright, & Brag, 2004).

In addition to greater social responsibility shown by NPO collaboration toward a health cause, third parties can benefit within the organization by enhanced employee culture,increased morale, and improved recruitment and retention of key employees (Xue-ying & Wen-wen, 2008). For example, if employees participate in a given collaboration with a NPO, it can increase loyalty and a sense of belonging for them which aids increasing work efficiency. Community service expectations for employees can foster an environment of empathy that reinforces a service-oriented mentality (Austin, 2000). Partnering with an NPO and giving back to the community also can be a strategic move for organizations and enrich the company's own aims and vision through service outreach and philanthropy. In short, there are several gains that may be realized through NPO–corporate collaborations and they stand to benefit employee culture, company image, and ultimately profit margins.

From the NPO perspective, there are clear motivations that drive partnerships with corporations. The most obvious motivation is financial investment when corporations donate generously to the NPO through cause-related marketing or philanthropy (Wymer & Samu, 2003). The collaboration can bring additional resources and promotional activities that benefit the cause. While these collaborations require a certain amount of calibration and oversight, they can become long-term partnerships that bring gains to the NPO directly in addition to greater attention and support for the cause itself.

Other underlying motivations for NPOs to collaborate include synergies, reputation enhancement, and other non-financial gains. Stated more plainly, together the groups achieve more working collaboratively than if each worked independent of one another in health promotion. Xue-ying and Wen-wen note, "they come together to assemble sufficient collective confidence, knowledge, skills, financial resources, or political power to enable them to be effective" (2008, p. 518). Reputation is an important social asset for NPOs as reputation enhances their ability to attract and retain employees, public donations, volunteers and partners (Deephouse & Carter, 2005), along with increasing or maintaining organizational credibility, and ability to overcome hardship (Milne, Iyer, & Gooding-Williams, 1996). Lastly, non-financial resources are also a motivation for collaboration. Technology, expert assistance, and labor are considered as critical resources corporations can provide NPOs with to reach their organizational and social objectives.

The next section discusses the communication challenges facing both NPOs and third-party groups in relation to health promotion. A convenient method to organize these challenges is to use Figure 19.1 to direct the discussion around communication processes in health promotion. An important consideration is the need to influence targeted individuals in relation to a given cause. This explains why Path F is designated on Figure 19.1 to indicate the relationship between individuals and the given health cause. For example, cancer prevention through increased colorectal screening is an important goal (e.g., Feeley, Cooper, Foels, & Mahoney, 2009) and the specific aim is to influence *individuals* to undergo screening. And this aim is accomplished through strategic health communication campaigns that stand to benefit from collaborations with NPOs (e.g., Feeley & Yang, 2013).

Communication Considerations

Forming the Partnership

The collaboration between a given NPO and third party groups (i.e., Path A in Figure 19.1) or organizations requires initiation and maintenance. Communication strategies are required to forge and sustain relationships with organizations. Any strategy used by NPOs must communicate the aims of the organization and the potential forms collaboration might take. A persuasive strategy to encourage collaboration is to use *social proofs* to show the value of collaboration; that is, show examples of other collaborations with like-minded companies or groups. Social proofs provide legitimacy to a given idea or practice by the use of evidence. An example of social proofs is the use of 'salted' tip jars for bartenders—customers' witness others recently tipped for service and thus make the practice appear normative. An organization showing evidence of other successful collaborations with the NPO (or with similar NPOs) may feel an even greater social responsibility to support the cause.

Once established, the collaborative agreement between NPOs and organizations must be sustained and perhaps strengthened via communication. Using the influence principle of *commitment and consistency*, the NPO may seek to strengthen the level of giving or support by the organization (see Cialdini, 1984). Commitment and consistency works by securing an initial level of commitment and then requesting a larger level of commitment in the future. Once committed, the individual, group or organization feels impelled to act consistently with their initial agreement. The appearance of inconsistency or hypocrisy may be undesirable to an organization. Also, organizations (or NPOs) may now require internal or external justification for their initial level of commitment of time, resources, or manpower.

Two factors impinge upon the commitment–consistency relationship: size of initial commitment and the public or private nature of the initial level of commitment. This morning I saw a poster at Manhattan Bagel advertising their cause-related campaign with American Cancer Society (ACS) where for one month they will donate 10 cents for every cup of coffee purchased. This poster publicly communicates their level of commitment to ACS and depending on how much accounting is required for the marketing campaign; the cost of initial commitment may be minimal. Greater levels of commitment coupled with the public nature of the commitments (e.g., through advertising) strengthen a third party's resolve to appear consistent and NPOs may be well served to remind organizations (and communicate their appreciation) of their earlier commitment(s) to the cause and ask for a higher level of participation. Thus, strategic communication on the part of NPOs can encourage new collaborations and also strengthen existing relationships that benefit the given health cause.

The majority of NPOs in health are dedicated to health prevention or detection and educating the general public or a given target audience about the prevalence and importance of the cause. Early models of prosocial intervention, such as Latane and Darley's (1970) bystander intervention model (see also Anker & Feeley, 2011), indicate individuals' need to *notice the event* and in turn *take responsibility for action* before helping occurs. Thus campaigns seek to increase the salience of the health cause through creative messaging and repetition.

Targeting the Cause and the Audience

The relationship between the target audience and the cause is another important consideration in collaboration. How relevant is the cause to an audience or, using the language of bystander intervention, how likely are targeted individuals to *interpret the cause as an emergency*? One might resolve they will quit smoking later in life or delay breast cancer screening till their forties. Certainly NPOs and organizations target individuals but messaging, if it is to be successful, must be sensitive to the audience–cause relationship (i.e., Path F).

Audiences with more direct experience or involvement with a cause will be more likely to attend to messaging and its message content. The messaging must also consider the costs and benefits associated with the health cause. The level of *self-efficacy* to perform the required action is an important consideration typically in health campaigns (Bandura, 1977). Thus, messages must communicate the relative ease and value of a given health practice or procedure. For example, oral hygiene is as easy as brushing your teeth twice per day to avoid cavities or worse conditions. Clearly there are health prevention measures that are perceived as higher in costs, such as colon cancer screening or yearly mammograms, that require creative messaging to recalcitrant individuals.

The relationship between the organization and the cause is an important consideration (Path E). It may not be patently clear that cancer prevention and bagels are associated, so it is imperative for Manhattan Bagel to create this association to shape customers' perception of the corporation–cause relation (C–C).

The greater the perceptions of the C–C link among customers, the higher the return on investment for the corporation in the form of customer loyalty (Andreason, 1996). Communicating an organization is civic-minded and dedicated to helping causes related to public health is an important and strategic message. What is more, the NPO can assist in promoting the C–C relation by promoting joint-related campaigns or other collaborative arrangements.

The amount of profits for the nonprofits in collaborating with outside organizations and groups can be many and these collaborations need not be 'one and done' in nature. Instead, yearly campaigns or functions can become important to an NPO's specific aims to promote public health in a given region. The next section seeks to bring some of these concepts to light through a specific case study involving the promotion of organ donation in the past decade or so. Before detailing the various collaborative arrangements between NPOs and outside groups, it is first important to detail the nature of the public health problem in relation to organ donation.

Case in Point: Collaborative Promotion of Organ Donation

Organ donation has represented nothing short of a medical marvel since the first kidney transplant in 1954 between identical twins in South Africa (Tillney, 2003). Transplanted organs extend the lives of thousands of Americans yearly, and for many represent the only life-saving treatment for organ failure. The national scale of the problem indicates there are currently 123,882 individuals on the active waiting list (www.unos.org) and this number increases exponentially yearly. At the same time the number of organ donors and transplants has remained steady for the past decade—in 2013 there were 14,256 donors while in 2004 there were 14,154 donors. Of note, a deceased donor typically provides three to four viable organs for transplant recipients and deceased donors represent 55–60% of all donors (living donors make up the remainder of the donors). Thus there is an increasing gap between the actual number of donors and the number of donors needed to significantly reduce the size of the waiting list.

So that you have a better understanding of what the Organ Procurement Organizations (OPOs) do, we briefly describe the process of organ donation. The typical manner for deceased donation to occur requires an individual to experience brain death in a hospital and be kept breathing on a ventilator so the organs are still viable.[1] The OPO is contacted by the hospital and an OPO coordinator works with hospital clinical staff to determine eligibility. If brain death is determined, OPO staff approach families to discuss donation options. In some cases, the decedent's wishes are known in relation to organ donation and optimally his or her wishes were communicated to next-of-kin directly. In other cases, one's intentions are made known through state-operated registries that are *first-person consent* and the coordinator and staff may lawfully recover the organ(s), as this type of registry is legally binding (as opposed to a registry of intent).

The NPOs: Organ Procurement Organizations

The organizations charged with increasing the pool of suitable donors are called Organ Procurement Organizations (OPOs) and they number 58 in the United States. Since 1984, OPOs have been federally designated agencies assigned regionally to address organ donation in a number of important ways. OPO staff members provide clinical services in terms of screening and authorizing donation for eligible patients. In terms of deceased donation, OPO coordinators identify the decedent's wishes (via the state registry) and approach next-of-kin in relation to donation. The donation decision and request is the purview of the OPO and is thus decoupled with the medical care team whose job is to treat the patient. OPOs also provide services to the donor family before, during, and long after donation occurs.

Additionally, OPOs are charged with hospital development of health professionals and public education about transplantation. This last responsibility of OPOs, public education, is the focus of the current chapter, and is considered as their main social objective as discussed earlier in the chapter. Hospital development and public education positively influence the main cause of the OPOs, organ donation. Specifically, OPOs often partner with third party organizations (e.g., hospitals, corporations, universities) to promote donation in the surrounding community (see Figure 19.2 for the application of our model of collaborations to the OPO setting). Educating selective audiences about organ donation and transplantation is no small task as studies indicate the general public report a lack of understanding about transplantation, and the popular media do little to help with sensationalized accounts of donation failures and fictional portrayals of the transplant process (Harrison, Morgan, & Chewning, 2008; Morgan, King, Smith, & Ivic, 2010).

Target Audience

OPOs have a direct link (Figure 19.2, Path C) to the cause of donation and work directly with organ donation promotion and recovery. What is also in their purview is public education of donation—this link (Path B) is what typically forms the OPO–third party relationship. That is, OPOs are required to educate the general public about transplantation and typically have a limited budget and limited staff to achieve this mandate. The challenge OPO staff face is to reach the general public with messages that influence their understanding and ultimately their decision-making surrounding donation intentions, declared through joining an organ donor registry (Feeley & Yang, 2013). One key difference from our more general model is that there is no direct link between OPO partner organizations and organ donation. This is because they work with OPOs to educate and register potential donors, not engage in actual transplantation—a process that is handled directly by the OPO, transplant team, and the United Network of Organ Sharing (UNOS). As such, their link to the cause is mediated through the target audience of potential donors.

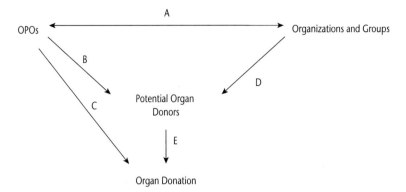

FIGURE 19.2   Organ Procurement Organizations' (OPOs) Collaboration to Promote Organ Donation.

The importance of filling the registry cannot be overstated as donation consent is made prior to eligibility and changes the conversation between coordinators and family members from an "ask" to a "tell" scenario. There are primarily three methods to register one's organ donation intentions: through certain Department of Motor Vehicles (DMV) transactions (e.g., license renewal), through a dedicated enrollment form, or through a state's online registry. To date, the DMV method is most common and this method has its own challenges due to long lapses in license renewals and reluctance of DMV clerks to discuss donation (Feeley, Reynolds-Tylus, Anker & Evans, 2014). The net effect is approximately 50% of adults nationally have formally registered their intentions (Gallup, 2012). Thus, there is a large target group that is still unregistered and in some cases those who are registered must re-register when they are required to renew their license or when DMVs change their registry systems.

The constellation of beliefs and emotions surrounding donation is a complicated mix of positive sentiment, uncertainty, and a certain level of squeamishness in many individuals. The sentiment in the academic literature indicates adults generally are in favor of organ donation as an overall concept (e.g., Feeley, 2007). However, when studies probe further (e.g., Pomerantz, 2010; Morgan et al., 2008), the beliefs surrounding donation are more sophisticated and, when the question is more personalized, individuals appear less comfortable about themselves donating compared to *others* donating. Anker and Feeley (2011) likened the donation decision to a bystander effect (Darley & Latane, 1968) wherein individuals fail to recognize the organ shortage problem and also do not take responsibility in helping the public health cause.

A challenge for NPOs and their partners is debunking false beliefs surrounding transplantation that are propagated through popular media (Morgan et al., 2007; Feeley, O'Mally, & Covert, in press). Three popular myths include a belief one's health care will be compromised if one is known to be a registered donor ("they will pull the plug earlier"), the myth that one is too old or unqualified to donate, and belief in unfair organ allocation process ("someone wealthy will get my organs"). Also, many individuals have non-cognitive beliefs about donation, that Morgan et al. (2008) term the "ick factor."

Related to the current chapter, nonprofits and their collaborators must educate individuals about the importance of organ donation and at the same time impress upon individuals the importance of registering one's intentions through enrollment and family notification (Feeley & Servoss, 2005). The forms of organ donation promotional activities will be taken up shortly in relation to nonprofit–third party arrangements. The content of messages typically consists of two important messages: (a) messages communicating the value of donation, and (b) messages communicating the facts about donation and transplantation.

Collaborative Arrangements in Organ Donation Promotion

OPOs have wisely collaborated with organizations to reach social objectives, to get the message out, and to ultimately increase the number of individuals who consent to donation through state registries. There are at least three types of organizations that OPOs have allied with to promote donation to targeted groups—enterprise organizations, college or university campuses and motor vehicles offices. Each organization represents a different collaborative arrangement and the dynamics of each arrangement are documented below.

Enterprise Organizations

Morgan, Miller, and Arasaratnam (2002) detailed the elements of a communication campaign to promote organ donation in two United Parcel Services (UPS) sites in the United States. The authors used one site as control and one as intervention, testing the efficacy of mass media appeals (e.g., billboards, newspaper articles, PSAs) and interpersonal appeals (e.g., tabling, educational sessions) on employees' intent to sign the organ donor registry and willingness to discuss donation with next-of-kin. The results indicated meaningful increases on several important factors antecedent to donation signing, such as knowledge, attitudes and subjective norms. Using the typology of potential collaborative arrangements listed earlier, the UPS–OPO (Kentucky Organ Donor Affiliates) arrangement can be considered a *volunteer program* wherein UPS permitted the OPO to use company media and employee time to promote the cause.

A second illustration of an OPO–organization agreement is reported by Morgan, Harrison, Chewning, DiCorcia, and Davis (2010) and represents a campaign spanning 45 organizations in New Jersey. These "worksite campaigns" (p. 341) varied the intensity of the campaign to identify differences in registrations rates from pre-test to post-test. The high intensity campaigns (i.e., campaigns that combined media and interpersonal channels in promotion) yielded higher registration rates when compared to low-intensity campaigns (i.e., media only) and no campaigns. The volunteer nature of collaboration was relatively low cost to organizations, which varied in size. Specifically, the costs to organizations included providing phone lists to researchers to conduct surveys to test the efficacy of the campaign, and access to OPO staff to promote donation on site for limited engagements (e.g., tabling in high traffic areas, such as cafeterias, email blasts, and posters).

University Partnership

A second form of collaboration is between OPOs and universities in the promotion of donation. Universities' motivation to partner with OPOs is usually driven by the value-added nature of collaborations in relation to service learning. Service learning opportunities provide a context for students to learn experientially in the community. Bringle and Hatcher (1996) summarize service learning as:

> A credit-bearing educational experience in which students participate in an organized service activity that meets identified community needs and reflect on the service activity in such a way as to gain further understanding of course content, a broader appreciation of the discipline, and an enhanced sense of civic responsibility.
>
> *(p. 222)*

Feeley, Williams, Anker and Vincent (2010) detail several years of OPO–university collaborations wherein students in public relations courses were hired by the OPO to promote donation on campus and in the campus community through media and other outreach efforts such as tabling and classroom presentations (see also Weber & Martin, 2012). A second illustration of OPO–campus collaboration is the use of student groups with team leaders to promote donation through social media or through offline methods (presentations, face-to-face approach) to their peers (Feeley et al., 2009, 2010; Stefanone, Anker, Evans & Feeley, 2012).

The benefits to students who campaign on behalf of donation are many—they learn the challenges of conducting a real promotional campaign versus reading about one in a textbook or in lecture. Second, students are usually given goals in terms of outreach (e.g., web hits, facebook likes) or results (e.g., number of signed organ cards) and must justify their activities in a time-sensitive project and present these activities to the client (the OPO).

Department of Motor Vehicles Collaboration

A somewhat obvious collaboration is between Department of Motor Vehicles (DMV) offices and OPOs. This type of partnership can be considered a *sponsorship of causes*. DMVs represent an ideal partner with OPOs as the majority of new organ donor registrants come from DMV transactions. The forms of collaborations between OPOs and DMVs vary from low-intensity media campaigns (e.g., posters, brochures, streaming video) to OPO staff discussing the donation decision with customers (Feeley et al., 2014, Harrison et al., 2010, 2011, Rodrigue et al., 2013). DMVs also provide the staff (employees to clerks) to make these campaigns possible. The motivation for DMV offices to collaborate is to partner with a community partner to help educate clerks and customers about donation (e.g., Harrison, Morgan, & DiCorcia, 2008). A second, perhaps less noble motivation, is to appease county clerks or community leaders who require DMV participation. The campaigns listed above are all examples of successful campaigns and collaborations between OPOs, universities, and DMVs to promote organ donation.

Summary

Nonprofits can benefit from collaborative arrangements with enterprise organizations in their community who seek to promote community health and welfare. This type of partnership aids NPOs in meeting their organizational objectives. While there are certain costs to establishing and maintaining these collaborations, the benefits to supporting nonprofits' bottom line can be many, such as an important revenue stream and assistance with joint-issue promotion. Some health issues might involve health prevention (e.g., colon cancer screening) and some may involve detection (e.g., mammography) while other health issues might be related to health promotion (e.g., blood drives).

An illustration of one type of collaboration between OPOs and their community partners in the form of universities, DMV offices and enterprising organizations was described. Space prevents a more expansive discussion of how OPO–third group collaborations come to fruition, as seldom do groups or organizations come knocking at the proverbial nonprofit door. These important relationships must be initiated by nonprofit public communications staff and nurtured over time. The hallmark of a successful collaboration is one that is sustained over time and the contributions to public health increase yearly as organizations increase their commitment to helping the public good.

DISCUSSION QUESTIONS

1. Name two for-profit and NPO collaborations that you are aware of and describe their relationship. What made you aware of these relationships?
2. Can you think of any other companies (for profit or nonprofit) that OPOs might collaborate with to achieve their social objective of building awareness for organ donation?
3. Create your own case study by thinking of some partnerships between other NPOs and for-profit companies that can fit one of the collaborations mentioned in this chapter. List what motivations are for both sides. List the benefits of collaboration for both sides.

Note

1 There is also donation after cardiac death (DCD)—donors who suffer devastating and irreversible brain injury and may be near death, but do not meet formal brain death criteria. In these cases, the family may decide to withdraw care. When the patient's heart stops beating, the organs are then recovered in the operating room.

Suggested Reading

Morgan, S. E., Harrison, T. R., Chewing, L. V., DiCorcia, M. J., & Davis, L. A. (2010). The effectiveness of high- and low-intensity worksite campaigns to promote organ donation: The workplace partnership for life. *Communication Monographs, 77*, 341–356.

Morgan, S. E., Miller, J., & Arasaratnam, L. A. (2002). Signing cards and saving lives: An evaluation of the worksite organ donation promotion project. *Communication Monographs, 69*, 253–273.

References

Andreasen, A. R. (1995). Profits for nonprofit: Find a corporate partner. *Harvard Business Review, 74*(6), 47–50.

Anker, A. E. & Feeley, T. H. (2011). Are nonparticipants in prosocial behavior merely innocent bystanders? *Health Communication, 26*, 13–24.

Austin, J. E. (2000). Strategic collaboration between nonprofits and business. *Nonprofit and Voluntary Sector Quarterly, 29*, 69–97.

Bandura, A. (1977). Self-efficacy: Toward a unifying theory of behavior change. *Psychological Review, 84*, 191–215.

Berger, L. P., Cunningham, P., & Drumwright, M. (2004). Social alliances: Company/nonprofit collaboration. *California Management Review, 47*, 58–90.

Bringle, R. G. & Hatcher, J. A. (1996). Implementing service learning in higher education. *Journal of Higher Education, 67*, 221–239.

Cialdini, R. B. (1984). *Influence*. New York, NY: Quill.

Coy, J. (1996). Redesigning corporate philanthropy. In L. Dennis (Ed.), *Practical public affairs in an era of change* (pp. 143–156). Lanham, MD: University Press of America.

Darley, J. M. & Latane, B. (1968). Bystander intervention in emergencies: Diffusion of responsibility. *Journal of personality and social psychology, 8*(4p1), 377.

Deephouse, D. L. & Carter, S.M. (2005). An examination of differences between organizational legitimacy and organizational reputation. *Journal of Management Studies, 42*, 329–360.

Feeley, T. H. (2007). College students' knowledge, attitudes, and behaviors regarding organ donation. *Journal of Applied Social Psychology, 37*, 243–271.

Feeley, T. H., Anker, A. E., Watkins, B., Rivera, J., Tag, N., & Volpe, L. (2009). A peer-to-peer campaign to promote organ donation among racially diverse college students in New York City. *Journal of National Medical Association, 101*, 1154–1162.

Feeley, T. H., Anker, A. E., Williams, C. R., & Vincent, D. E. (2010). A multi-campus classroom intervention to promote organ and tissue donation. In E. Alvaro & J. Siegel (Eds.). *Understanding organ donation: Implementing and evaluating health behavior interventions* (pp. 200–220). Malden, MA: Wiley-Blackwell.

Feeley, T. H., Cooper, J., Foels, T., & Mahoney, M. C. (2009). Efficacy expectations in colorectal cancer screening: The perspectives of the patient and the clinician. *Health Communication, 24*, 304–315.

Feeley, T. H., O'Mally, A. K., & Covert, J. M. (in press). A Content Analysis of Organ Donation Stories Printed in United States' Newspapers: Application of Newsworthiness. *Health Communication.*

Feeley, T. H., Reynolds-Tylus, T., Anker, A. E., & Evans, M. (2014). Reasons for (not) signing the state registry: Surveying Department of Motor Vehicles customers in New York State. *Progress in Transplantation, 24,* 97–105

Feeley, T. H. & Servoss, T. J. (2005). College students as potential organ donors: Reasons for low signing rates. *Journal of Health Communication, 10,* 237–250.

Feeley, T. H. & Yang, Z. J. (2013). Promoting organ donation through communication campaigns. In M.A. Lauri (Ed.), *Organ donation and transplantation: An interdisciplinary approach* (pp. 263–278). New York, NY: Nova Biomedical.

Gallup. (2012). 2012 national survey of organ donation attitudes and behaviors. Retrieved from www.organdonor.gov/dtcp/nationalsurveyorgandonation.pdf.

Gidiron, B., Kramer, R. M., & Salamon, L. M. (1992). *Government and the third sector.* San Francisco, CA: Jossey-Bass.

Gourville, J. T. & Rangan, V. K. (2004). Valuing the cause marketing relationship. *California Management Review, 47,* 38–56.

Grobman, G. M. (2008). The nonprofit handbook: Everything you need to know to start and run your nonprofit organization. Harrisburg, PA: White Hat Communications.

Harrison, T. R., Morgan, S. E., & Chewning, L. V. (2008). Social marketing for health meets the marketing for entertainment: The case of organ donation. *Health Marketing Quarterly, 25,* 33–65.

Harrison, T. R., Morgan, S. E., & DiCorcia, M. J. (2008). The impact of organ donation education and communication training for gatekeepers: DMV clerks and organ donor registries. *Progress in Transplantation, 18,* 301–309.

Harrison, T. R., Morgan, S. E., King, A. J., DiCorcia, M. J., Williams, E. A., Ivic, R. K., & Hopeck, P. (2010). Promoting the Michigan Organ Donor Registry: Evaluating the impact of a multi-faceted intervention utilizing media priming and communication design. *Health Communication, 25,* 700–708.

Harrison, T. R., Morgan, S. E., King, A. J., & Williams, E. A. (2011). Saving lives branch by branch: The effectiveness of driver licensing bureau campaigns to promote organ donor registry sign-ups to African Americans in Michigan. *Journal of Health Communication, 16,* 805–819.

Jang, H. S. & Feiock, R. C. (2007). Public versus private funding of nonprofit organizations. *Public Performance & Management Review, 31,* 174–190.

Latane, B. & Darley, J. M. (1970). *The unresponsive bystander: Why doesn't he help?* Englewood Cliffs, NJ: Prentice Hall.

Lefroy, K. & Tsarenko, Y. (2012). From receiving to achieving: The role of relationship and dependence for nonprofit organizations in corporate partnerships. *European Journal of Marketing, 47,* 1641–1666.

Lichtenstein, D. R., Drumwright, M. E., & Braig, B. M. (2004). The effect of corporate social responsibility of customer donations to corporate-supported nonprofits. *Journal of Marketing, 68,* 16–32.

Milne, G.R., Iyer, E. S., & Gooding-Williams, S. (1996). Environmental organization alliance relationships within and across nonprofit, business, and government sectors. *Journal of Public Policy and Marketing, 15,* 203–215.

Morgan, S. E., Harrison, T. R., Chewning, L. V., Davis, L., & DiCorcia, M. (2007). Entertainment (mis)education: The framing of organ donation in entertainment television. *Health Communication, 22*(2), 143–152.

Morgan, S. E., Harrison, T. R., Chewning, L. V., DiCorcia, M. J., & Davis, L. A. (2010). The effectiveness of high- and low-intensity worksite campaigns to promote organ donation: The workplace partnership for life. *Communication Monographs, 77*, 341–356.

Morgan, S. E., King, A. J., Smith, J. R., & Ivic, R. (2010). A kernel of truth? The impact of television storylines exploiting myths about organ donation on the public's willingness to donate. *Journal of Communication, 60*, 778–796.

Morgan, S. E., Miller, J., & Arasaratnam, L. A. (2002). Signing cards and saving lives: An evaluation of the worksite organ donation promotion project. *Communication Monographs, 69*, 253–273.

Morgan, S. E., Stephenson, M. T., Harrison, T. R., Afifi, W. A., & Long, S. D. (2008). Facts versus "feelings": How rational is the decision to become an organ donor? *Journal of Health Psychology, 13*, 644–658.

Pomerantz, A. (2010). The value of qualitative studies of interpersonal conversations about health topics: A study of family discussions about organ donation and illustrations (pp. 272–291). In E. Alvaro & J. Siegel (Eds.), *Understanding organ donation: Implementing and evaluating health behavior interventions.* Malden, MA: Wiley-Blackwell.

Rodrigue, J. R., Krouse, J., Carroll, C., Giery, K. M., Fraga, Y., & Edwards. E. (2013). A department of motor vehicles intervention yields moderate increases in donor designation rates. *Progress in Transplantation, 22*, 18–24.

Starbucks Foundation (n.d.). Retrieved from http://www.starbucks.com/responsibility/community/opportunity-youth.

Stefanone, M., Anker, A. E., Evans, M., & Feeley, T. H. (2012). Click to "like" organ donation: The use of online media to promote organ donor registration. *Progress in Transplantation, 22*, 168–174.

Tilney, N. L. (2003). *Transplant: From myth to reality.* New Haven, CT: Yale University Press.

Varadarajan, P. R. & Menon, A. (1988). Cause-related marketing: A coalignment of marketing strategy and corporate philosophy. *Journal of Marketing, 52*, 58–74.

Weber, K. & Martin, M. M. (2012). Designing and evaluating the campus organ donor project. *Communication Quarterly, 60*, 504–519.

Wymer Jr., W. W. & Samu, S. (2003). Dimensions of business and non-profit collaborative relationships. *Journal of Nonprofit & Public Sector Marketing, 11*(1), 3–22.

Xue-ying, T. & Wen-wen, S. (2008). Motivation and form of the collaboration between enterprise and nonprofit organization. *International Seminar on Business and Information Management.*

20

LEADING INTERORGANIZATIONAL HEALTH COLLABORATIONS

The Importance of Multi-Dyadic Relationships

Elizabeth A. Williams

Health initiatives often require collaborations between multiple organizations. For example, disease outbreaks create the need for partnerships between large government organizations (e.g., the Centers for Disease Control and Prevention [CDC], the World Health Organization [WHO]), local health departments, hospitals, and health providers. Another example of these partnerships is when organizations partner to address a health concern—for instance oftentimes governmental organizations (e.g., the National Institutes of Health) provide funding to university researchers who then collaborate with various organizations with aims of promoting some type of health behavior (e.g., cancer screening, organ donation, vaccinations) or encouraging research on a health issue (for an exemplar of this, see Silk & Smith, this volume). These interorganizational collaborations are complex because although all parties share the same overarching goal, each organization has multiple additional goals. These goals may compete with the larger goal that seeks to unite the organizations. Additionally, oftentimes these partnerships are caused by some environmental exigency (e.g., a disease outbreak) and bring together organizations that may or may not have relational histories.

In this chapter, I argue that coordination *between* positional leaders in organizations is central to the success of these collaborations. To do so, I explore how relationships among leaders of component organizations (i.e., those organizations involved in the larger system), and subsequently among those leaders and their organizational members, can facilitate or constrain organizing processes and goal achievement in interorganizational health collaborations. Specifically, I draw from exchange theories of leadership to understand the influence of these multi–dyadic relationships on organizational partnerships and consequently on the success of health initiatives by exploring both a recent example from media coverage of the Ebola epidemic in West Africa and an empirical study of a multiteam system. To do so, I first position health collaborations as functioning multiteam systems (MTSs; see also Real & Poole, this volume). I then examine how leadership has been explored in health collaborations broadly and in MTSs specifically. I subsequently make the argument that, in order to fully understand the functioning of health MTSs and to adequately harness the power of multiple teams working together, exchange theories of leadership, and specifically recent advancements of this theoretical tradition, are a particularly well-suited framework to guide leadership of health collaborations. To make this argument, I delineate the communicative components of exchange theories of leadership, and offer specific ways the theory may be operationalized.

Multiteam Systems

One way to conceptualize the organization of large-scale health collaborations is by using an MTS framework. A theory of MTSs was first proposed by Mathieu, Marks, and Zaccaro (2001) who offer the following definition:

> Multi-team systems are two or more teams that interface directly and interdependently in response to environmental contingencies toward the accomplishment of collective goals. MTS boundaries are defined by virtue of the fact that all teams within the system, while pursuing different proximal goals, share at least one common distal goal; and in so doing exhibit input, process, and outcome interdependence with at least one other team in the system.
>
> *(p. 290)*

From this definition four important elements of MTSs can be identified: (a) they consist of multiple teams; (b) these teams rely on one another to complete tasks and achieve goals; (c) they share a collective goal; and (d) the teams negotiate a variety of organizational and team boundaries. Mathieu and colleagues (2001) offer one additional defining characteristic of MTSs: (e) they are an open system that stems from and responds to environmental needs. The remainder of this section walks through an example of a health collaboration and highlights how it exemplifies the elements of MTSs.

An example of a health collaboration that could be framed as an MTS is the international response to the Ebola outbreak. The outbreak which began in West Africa in March of 2014 and is an ongoing threat at the time this chapter was written has affected over 23,000 people and resulted in just under 10,000 deaths as of February, 2015 (CDC, 2015a). Indeed, this outbreak is one of monumental proportions and has required the coordination and collaboration of multiple teams. Considering the above definition, the international response to this outbreak provides a clearer understanding of the nuances of MTSs.

In this MTS, there are countless individual component teams—local health departments, hospitals, non-governmental international aid organizations (e.g., Doctors Without Borders or the Young Men's Christian Association (YMCA)—an organization whose response to the Ebola epidemic is discussed in Taylor and Kent, this volume), international governmental agencies (e.g., the U.S. CDC); and multi-nation collaborative organizations (e.g., the WHO). These teams must coordinate activities with one another to achieve their collective goal: stopping the spread of Ebola. Although eradicating the virus is the superordinate goal, each team may also have different proximal goals. In MTS research, proximal goals refer to those immediate goals that the component teams have and distal goals are those superordinate goals of the system (Zaccaro, Marks, & DeChurch, 2012). These proximal goals are often organized into a goal hierarchy in which certain goals must be met prior to other goals being accomplished. For example, in this MTS medical professionals' proximal goal is to care for the ill; however, before that happens, public health officials have to convince the ill to come to the clinic for care and then there has to be a transportation infrastructure to get the ill to the Ebola treatment units or hospitals. This was one of the main issues at the onset of the crisis—infected patients believed that Ebola treatment centers were "death traps . . . even desperately ill patients devoted their waning strength to avoiding them" (Sack, Fink, Belluck & Nossiter, 2014, para. 11).

Some of the messages initially disseminated both by local governments and by well-meaning aid organizations did little to ease those fears as they did not take into account the local culture and customs. Additionally, the local government, at least in Guinea, is reported to have had the competing goal of ensuring "'positive communication' so as not to scare away airlines and mining companies" (Sack et al., 2014, para. 68). Indeed, a major factor in the spread of the disease was that public outreach was not able to encourage the infected to seek treatment and instead those who were ill and highly contagious remained in their communities, exposing others to the virus. In this example, the two proximal goals—to encourage the ill to seek care and to care for them—are organized into a hierarchy in which one goal must be accomplished before progress on the next begins (i.e., in cultures highly suspicious of biomedical health care, the first step is gaining trust so that the ill seek care). The existence of this goal hierarchy is believed to result in cooperation among component teams as it creates interdependence among the teams. That is, one group cannot complete their task without the other group completing theirs, and likewise no group can see the task through to completion without the involvement of at least one other team—neither world-class care nor culturally sensitive messaging can be effective at stopping the spread of the virus without the other.

In addition to a range of proximal goals, various degrees of functional interdependence also exist among teams. Functional interdependence is defined as "a state by which entities have mutual reliance, determination, influence, and shared vested interest in processes they use to accomplish work activities" (Mathieu et al., 2001, p. 293). Three types of functional interdependence are identified in the MTS literature: intensive, reciprocal, and sequential. Intensive independence is when system members are working side by side on a particular task. For example, CDC officials work with health department personnel from various affected countries to develop procedures for checking individuals for Ebola symptoms at the country's points of entry (e.g., airports, CDC, 2015b). Next, reciprocal interdependence is when system members hand tasks back and forth. An example of this would be medical personnel handing off the care of patients as individuals can spend only 45 to 60 minutes in the protective gear required to be worn when caring for the ill (Sack et al., 2014). Finally, sequential interdependence is marked by system members completing their portion of the task and then other component teams taking over to complete their assignment. For example, Doctors Without Borders often transitions projects to local organizations when the need for continued intervention is not acute and local individuals have received adequate training to continue to provide care (Doctors Without Borders, 2015). As we see from the examples of the various types of interdependence, no one type of interdependence is more or less important. In order to stop the outbreak of the disease all forms of interdependence between the multiple teams and agencies responding are significant.

Next, teams in MTSs negotiate a variety of borders or boundaries. These teams may all exist within the same organization or they may come from a variety of organizations. In the example above, not only are there various organizations (i.e., international aid organizations, hospitals, local health departments) but there are also larger entities to which some of these teams belong (e.g., the CDC has had a large presence in Africa during the epidemic and is a U.S. governmental agency). Additionally, not all members of the individual organizations are a part of the MTS. For instance, despite the large amount of CDC resources going towards Ebola, not all members of the organization have participated in the Ebola response. These boundaries may be fluid, negotiated, and contested.

Moreover, Mathieu and colleagues (2001) contend that an additional defining characteristic of MTSs is that they are an open system that stems from and responds to environmental needs. Certainly, in this example we see an open system at work. As the need for assistance became acute, various organizations have sent assistance. Organizations come into the system and leave the system. The teams and organizations that are participating in providing care and resources are fluid and, while it is likely that many of these organizations have worked together before, they typically come together only when there is a need—an exigency such as a health epidemic.

With these five MTS features in mind, we can begin to understand why leadership in this scenario is so important. Specifically there is a need for strong leadership *within* individual teams as these groups must define their goals and coordinate activity to achieve those goals as any team must do. However, in MTSs there is also a need for *between* team leadership as the goal of these teams coming together is to harness the various strengths and abilities and to coordinate the activity of the multiple teams in order to address a problem that is too big for any one team—to "facilitate a degree of effective synergy and coordination among component teams in the MTS" (Zaccaro & DeChurch, 2012, p. 264; see also DeChurch, Burke, Shuffler, Lyons, Doty & Salas, 2011; DeChurch & Marks, 2006).

Leadership in Health Collaborations and Multiteam Systems

The study of leadership in health collaborations has existed largely outside of the communication discipline. Indeed, a search for "leadership" in the flagship health communication journals (i.e., *Journal of Health Communication, Health Communication*) returned few, if any, articles explicitly examining leadership processes. In addition, while paying attention to several organizational factors in the delivery of health care, the *Routledge Handbook of Health Communication* (Thompson, Parrott, & Nussbaum, 2011) also neglects to explore leadership or the communication among and from leaders as a central force in the delivery of health care.

Indeed, the examinations of health leadership that do exist come from scholars outside of the communication discipline who are interested in the collaborative nature of health care (e.g., Alexander, Comfort, Weiner, & Bogue, 2001; Currie & Lockett, 2011; VanVactor, 2012; White, Currie, & Lockett, 2014). These pieces have theorized that collaborative leadership is necessary for successful health care management and that the ability of leaders to foster collaborative relationships with multiple stakeholders is paramount. For example, in VanVactor's model the role of the leader is to encourage discussion among the multiple stakeholders. Indeed, according to VanVactor (2012) "openly sharing knowledge and experiences stimulates resolutions and problem solving which can often mitigate complexity in health care organizations" (p. 560). Similarly, White and colleagues (2014) examine how plural leadership, or leadership that is conceived as being distributed throughout and across organizational hierarchies, can spread between people, both intra- and interorganizationally in a health and social care network of organizations, suggesting:

> Formal leaders have agency as to how institutional influences may channel the enactment and spread of plural leadership, and so need to be attuned to how they are best able to do so in order to achieve their desired goals.
>
> *(p. 742)*

Currie and Locket (2011) offer a model of how power is distributed in interorganizational collaborations, suggesting that professional hierarchy and power relationships influence the enactment of distributed leadership, or leadership in which there is joint action and agency. Alexander and colleagues (2001) echo these sentiments, suggesting that effective leadership in health collaborations, or what they call partnership leadership:

> recognizes the need for balance—between power sharing and control, between process and results, between continuity and change, between interpersonal trust and formalized procedures. The ability of partnership leaders to walk a fine line often distinguishes truly effective leadership from mere management.
>
> *(p. 174)*

In these examinations of health leadership, communication is acknowledged but it is not treated as a central factor and theories are not employed to examine the communication from and among leaders. Indeed, the influence of communication between leaders in health contexts remains underdeveloped theoretically, empirically, and pragmatically.

Similarly, the examination of leadership in MTSs is in its nascent stages and treats communication as a variable rather than a constitutive force of the collaboration needed between teams. In their 2012 review of leadership in multiteam systems, Zaccaro and DeChurch, note only two empirical studies of leadership processes in MTSs (i.e., DeChurch et al., 2011; DeChurch & Marks, 2006) and since then few studies have joined that body of work. DeChurch and Marks (2006) found that interteam coordination fully mediated the effect of MTS leadership on MTS performance. This study utilized undergraduate participants and those who were assigned to a leadership role were trained on methods of interteam coordination. This training improved MTS performance, which, as DeChurch and Marks (2006) point out, is "more than just the sum of the parts, individual team processes and performance levels" (p. 326). In this study, MTS performance was measured by how well the system functioned together and coordinated individual team activities. The other study by DeChurch and colleagues (2011) analyzed 110 previous critical incidents in which MTSs had been employed (primarily examining case studies from provincial reconstruction teams and cross-regional hurricane response teams—both of which have securing the health of local citizens as a goal) to arrive at a taxonomy of leadership behaviors. These behaviors revolved around strategy and coordinating behaviors and highlighted within team, between team, and across system collaboration. The result of this study was a set of propositions to spur further research. Bienefeld and Grote (2014) took up this call, echoing that leadership training in MTSs should focus on shared leadership or the "dynamic, interactive influence process among individuals in groups for which the objective is to lead one another to the achievement of group goals" (Pearce & Conger, 2003, p. 3; see also Friedrich, Vessey, Schuelke, Ruark, & Mumford, 2009). In their article, Bienfeld and Grote (2014) argued that individuals who spanned team boundaries are critical. To summarize, empirical and theoretical examinations of leadership in MTSs have (a) established leadership to be an important factor in MTS effectiveness; (b) highlighted the need to examine leadership functions within teams, between teams, and external to the system; and (c) conceptualized MTS leadership as being able to take a vertical form (i.e., top-down leadership) or a shared form (Zaccaro & DeChurch, 2012).

Despite multiple calls for further research on MTSs, much of the extant literature remains at the theoretical level (e.g., Connaughton, Shuffler & Goodwin, 2011; Zaccaro & DeChurch, 2012). The scant empirical research on MTSs has shown that between-team processes are important and that leaders play a vital role in the coordination of these processes. However, little is known about how coordination and communication among leaders helps shape MTSs and, furthermore, how interactions among leaders and component team members create perceptions of the system for component team members. I argue that communication scholars are uniquely positioned to fulfill the need for empirical studies of leadership in MTSs. In an effort to spur this research, I turn to exchange theories of leadership, specifically leader–leader exchange theory, and suggest that employing a communicative approach to exchange theories of leadership within a framework of MTSs will be particularly useful for understanding interorganizational health collaborations.

Exchange Theories of Leadership

When one mentions leadership, an abundance of theories come to mind. From trait theories to theories of transformational and servant leadership, a wealth of perspectives and frameworks exist. Thayer (1988) argues that the way leadership has traditionally been viewed is not productive and suggests a new approach— "one that does not assume the characteristics of a leadership situation are separable from that situation, *nor* that the characteristics of leaders and followers are separable from those persons in that place and that time" (p. 238). A new approach provides a holistic view—it focuses not only on the leader, but also the follower(s) and, the relationship between leader and follower, as well as the situation. Fairhurst (2001) echoes these sentiments as she challenges communication research to go beyond the uni-dimensional approach of considering either the leader or the system. Rather, she urges scholars to consider the individual *and* the system. This chapter argues that using exchange theories of leadership allows us to do just that in complex health collaborations—considering the larger interorganizational system, the individuals that assume leadership roles within that system, and those led by the multiple leaders.

Leader–Member Exchange Theory

This chapter approaches leadership from the leader–member exchange (LMX) tradition (Dansereau, Graen, & Haga, 1975; Graen & Scandura, 1987; Graen &

Uhl-Bien, 1995). An LMX framework places relationships at the fore. Leadership in the LMX framework portrays effective leadership as incremental influence as "'leadership' relationships develop because there is mutual trust, internalization of common goals, extra-contractual behavior and the exchange of social resources, support, and mutual influences" (Fairhurst, 2001, p. 413). Leadership, in this model, develops as the leader and member foster a relationship (Graen & Uhl-Bien, 1995). In what has been modeled as a three-step process, the relationship can move through stages, from that of strangers, to acquaintances, and finally to maturity. When the relationship has reached maturity there is reciprocity between the leader and the organizational member. At this time, the member has developed a concern for organizational interests because this is what the leader desires. According to LMX, a member who has a high-quality relationship with the leader will be more apt to make decisions which will further the interests of that leader, often paralleling the interests of the organization. Relationships from an LMX framework are characterized as having high-, medium-, and low-exchange, with high-LMX relationships being those that have reached maturity.

Communication scholars have explored the interplay between LMX relationships and communication, specifically looking at the influence of various levels of LMX relationships (i.e., high-, medium-, and low-LMX). For example, research has explored how individuals discursively frame differences in LMX relationships (Sias, 1996), how LMX influences cooperation and perceptions of distributive and procedural justice (Lee, 2001), and the various communicative tactics leaders employ in various situations within various LMX-level relationships (Campbell, White, & Durrant, 2007; Lee & Jablin, 1995). Other communication theorists have examined patterns of interaction influencing LMX quality (Fairhurst, 1993) and how the differences in conversations between a leader and members at the high-, medium-, and low-LMX levels reflect differences in the influence the member has in decision-making and latitude, as well as the autonomy given to the member (Fairhurst & Chandler, 1989). What is clear from these various studies is that exchange theories offer a valuable framework for exploring the relationships that exist between leaders and members and the influence of these relationships on a variety of within-team factors.

Advances in LMX

Scholars are continually theorizing and empirically testing what is known about LMX. Graen and Uhl-Bien (1995) offer a summary of LMX theory and divide the study of leader–member relationships into four research stages. The first of these phases was marked by a departure from traditional leadership theories that did not differentiate between a leader's relationships with various members—all followers were seen as equal. LMX theory proposed that relationships did in fact differ among members and these differences were grounded in the various material and social exchanges between members and leaders (Dansereau et al., 1975).

The second stage of LMX research sought to explore these differences, their antecedents and their organizational outcomes. The third phase shifted from a descriptive approach to a prescriptive approach—trying to teach leaders how to develop high-LMX relationships with subordinates, resulting in the proposal of the LMX life-cycle model showing the progression of leader–member relationships (Graen & Uhl-Bien, 1991; Uhl-Bien & Graen, 1993). The fourth, and most salient for this chapter, stage of LMX research is marked by a shift in the level of analysis from the dyad to the collective. In this phase, networks are seen as "aggregations of dyads" (Graen & Uhl-Bien, 1995, p. 225). In other words, all organizations are comprised of networks of dyadic relationships (Graen & Scandura, 1987). This shift has brought to the fore the interplay between various organizational relationships and the influence that these relationships have on LMX and has created the opportunity to use exchange theories interorganizationally.

The recognition of the influence of multiple dyadic relationships has made a mark on current LMX research. Indeed, there are suggestions that the relationships among leaders, the relationships among coworkers, and both the leader and member's location within the larger social network may influence the LMX relationship. While much of the literature on these links is theoretical, empirical studies are beginning to provide support for these hypothesized effects. The following summarizes the extant empirical studies.

First, the relationship between the leader and his/her supervisor (leader–leader exchange; LLX) has been found to correlate to the leader–member relationship. A study by Tangirala, Green, and Ramanujam (2007) showed that a high LLX was correlated with the LMX relationship and had both positive and negative effects. That is if a leader had a high LLX with his/her supervisor and a positive LMX relationship with an employee, that member reported greater organizational identification and perceived organizational support. However, if the LMX relationship was not as strong, the employee did not experience these feelings. Interestingly, Sluss, Klimchak, and Holmes (2008) found that a high-LLX relationship weakened the link between LMX and members' perceived organizational support. Sluss et al. point to contextual and gender differences between the two studies to explain the discrepancies in findings. Nonetheless, both studies point to a correlation between LLX and LMX.

Other dyadic studies have focused on the relationship among members and the link to LMX. Specifically, Sherony and Green (2002) explored coworker exchange relationships (CWX). Their study found that coworkers with a high CWX tend to have similar LMX relationships with the leader (i.e., they both have high LMX or low LMX). However, if the coworkers have different LMX relationships with the leader, they have lower CWX. In similar research, Schyns (2006) found that consensus in the perceptions of LMX relationships across team members led to specific outcomes, including job satisfaction and commitment.

Finally, other researchers have focused on the leader's and member's location within the organizations' social network and how this influences or is influenced by the LMX relationship. A study by Venkataramani, Green, and Schleicher (2010) found that a leader's centrality and influence in his/her peer network influenced LMX relationships. However, this correlation was moderated by the member's centrality in his/her network. This suggests that when the member has alternative access to resources, the LMX relationship may not be as salient. Similarly, Sparrowe and Liden (2005) found that a member's advice centrality and influence was correlated to LMX but this relationship was moderated by sponsorship and the leader's advice centrality. Indeed, both of these studies provide a model of highly nuanced interplay among various dyadic relationships within organizations.

One way that networks of relationships transform theorizing about LMX relationships is in considering what relationships matter interorganizationally. As Graen and Scandura (1987) suggest, "drawing limits around the boundaries of the network may be problematic" (p. 202). While distant linkages do not influence LMX relationships as strongly, some interorganizational relationships have just as much influence as intra-organizational relationships. Tangirala and colleagues (2007) begin to expand the network of organizational actors when they examine the influence of LLX and LMX on customer care. However, in their study, the customer is treated as an outcome (i.e., customer satisfaction) rather than an actor who might influence LLX and LMX relationships.

Indeed, exchange theories provide a fruitful lens to use when exploring MTSs, and specifically interorganizational health collaborations as these systems are comprised of a complex network of dyadic relationships with varying degree of interdependencies. It may seem counter-intuitive to look at relationships between leader and member in an organizational structure that highlights *inter*-team processes. However, the complex nature of this system is precisely why dyadic relationships are important. As individuals work within the system they rely on what they know about the distal and proximal goals. One source for information and guidance on how to interact comes from the relationship that the member has with his/her component team leader. In addition, it is also possible that members observe the interactions among leaders and between their leader and coworkers. Based on these observations, individuals may come to conclusions about the leader's perceived influence in the system and use this information as another resource for interacting (Harrison & Williams, 2010).

Exchange theories are also an appropriate framework for studying MTSs as constituted by communication. As Fairhurst (2007) explains, exchange theories have narrative roots. That is, certain discursive resources become available through the relationship that is fostered between a leader and member. For example, one set of resources that may become available to members is knowledge of the system and their team's role in the system. In other words, the communicative exchanges between the leader and the member, as well as the communicative exchanges that the member perceives among the leader and other leaders, and the exchanges that he/she has with other system members creates the system.

The Importance of the Communicative

A communicative approach to leadership in MTSs can be seen in Williams' (2011) study of an emergency response system—a system that at its core is concerned with the health and safety of the community and the members of the system. Specifically, the study heeded Fairhurst's (2007) call to look at both the macro-Discourse in the organization and the micro-discourse—that is, it looked at the larger communicative themes driving the system and how those themes translated into communicative acts.

In this study leaders were found to be the driving force of coordination in MTSs and the privileging of certain D/discourses (i.e., larger cultural ideas and assumptions and how those are represented in everyday talk) by leaders in the MTS set the tone for coordination and shaped the various relationships within the system. Specifically, participants, both leaders and "rank-and-file employees", in this study pointed to an overarching Discourse of interagency cooperation among leaders. Despite this larger Discourse of cooperation, two underlying discourses existed. First there was an underlying discourse of deferring to individual organizational interests and second there was a discourse of material constraints. At first blush, the Discourse of cooperation seems at odds with discourses of organizational interests and material constraints. Indeed, tensions may exist between doing what is best for the system and what is best of possible for the individual organization. However, upon further examination, it appears that they may actually work in tandem. To explain, emergency response organizations are extremely paramilitary in nature—members of the various component teams are trained to defer to the chain of command. This emphasis on one's own organization and following its chain of command could undermine the larger goals of the system. But, because this particular system was self-described as having strong leader–leader relationships and there was widespread knowledge of the strength of these relationships, there was an understanding that the direction of the organization, most likely, mirrored the direction of the larger system. This gave system members the ability to talk about working towards larger system goals while focusing on their own organizational goals. Similarly, while leaders talked about doing whatever they could to contribute to the system and to help other organizations within the system, there was also a consistent acknowledgment of the economic and time constraints facing the organizations. This discourse seemed to open up a space for leaders to do what they deemed best for their own organization while still maintaining system relationships.

This study represents an important look at a bona fide MTS and highlights the constitutive nature of communication within the system. Indeed, the way leaders talk about issues, how they frame their communication with other leaders, and their leader–member relationships within their teams all play a part in system success. When system members have varying degrees of interaction with the larger system, the ability of leaders to frame the interdependencies of the system and to clarify individual members' roles in achieving system goals is paramount.

If we apply this lens to the Ebola crisis used as an exemplar above, we can see how leader–leader relationships that may have influenced the d/Discourse about the epidemic in a variety of ways. An example of this is the interactions between leaders of two key agencies responding to the Ebola Crisis: the WHO and Doctors Without Borders. The WHO "took a decidedly anti-alarmist approach" at the beginning of the epidemic (Sack et al., 2014, para. 59). When the outbreak was announced, the WHO spokesman, Gregory Härtl, used social media to assure individuals that "there has never been an #Ebola outbreak larger than a couple of hundred cases" and "Ebola has always remained a very localized event" (Sack et al., 2014, para. 60). Meanwhile, the coordinator of a Doctors Without Borders Ebola clinic in Guinea declared in a news release, "We are facing an epidemic of a magnitude never before seen in terms of the distribution of cases in the country" (Sack et al., 2014, para. 62). According to Sack et al. (2014) this perpetuated a "three-day Twitter war" between the two agencies (para. 63). While not privy to the discourse that occurred between the leaders of these organizations and their members, we can see from this example the magnitude of the difference in the Discourse surrounding the threat of Ebola. Findings from Williams' (2011) study would suggest that this contentious relationship between the leadership of the two organizations would impact how organizational members interacted and how the members perceived system level goals and their organization's role in fulfilling the goals. Indeed, we can imagine the sense of urgency that existed for those members of Doctors Without Borders based on the communication from their leader. The response at the WHO was to attempt not to, as Mr. Härtl contended, "overblow something which is already bad enough" (Sack et al., 2014, para. 64). In fact, it was not until July 2014, that the WHO set up a regional coordinating center in Guinea (Sack et al., 2014)—4 months after the initial outbreak and after the virus had already claimed over 300 lives in Guinea alone (CDC, 2015a). At a time when coordination between the various component teams of the system was paramount, communication from leaders instead highlighted strained relationships.

Practical and Theoretical Considerations

Considering Williams' (2011) study and the theoretical explanation of both MTSs and exchange theories of leadership, three propositions about communication and leadership in interorganizational health collaborations are advanced. These propositions supplement those advanced by Zaccaro and DeChurch (2012) in their chapter on leadership in MTSs. The goal of these propositions is to offer pragmatic considerations grounded in theoretical conceptions of MTSs and leadership for practitioners involved in interorganizational health collaborations. At the same time, these propositions provide heuristic value as little empirical research exists on leadership in MTSs.

First, leaders in interorganizational health initiatives should be mindful of both their relationships with other leaders and how they are talking about those relationships with the members of their organization. As Williams (2011) noted, both the relationship among leaders and how that relationship is framed helps members make sense of the system and their role in it. This is consistent with LLX research (e.g., Tangirala et al., 2007; Venkataramani et al., 2010). In the Ebola example, we can imagine a scenario in which teams have different subordinate goals emerging from their multiple cultural perspectives (both organizational and national; see Connaughton & Shuffler, 2007). From the example above, while the WHO has been critiqued for their slow response, they were operating under "recessionary cutbacks and [were] strained to its limits by concurrent emergencies and outbreaks" (Sack et al., 2014, para. 38). In this situation, coordination with other agencies, such as Doctors Without Borders, may have best been achieved at the leader level with the various organizations being upfront about the resources they had to commit to the response. Furthermore, the leaders may have discursively constructed the solutions to their individual teams in ways that made sense to that team's reality but also fit within the larger system Discourse of preventing the spread of the disease. Knowing that relationships exist between leaders frees members to focus on their local tasks.

Second, while building an overarching Discourse of collaboration, leaders are able to employ competing discourses that allow their individual organizations to maintain agility and responsiveness. As the previous example suggests, and Williams' (2011) study highlights, a leader's role is often to negotiate the tensions inherent in between-team activities. By being mindful of how they communicate about opportunities for collaboration and constraints in these collaborations, they may open up space for coming up with unique solutions. For instance, if the leader of the WHO in the above example is able to discursively construct the material financial constraints they face, other leaders may be able to help them find work arounds or help them secure the necessary funding. By opening up the space for individual organizations to identify what they are and are not able to do, the system is able to become more agile and responsive to the ever changing needs of the situation.

Third, leadership training must occur before environmental stimuli create the need for an MTS and should focus on building leader–leader and leader–member relationships. Studies by DeChurch and Marks (2006) and Bienefeld and Grote (2014) both highlight the importance of training for leaders in MTSs. While it is impossible to hypothesize the multiple leader–leader relationships that might come into play in an MTS, it is possible to train leaders on how to communicate across teams and cultures and to help them foster relationships within teams.

Research has shown that cross-team processes are more important to MTS success than within-team processes and that the influence of these between-team processes is more profound when there are higher levels of interdependence among the teams (Marks, DeChurch, Mathieu, Panzer, & Alonso, 2005). Leaders are central agents in these cross-team processes and are key to how cross-team processes are translated to individual team action. This chapter has attempted to extend the theorizing on leadership in MTSs by adopting a communicative perspective on relationships among leaders and situating them within the rich tapestry of relationships that exist in interorganizational collaborations. Indeed, these relationships may serve as predictors for interorganizational health collaboration effectiveness and as such, are deserving of further empirical study.

DISCUSSION QUESTIONS

1. Have you been part of an MTS? What was leadership like in that MTS? How did leaders communicate in that MTS?
2. This chapter highlights the importance of communication *among* leaders—what are ways that we can design systems that encourage this?
3. This chapter proposes that communication about relationships among leaders helps highlight a component team's role in the larger system. How can leaders facilitate these discussions with their subordinates?
4. What are additional *between*-team challenges that leaders may encounter when they are operating in an MTS? How might they tackle these challenges from a communicative perspective?
5. What are additional *within*-team challenges that leaders may encounter when they are operating in an MTS? How might they tackle these challenges from a communicative perspective?

Suggested Reading

Fairhurst, G. T. (2007). *Discursive leadership: In conversation with leadership psychology.* Los Angeles, CA: Sage.

Graen, G. B. & Uhl-Bien, M. (1995). Relationship-based approach to leadership: Development of leader–member exchange (LMX) theory of leadership over 25 years: Applying a multi-level multi-domain perspective. *Leadership Quarterly, 6*, 219–247.

Zaccaro, S. J. & DeChurch, L. A. (2012). Leadership forms and functions in multiteam systems. In S. J. Zaccaro, M. A. Marks, & L. A. DeChurch (Eds.), *Multiteam systems: An organization form for dynamic and complex environments* (pp. 253–288). New York, NY: Routledge.

References

Alexander, J. A., Comfort, M. E., Weiner, B. J., & Bogue, R. (2001). Leadership in collaborative community health partnerships. *Nonprofit Management and Leadership, 12*, 159–175.

Bienefeld, N. & Grote, G. (2014). Speaking up in ad hoc multiteam systems: Individual-level effects of psychological safety, status, and leadership within and across teams. *European Journal of Work and Organizational Psychology, 23*, 930–945.

Campbell, K. S., White, C. D., & Durant, R. (2007). Necessary evils, (in)justice, and rapport management. *Journal of Business Communication, 44*, 161–185.

CDC (2015a, February 27). 2014 Ebola outbreak in West Africa. Retrieved from http://www.cdc.gov/vhf/ebola/outbreaks/2014-west-africa/index.html.

CDC (2015b, March 1). Travelers' health. Retrieved from http://wwwnc.cdc.gov/travel/page/ebola-outbreak-communication-resources.

Connaughton, S. L. & Shuffler, M. (2007). Multinational and multicultural distributed teams: A review and future agenda. *Small Group Research, 38*, 387–412.

Connaughton, S., Shuffler, M., & Goodwin, G. F. (2011). Leading distributed teams: The communicative constitution of leadership. *Military Psychology, 23*, 502.

Currie, G. & Lockett, A. (2011). Distributing leadership in health and social care: Concertive, conjoint or collective? *International Journal of Management Reviews, 13*, 286–300.

Dansereau, F., Jr., Graen, G., & Haga, W. J. (1975). A vertical dyad linkage approach to leadership within formal organizations: A longitudinal investigation of the role making process. *Organizational Behavior and Human Performance, 13*, 46–78.

DeChurch, L. A., Burke, C. S., Shuffler, M. L., Lyons, R., Doty, D., & Salas, E. (2011). A historiometric analysis of leadership in mission critical multiteam environments. *The Leadership Quarterly, 22*, 152–169.

DeChurch, L. A. & Marks, M. A. (2006). Leadership in multiteam systems. *Journal of Applied Psychology, 91*, 311–329.

Doctors Without Borders (2015, March 1). Closing a project. Retrieved from http://www.doctorswithoutborders.org/closing-project.

Fairhurst, G. T. (1993). The leader-member exchange patterns of women leaders in industry: A discourse analysis. *Communication Monographs, 60*, 321–351.

Fairhurst, G. T. (2001). Dualisms in leadership research. In F. M. Jablin & L. L. Putnam (Eds.), *The new handbook of organizational communication: Advances in theory, research, and methods* (pp. 379–439). Thousand Oaks, CA: Sage.

Fairhurst, G. T. (2007). *Discursive leadership: In conversation with leadership psychology.* Los Angeles, CA: Sage.

Fairhurst, G. T. & Chandler, T. A. (1989). Social structure in leader-member interaction. *Communication Monographs, 56*, 215–239.

Friedrich, T. L., Vessey W. B., Schuelke M. J., Ruark G. A., Mumford M. D. (2009). A framework for understanding collective leadership: The selective utilization of leader and team expertise within networks. *Leadership Quarterly, 20*, 933–958

Graen, G. B. & Scandura, T. A. (1987). Toward a psychology of dyadic organizing. In L. L. Cummings & B. M. Shaw (Eds.), *Research in organizational behavior* (pp. 175–209). Greenwich, CT: JAI Press.

Graen, G. B. & Uhl-Bien, M. (1991) The transformation of work group professionals into self-managing and partially self-designing contributors: Toward a theory of leadership-making. *Journal of Management Systems, 3*, 33–48.

Graen, G. B. & Uhl-Bien, M. (1995). Relationship-based approach to leadership: Development of leader-member exchange (LMX) theory of leadership over 25 years: Applying a multi-level multi-domain perspective. *Leadership Quarterly, 6*, 219–247.

Harrison, T. R. & Williams, E. A. (2010). Structural links, communication, and conflict in three inter-organizational virtual collaborations. In S. D. Long (Ed.), *Communication, relationships, and practices in virtual work* (pp. 26–45). Hershey, PA: IGI Global.

Lee, J. (2001). Leader-member exchange, perceived organizational justice, and cooperative communication. *Management Communication Quarterly, 14*, 574–589.

Lee, J. & Jablin, F. M. (1995). Maintenance communication in superior-subordinate work relationships. *Human Communication Research, 22,* 220–257.

Marks, M. A., DeChurch, L. A., Mathieu, J. E., Panzer, F. J., & Alonso, A. A. (2005). The importance of goal hierarchies and teamwork processes for multi-team effectiveness. *Journal of Applied Psychology, 90,* 964–971.

Mathieu, J. E., Marks, M. A., & Zaccaro, S. J. (2001). Multiteam systems. In N. Anderson, D. S. Ones, H. K. Sinangil, & C. Viswesvarin. *Handbook of industrial, work and organizational psychology* (pp. 290–313). Thousand Oaks, CA: Sage.

Pearce, C. L. & Conger J. A.*(2003). Shared leadership: Reframing the how's and why's of leadership.* Thousand Oaks, CA: Sage.

Sack, K., Fink, S., Belluck, P., & Nossiter, A. (2014, December 29). How Ebola roared back. *The New York Times.* Retrieved from http://www.nytimes.com/2014/12/30/health/how-ebola-roared-back.html?_r=0.

Schyns, B. (2006). Are group consensus in leader-member exchange (LMX) and shared work values related to organizational outcomes? *Small Group Research, 37,* 20–35.

Sherony, K. M. & Green, S. G. (2002). Coworker exchange: Relationships between coworkers, LMX, and work attitudes. *Journal of Applied Psychology, 87,* 542–548.

Sias, P. M. (1996). Constructing perceptions of differential treatment: An analysis of coworker discourse. *Communication Monographs, 63,* 171–187.

Sluss, D. M., Klimchak, M., & Holmes, J. J. (2008). Perceived organizational support as a mediator between relational exchange and organizational identification. *Journal of Vocational Behavior, 73,* 457–464.

Sparrowe, R. T. & Liden, R. C. (2005). Two routes to influence: Integrating leader–member exchange and social network perspectives. *Administrative Science Quarterly, 50,* 505–535.

Tangirala, S., Green, S. G., & Ramanujam, R. (2007). In the shadow of the supervisor's boss: How supervisors' relationships with their bosses influence frontline employees. *Journal of Applied Psychology, 92,* 309–320.

Thayer, L. (1988). Leadership/communication: A critical review and a modest proposal. In G. M. Goldhaber & G. A. Barnett (Eds.), *Handbook of organizational communication* (pp. 231–263). Norwood, NJ: Ablex.

Thompson, T. L., Parrott, R., & Nussbaum, J. F. (2011). *The Routledge Handbook of Health Communication.* New York, NY: Routledge.

Uhl-Bien, M. & Graen, G. B. (1993). Leadership-making in self-managing professional work teams: An empirical investigation. In K. E. Clark, M. B. Clark, & D. P. Campbell (Eds.), *The impact of leadership* (pp. 379–387). West Orange, NJ: Leadership Library of America.

VanVactor, J. D. (2012). Collaborative leadership model in the management of health care. *Journal of Business Research, 65,* 555–561.

Venkataramani, V., Green, S. G., & Schleicher, D. (2010). Well-connected leaders: The impact of leader's social network ties on LMX and members' work attitudes. *Journal of Applied Psychology, 95,* 1071–1084.

White, L., Currie, G., & Lockett, A. (2014). The enactment of plural leadership in a health and social care network: The influence of institutional context. *The Leadership Quarterly, 25,* 730–745.

Williams, E. A. (2011). *Towards an understanding of multiteam systems: Theorizing about identification, leadership, and communication in an emergency response system* (Doctoral dissertation). Purdue University, West Lafayette. Available from ProQuest Digital Dissertations. (AAI No.3481172).

Zaccaro, S. J., Marks, M. A., & DeChurch, L. A. (2012). Multiteam systems: An introduction. In S. J. Zaccaro, M. A. Marks, & L. A. DeChurch (Eds.), *Multiteam systems: An organization form for dynamic and complex environments* (pp. 3–32). New York, NY: Routledge.

Zaccaro, S. J. & DeChurch, L. A. (2012). Leadership forms and functions in multiteam systems. In S. J. Zaccaro, M. A. Marks, & L. A. DeChurch (Eds.), *Multiteam systems: An organization form for dynamic and complex environments* (pp. 253–288). New York, NY: Routledge.

21

USING SOCIAL CAPITAL TO BUILD GLOBAL HEALTH INITIATIVES

Connecting Organizations and Citizen-Stakeholders Through Social Media

Lisa V. Chewning

Social capital has been linked to community building, collective action, and crisis recovery, on both individual and system levels (Doerfel, Lai, & Chewning, 2010; Putnam, 1993). Regarding health, social capital can lead to positive outcomes, in terms of obtaining information, access to resources, and formal or informal support (Rocco & Suhrcke, 2012). Generally, the coordinated action motivated by social capital takes place within a localized geographic area, or by connecting with established partners. However, social media offers opportunities for engagement and capital building across geographic boundaries, allowing for larger networks and, therefore, greater benefits. Organizations are harnessing this power as for-profit businesses connect with nonprofit and community based organizations to promote better health. The utilization of social media allows for the inclusion of a third party: individuals. Individuals become citizen-stakeholders as they act on behalf of the organization to further its cause. This chapter examines how social capital both facilitates and is created by this three-way interaction, with the potential of leading to better health outcomes in a global community.

To some, the idea of citizen-stakeholders might seem problematic, as citizens are generally associated with a democratic (public) process and stakeholders are linked to organizational (private) processes. While recognizing this tension, this chapter lays out a model through which organizations can, and are, generating and sharing capital for better social outcomes. Citizenship comes into play in two ways in the citizen-stakeholder model: corporate citizenship, or the idea that corporations are "legal entities with rights and duties, in effect 'citizens' of the states within which they operate" (Marsden, 2000, p. 11), and the idea that, via the social capital shared between stakeholders and organizations, stakeholders can be engaged into action, thus becoming better citizens in the process. This dual notion of citizenship flips the idea that stakeholders can pressure organizations to do good by positing that organizations can persuade stakeholders to do good. It has been argued that organizations can genuinely engage with stakeholders to enact change (Taylor, 2011), and that organizations can help promote civil society and positive health outcomes (Taylor, 2009). This chapter builds on such arguments, contextualizing social capital in a global and technologically networked society, and developing a model of capital sharing through which global health networks are built and better health outcomes can be generated.

Social Capital

Social capital is the "resources embedded in a social structure which are accessed and/or mobilized for purposive action" (Lin, 2001a, p. 13). As a theory, social capital has been used to explain how participation and position in social networks provide benefits that could not be accrued without these connections. Such benefits can be assessed in terms of the individual or on a collective level, and therefore can be assessed in terms of one actor's participation in a network or the resources embedded in a network as a whole. Social capital is different from other forms of capital (financial, human) in that it resides not in physical place, but rather, in the connections between and among actors. If human capital leads to better outcomes for more capable individuals, social capital leads to better outcomes for more connected individuals (Burt, 2000, p. 347).

Social capital is inextricably linked with the organizing process, in that it "represents resources that social contacts hold as well as the structure of contacts in a network" (Doerfel, Lai, & Chewning, 2010, p. 129). It is created, shared, and maintained through the connections that make up the social structures in which we are embedded. Coleman (1988) argues that while social capital can vary across contexts, it has two constants: the presence of some aspect of social structures and the facilitation of certain action of actors within a structure. However, Lin (2001b) argues that a network alone is not social capital; it is the resources embedded within the network, and the activation of those resources, that create social capital. Arguably, the value of a network can be conceptualized in terms of the social capital it contains, and therefore, it is reasonable to assume that actors will create networks based upon the potential for access to social capital.

To this end, social capital has been conceptualized in terms of two different structures: bonding and bridging. Bonding social capital is found in closed, cohesive networks where there are high levels of trust, but lower levels of diversity (Putnam, 2000). Closed networks are those in which members are reciprocally connected, and "everyone knows your name." Therefore, bonding social capital will create strong norms, which will likely facilitate coordinated action and sharing of financial or other resources. Indeed, Doerfel, Lai, and Chewning (2010) found that in times of crisis, business owners turned first to their personal networks, composed of family and friends, activating the bonding social capital that led to quick and easy access of needed resources. Bridging social capital is based on what Burt (2000) calls "brokerage opportunities," for parties that can fill missing or weak links in a network called structural holes. Structural holes create opportunities for social capital on both the individual and network level, in that parties that fill the holes, and connect otherwise unconnected networks, control the flow of information and resources between the formerly unconnected structures. Therefore, these parties hold power and have access to diverse resources. Additionally, connecting formerly unconnected networks can lead to access of more diverse, non-redundant, and even more plentiful resources.

So, linked to the organizing process is social capital, which has been hypothesized as the glue that undergirds social participation and democracy (Putnam, 1995, 2000). Putnam (1995) posits social capital in terms of participation in civic clubs, and argues that social capital is diminishing because we do not have the same opportunities to discuss, debate, and participate. However, in a global society, where we have disembedded from our geographic communities and reembedded in interest-based communities, our sense of belonging may be no less strong, and our conversations no less real. While Putnam (1995) argues that technology, specifically television, has caused us to lose interest in civic organizations and participation in a civil society, it may be that in a society in which networks are no longer based on geographic proximity, technology is actually what helps us to build social capital. For example, face-to-face relationships can be maintained and strengthened in the absence of physical proximity via Skype or family blogs. Online social support communities provide support to similarly afflicted individuals across the globe. Facebook and Twitter can be used to renew the social capital from older relationships in which individuals had lost touch, or even to create prayer networks and galvanize donations for people in need through sites such as Give Forward.

Thus, in a globalized and technologically networked society, we can reconceptualize social capital in terms of the networks created and maintained through a combination of on- and offline networks. While this is a departure from what Putnam (1995, 2003) describes as social capital, it builds on the work of scholars such as Lin (1999, 2001b) and Burt (2000), who consider resources and structure as measures of social capital. As the concept of social capital is broadened to include those relationships built and/or maintained virtually, is can arguably be expanded to include alternative relational partners, as well.

Coleman (1988) argued that as society changes, we might have to substitute formal organizations for the spontaneous social organization that has, in the past, been a major source of social capital (p. 117). In a time of Globalization, when we are disembedding and reembedding in communities, some argue that organizations are increasingly undertaking the "protecting, facilitating, and enabling of citizen's rights" (Crane, Matten, & Moon, 2004, p. 109). As this happens, there is a call for "the creation of partnerships between organizations and civil society designed to build trust" in which organizational communication and action is employed for societal good (Willis, 2012, p. 116). Such a practice is commonly known as Corporate Citizenship, or the idea that organizations are citizens of the community (local or global) in which they operate, thus engendering certain rights and responsibilities toward that community (Crane, Matten, & Moon, 2004, p. 108).

One way this is being enacted is through the institutionalized practice of Corporate Social Responsibility (CSR), through which for-profit organizations serve as lynchpins between nonprofit organizations, capital-deficient populations, and organizational stakeholders in order to create support networks. In the context of health, these networks, rich with bridging social capital, can leverage access to needed resources, creating better health outcomes for the affected community, better access for nonprofits, and strengthen the sense of engagement between for-profit organizations and stakeholders.

Organizations, Health, and Social Capital: Creating Citizen Stakeholders and Global Health Communities

Organizational engagement in pro-social arenas has arguably become a standard "global business ethic" (Jackson, 2004, p. 3). Business is undergoing a paradigm shift in values, which "presupposes and expresses timeless principles and values—human rights, responsible citizenship, corporate credibility and character" (Jackson, 2004, p. 3). Both for-profit and nonprofit organizations have been filling this role for years, but from opposite sides of the coin. For-profit organizations have been filling this role for years through CSR, or the "social responsibility [of organizations] to pursue those policies, and to make those decisions, or to follow those lines of action that are desirable in terms of the objective and values of our society" (Bowen, 1953, p.6). On the other side of the coin, nonprofits, due to the nature of their mission, serve to fill the resource gaps in a community. While CSR has been around in some form since the early twentieth century (see also May, this volume), the values that are the foundation of CSR are now becoming industry standards as organizations strive to become good global citizens.

One area in which this could have a great impact is world health. Research has shown that social capital has a tremendous impact on health outcomes. Rocco and Suhrcke (2012) posit three mechanisms for the positive role of social capital on individual health: access to relevant information, informal care and support, and the ability to organize and lobby health-related causes. Repeatedly, the presence of social capital has been shown to positively affect health outcomes, with the converse also being true (Cattell, 2001; Cobb, 1976; Folland, 2007). Additionally, Stephens, Rimal, and Flora (2004) found that membership in community organizations (regarded by Putnam [2000] as a measure of social capital) explained greater variance in health outcomes than did general and health-specific media use or demographic factors. Thus, social capital is crucial in spreading health messages, creating health opportunities, and achieving positive health outcomes. While the majority of these studies look at how an individual's or community's social capital create better health outcomes for the individual or community, the citizen-stakeholder model looks at how individual or community social capital can help create better health outcomes for *other* individuals or communities.

For-profit organizations have a long history of working with nonprofit and community organizations to promote health-related goals (see also Feeley & O'Mally, this volume). Increasingly, these partnerships are extending past the local community and into the global community. For example, Johnson & Johnson supports Operation Smile with both fundraising and employee volunteers, to help surgically repair cleft conditions in children throughout Asia Pacific. Tom's Shoes created an in-house foundation, One-for-One, which partners with worldwide "Giving Partners" in order to support sustainable eye care and clean water. Their model differs from Johnson & Johnson, in that they engage the public, typically their consumers, in their giving efforts. For every pair of glasses or bag of coffee a stakeholder buys, Tom's provides an eye-care service or a week's worth of clean water. Essentially, in these models, employees *and* consumers are becoming citizen-stakeholders, as they move past connecting with for-profit organizations because of employment status or product, and lend their services or money to a larger cause.

Putnam (1995) proposed that increased social capital leads to a variety of social benefits, including improved governance and economic prosperity. That is, the mechanisms underlying the development of social capital, as described in the preceding section, are enough to get individuals to invest resources such as time, care, and money toward a common interest. The citizen stakeholder model posits that for-profit organizations can harness the social capital they share with stakeholders to create communities of interest that generate and share both social and economic capital with capital-poor communities. For-profit organizations would work to translate the reputational capital they have with stakeholders into social capital, and then prompt involved stakeholders to leverage their own social capital among friends and other relations. The capital created and shared would then be passed on to capital-poor communities, with the intent of changing social conditions that serve as an impediment to health. Such a model would crack open the ideas of "community," "trust," and even "social capital," and adapt them to a mediated and global environment.

Structural and Communication Mechanisms Behind Building Global Social Capital

As research has shown that communities with high social capital exhibit better outcomes in terms of both social action and health outcomes (Krishna, 2002;

Putnam, 1993), the citizen-stakeholder model posits social capital as important on three levels: between the organization and stakeholders, between stakeholders and their personal contacts, and among the organization, nonprofit community partners and capital-deficient communities. As research has shown that both bonding and bridging social capital are needed to achieve community-related aims (Marino & Starfield, 2001), the citizen-stakeholder model draws upon both. It also incorporates a third type of social capital known as linking social capital, which adapts the idea of bridging social capital specifically to vertical power differentials (Szreter & Woolcock, 2004). As social capital is built around two primary components, network structure and its content (Lee & Lee 2010), the citizen-stakeholder model considers both mechanisms across all three levels of capital building.

Organizational-Stakeholder Capital

As the primary focus of this chapter is on the how the relationship between organizations and stakeholders can contribute to global health, a good place to start is by identifying how social capital is built between these parties. Stakeholders interact with organizations for a variety of reasons, including products, services, and employment. While need and availability can determine whether or not a stakeholder interacts with an organization, enduring interaction often begins with reputation. Reputation is the "aggregate evaluation constituents make about how well an organization is meeting constituent expectations based on its past behaviors" (Coombs & Holladay, 2010, p. 168). Expectations are built on a variety of factors, including the identity of the organization, the values of the society in which it operates, and the values of the society to which a stakeholder belongs (often, but not always, the same as the organization).

Organizational identity, or how the organization perceives itself, is built around the shared values of society. Organizations act in a way that is in alignment with those values, and then communicate this behavior in a way that has meaning for stakeholders. Thus, when organizations act in accordance with stakeholder values, they generally develop a positive relationship with a stakeholder, which leads to a positive reputation (Coombs & Holladay, 2010). Reputations can be created along several dimensions, including functional (competence in relation to functional systems), social (good citizenship, in line with social norms and values), and expressive ("emotional attractiveness," or expressiveness and uniqueness) (Eisenegger, 2009). Therefore, reputation and subsequent reputational capital can be affected by more than just the goods or services that an organization offers, but also by how the organization "acts" in accordance with social values.

Reputation capital can generally be understood as the goodwill that an organization accumulates through the maintenance of a good reputation. Following, both internal and external stakeholders develop trust in the brand, which leads to loyalty, and therefore repeated interactions with the organization.

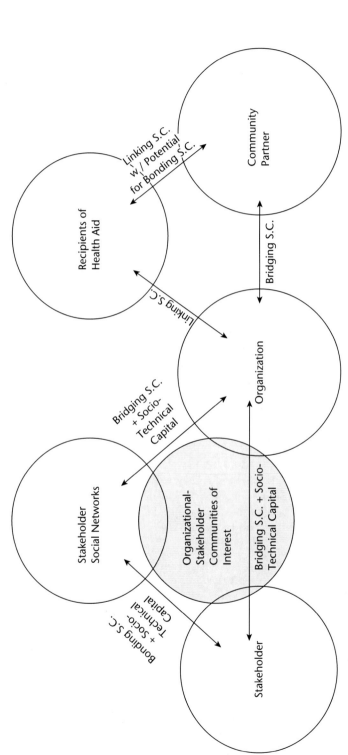

FIGURE 21.1 Structural Mechanisms for Social Capital in Citizen–Stakeholder Networks.

Arguably, when stakeholders and organizations repeatedly interact with each other on the basis of shared values, social norms, and trust, they are engaging. When this happens, reputation capital becomes a form of social capital. Barriers between the organization and stakeholders diminish as both parties participate in dialogue through which "organizations and publics can make decisions that create social capital" (Taylor & Kent, 2014, p. 384).

Taylor and Kent (2014) position social capital as both a precursor and outcome of engagement, as it builds upon capital that already exists between organizations and stakeholders, and is a result of the dialogue created via engagement. When done correctly, this engagement leads to a sense of identification and connection with the organization on the part of stakeholders. This connection binds the parties in a loosely coupled network that includes "organizations, stakeholders, and publics, as well as activists and stake seekers" in which real dialogue leads to engagement, which can serve as a precursor to participation (Taylor & Kent, 2104, p. 395). Considering Putnam, Leonardi, and Nanetti's (1993) definition of social capital as "features of social organization, such as trust norms, and networks that can improve the efficiency of society by facilitating action" (p. 167) these loosely-coupled networks based on organizational-stakeholder engagement can be considered legitimate social structures ripe for coordinated action.

Organizations that already engage with stakeholders on health-related topics are more likely to have built social capital with stakeholders who will be both more interested in, and inclined to act on, health initiatives. On both sides of the organizational/stakeholder relationship, there will be shared values that galvanize stakeholders to act on organizational initiatives. Likewise, if organizations have demonstrated expertise in the health field, they will have gained legitimacy in that domain. Arguably, organizations must be perceived as legitimate in their area of business, and in their genuine intent to do good, as well as in the social domain in which they are participating. Jackson (2004) identifies this as the organization's "moral signature," or "pursuing strategies that differentiate it from competitors" (p. 148). This, in turn, builds reputational capital, which, when reinforced, leads to social capital.

While such a conceptualization of social capital differs from what Putnam (2000) would describe, it encompasses the essential building blocks of social capital, including a network of relations based on shared norms, values, trust, and interaction. Essentially, the community's role is still present in the process, but the definition of community is expanded to include organizations and their stakeholder communities. The question of whether or not these are "real communities" with "real social capital" is one that is not necessarily new. For years, scholars have debated about alternate contexts for community and social capital, particularly in the online realm. As online media, particularly social media, is the main vehicle through which organizations and stakeholders engage, an examination of communication and social capital in mediated environments can shed light on how create a network of citizen-stakeholders, and then extend it into personal networks via the structural and communicative affordances of social media.

Building and Extending Social Capital Through Mediated Communication

The proliferation of online media, especially social media, has allowed organizations to extend their reach with both internal and external stakeholders, engaging in a more genuine way. Online media has led to an interconnectedness among individuals that transcends geography and time, allowing individuals to dis-embed and re-embed themselves in communities of others who share similar interests, or hold the information or resources that they are seeking. Such technology can be used to enable new forms of "togetherness" more amenable to the technologically and globally linked world in which we live, but only if we choose to use it in such a way.

Technology offers affordances, or "functional and relational aspects which frame, while not determining, the possibilities for agentic action in relation to an object" that both shape and are shaped by interaction with the object (Hutchby, 2001, p. 444). Often, affordances are enabled and constrained by the social context of both use and user, making affordances both a technological and social construct. In terms of supporting social capital, online technology removes barriers to interaction (i.e., space and time), expands interaction networks (i.e., enables more connections, thus increasing the potential for both incoming and outgoing information), restricts information flow (reduces communication cues, which can have both positive and negative effects on interaction), manages dependencies (creates a framework for communication), maintains history (creates repositories and easily accessible markers of a group/collective identity), and names (reifies roles and establishes identity) (Resnick, 2001). This allows for the creation of SocioTechnical capital, or the "productive combinations of social relations and information and communication technology" (Resnick, 2001, p.3).

Thus, online technology can be used to reconfigure social relations and create both community and social capital. Wellman, Haase, Witte, and Hampton (2001) suggest that internet based-communication has led to "community becoming embedded in social networks rather than groups and a movement of community relationships from easily observed public spaces to less accessible private homes" (p. 437). Wellman et al. (2001) found that rather than replacing face-to-face contact, internet use supplemented such contact, increasing communication among existing partners. Essentially, Wellman et al. (2001) found the internet to be a tool for building and maintaining social capital when used in a social way, but detrimental to social capital (as it draws people away from interaction) when used in an asocial way.

There has been success in using ICT to create social capital in the health domain. For example, research has found that online health social support communities support a variety of ties, ranging from weak, to intermediate, to strong. Such communities enable supportive communication among members, with the added benefit of connecting individuals who, because of physical or other limitations might not have received any such communication otherwise (Braithwaite, Waldron, & Finn, 2009; Loane & D'Allesandro, 2013; Wellman & Gulia, 1999). Arguably, online social support communities maximally utilize both bridging and bonding social capital, as they unite geographically disparate and unfamiliar participants around a common interest. Thus, participants are able to build relationships around a common need that is not being met in their face-to-face environments, while tapping into other differences (e.g., ethnic, geographic), also unavailable in their face-to-face environments. That is, the linking power of social media, combined with the ability of online communities to turn weak ties into strong ties, can harness both the emotional and material benefits of being connected to others and provide new opportunities for improved health.

Additionally, in terms of health promotion, Wallack (2001) argues that if mass media, including the internet, is used to relate to people as citizens who are valued for their potential participation, it can be used to create social capital. Such communication should emphasize: (a) increased capacity for participation in collective action, (b) the connection between problems/issues and broader social forces, (c) the creation of both bridging and bonding social capital, and (d) a social justice orientation (pp. 358–359). Communication invoking the idea of community and citizenry, or essentially *tapping into* the idea of social capital and community action, can be an effective way to promote health initiatives.

While these studies looked at health benefits accrued via online media in terms of the benefits shared by the participants, they demonstrate several principles relevant to the citizen-stakeholder model. First, discussion and promotion of health topics are acceptable in an online venue. Although health is often a personal issue, many people feel comfortable learning about, building relationships around, and acting on health-related information via online media. Second, people are willing to trust both information and individuals with sensitive health-related information in a mediated environment. Third, both the idea of social capital and social capital itself can be created online in order to engage people into action around a health related cause, either for themselves or others.

Combining Organizational and Personal Capital

Given the previously described capacity for social media to enable the building of social capital across time and geography, organizations arguably have the capacity to build connections not only between themselves and stakeholders, but also among stakeholders who connect on the organization's various media platforms. By building online communities, organizations can create a space for stakeholders to engage with each other, and to indirectly or directly link their conversation to personal contacts that they follow or like. In doing so, they promote the possibility of bonding social capital developing among formerly unconnected stakeholders, which would in turn strengthen the social capital in the online community. Additionally, as stakeholders become truly engaged with the organization and other stakeholders in the community, they are more likely to share the organization's message and initiative with their own personal networks, thus connecting their contacts with the organization.

For the communication shared in this place to be considered worth investing in, it should be genuine and transparent. Organizations should "relinquish any notion of control as building social capital is dependent on mutuality, collaboration and community" (Willis, 2012, p. 120). Good content will not only get speople to engage with the organization, but with each other, by "provid[ing] the discourses that construct issues and their resolutions" (Taylor, 2011, p. 437). To that end, organizations can create a sort of social commons, where discourse aimed at community engagement can be shared (Willis, 2012).

This commons can be created via social media platforms, web content, and even one-way messages including information about the health problem, the intended or ongoing initiative, and the organization's stance and record to date; as well as on the ground via connections with partners local to the health initiative. As informational use of media, as well as self-efficacy to take action, have been linked to social capital, providing information both about the cause, and what the individual can do about it, can be effective in generating interest and participation (Jeffres, Jian, & Yoon, 2013). Ideally, organizations would begin to engage with stakeholders via routine transactions and social media, converting reputational capital into social capital. Once stakeholders trust the organization on routine issues, they would then be more likely to extend that trust to other issues, particularly if that issue falls under the purview of the organization's operation (e.g., Johnson and Johnson working with Operation Smile). Within this community, content aimed at combining a sense of individual responsibility with communitarian responsibility (two ideas inherent to citizenship; e.g., Etzioni, 1995) could be effectively used to engage stakeholders to both take and share their actions.

Building on Gregory's research (2010), Willis (2012) emphasizes six communication principles for engaging stakeholders in a dialogue around social action: salience (will content stand out), empathy (does content relate to hopes and fears), timeliness (is it what they want to consider in this precise moment), accessibility (is the content, tone, style and place what they want or will respond to), credibility (does the organization have the appropriate authority or knowledge related to this issue) and feasibility (is what is being requested possible and/or desirable). Each of these principles can evoke a part of the decision-making process in order to get people involved: attention, emotion, relevance, trust, and self-efficacy. Further, utilizing technological attributes such as hashtags, liking, sharing, and posting will allow for the creation of a "common space," where engaged stakeholders can meet and communicate, and draw their own online connections into the health initiative. As indicated in Figure 21.2, this communication is

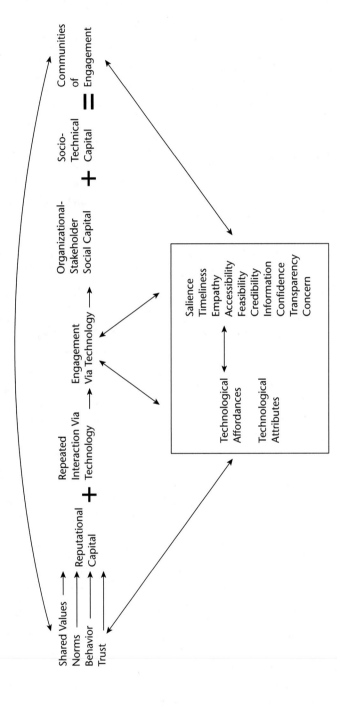

FIGURE 21.2 Communication Mechanisms for Social Capital in Citizen-Stakeholder Networks.

reinforced by the communicated values, norms, and trust that create and reinforce the social capital between the organization and the stakeholder. Once such a framework is set up, organizations and individuals can create a "communication intervention," in which websites, social media and mobile platforms can create a forum for discussion and also "strengthen interaction across social boundaries" (Jeffres, et.al, 2013, p. 556).

Sharing Capital Across Communities

The last area in which social capital comes into play in the citizen-stakeholder model is in sharing the capital generated via organization-stakeholder networks with capital-deficient communities, most likely via a nonprofit community partner. This side of the equation relies upon a combination of linking social capital, or "norms of respect and networks of trusting relationships between people who are interacting across explicitly formal or institutionalized power or authority gradients in society" (Szreter & Woolcock, 2004, p. 651), and bonding social capital. That is, for-profit organizations serve as macro-level organizing mechanism to generate and share capital to improve health. On the local-community level, this is accomplished as nonprofits and non-governmental organizations use the capital shared by the citizen-stakeholder networks and create community-based health programs specific to the local, geographic communities of which they are part.

The citizen-stakeholder model looks primarily at how for-profit organizations can use their tremendous capital to provide bridging and linking capital to capital-deficient areas. While the model acknowledges the role of community partners the equation, it does not explicitly detail how these partners, such as nonprofits and NGOs, will share this capital within affected communities, or use communication to foster the bonding capital that is often associated with health outcomes. This is largely because how nonprofits work with individual community partners is best determined by the practices of each community. Thus, while the citizen-stakeholder model provides an outline for the entire process, it only fills in the details for the first half. The following section provides examples to help visualize how this might look in practice.

The Citizen-Stakeholder Model: What It Might Look Like

The examples given earlier in this chapter of Johnson and Johnson's work with Operation Smile and Tom's Foundation, One-for-One, capture a preliminary view of what this model might look like. Each organization is building on reputational capital with stakeholders to create social capital through which stakeholders invest time or money in the organization's social cause. However, the citizen stakeholder model as envisioned in this chapter would take the idea a step further, by getting stakeholders to tap into their own social capital outside of the organizational relationship, at the behest of the organization, to further the cause.

The ALS ice-bucket challenge, popular during the summer of 2014, is an example of the way that individuals can harness their own social capital via their social networks in order to generate action toward a social cause. Different than what is discussed in this chapter, in that the challenge was not started for, or done on the behalf of, a specific organization, the principles of sharing social capital with a virtual community to create a collective effort is the basic premise of citizen stakeholders. Although there were many other factors at play, the way in which individuals contributed their time/effort/reputation/money in order to create positive health change, and engaged social capital via social networks to do so, is a reflection of the way that socio-technical capital can be used to activate social capital for a common cause.

In late 2014, Unilever launched "Project Sunlight," an initiative "made up of a community of people who believe it is possible to build a world where everyone lives well and lives sustainably" (Unilever, 2014). Working together with the nonprofit food bank Feed America, Unilever encourages individuals to share a meal, or commit an "act of sunlight" (donate or volunteer) via their online platform. While the initiative uses traditional media, such as television advertisements, it largely resides online, where individuals are encouraged to support Feeding America, tell why they #shareameal, and "join" Project Sunlight by signing up to receive updates. The official website of Project Sunlight is also abundant in content, both informative and social, including a social media wall that features feeds of Unilever's social media platforms.

Perhaps the best example of the principles present in this chapter is the way Change Heroes, a for-profit social enterprise, uses social networks to get people involved in providing access to education in developing countries, such as Uganda and Kenya. The basic premise involves getting 33 people to give $3.33/day, for three months. Individuals are recruited by friends to donate, and then in turn, take on the challenge of getting 33 of their friends to donate, and in turn, pass on the mission (http://www.changeheroes.com/howitworks/). Individuals solicit donations through semi-scripted brief videos that they create and send to friends via e-mail or social media. They support their communication through customized Facebook banners, and updates on the status of the project that they are funding. Change Heroes partners with a nonprofit; Free the Children, to undertake the logistical elements of the outreach in the Kenyan and Ugandan communities. While Change Heroes is a for-profit company, its sole mission is to engage donors via the 33/$3.33/3 formula. The simplicity of the Change Heroes mission puts it in a somewhat different category than organizations enacting CSR. However, their efforts represent a similar model to what is proposed here, particularly in terms of using social networks to create collective identification and action toward a health initiative that uses social capital to create social conditions amenable to healthy change.

Looking Forward: Future Theorizing and Potential Pitfalls

Although the citizen-stakeholder model articulates a useful way for harnessing and sharing social capital to improve health, elements of which are already at play in various formats and contexts, there are drawbacks to the model. From a theoretical point of view, there are two primary pitfalls. The basic premises of the model rely upon the reconceptualization of several standard ideas, including those of community, social capital, and citizenship. While there is data to support that these ideas can and should be altered to accommodate a world that is interconnected across geographic boundaries by computer networks, creating these new definitions will likely be a lengthy process of negotiation, not to be sorted out in the short term. This chapter represents one voice in that discussion. Another theoretical consideration regarding the creation and sharing of social capital online is that it will be hard to harness the face-to-face component of social capital building that much research still posits as part of the puzzle (Jeffres et al., 2013, Willis, 2012). However, when individuals engage others in their network of strong ties to join, it is likely that they are tapping into a relationship built on face-to-face communication. Whether or not this is enough to carry participation is a question for future research.

To that end, the idea of citizen-stakeholdership touches on the idea of whether or not the internet lives up to the often-quoted potential to unite and democratize (Morozov, 2011). Morozov (2011) argues that online giving makes it too easy to engage in superficial giving, and takes away from real philanthropy and engagement. He points out that people are able to donate and be publicly lauded for doing so, without the real commitment involved in community building. The danger, he argues, is that such "slactivists" will feel as if they have done their duty, and pass up "deeper" opportunities for volunteerism or giving. However, if online initiatives, such as those posited in this chapter (a) reach people who would not normally get involved, or (b) widen the scope of giving by reaching larger networks via both bridging and bonding social capital, then arguably, citizenship is being activated and help is being given. Future theorizing should tease out the dimensions of quantity versus quality of giving and citizenship, as well as the interplay between intention and action.

From an enactment point of view, the time and resources detailed as part of the citizen-stakeholder model are hard to realize. Funding and maintaining communities of engaged stakeholders around a health-related cause, as well as enacting the fulfillment of the initiative with nonprofit partners, can only be accomplished by an organization fully committed to the philanthropic initiative. Without this genuine enactment, organizations, and by proxy their initiatives and partners, could lose social capital, leaving the health initiative dead on arrival.

Conclusion

The citizen-stakeholder model, as presented in this chapter, provides an outline of how communication, social capital, and organizations can intersect to create better health outcomes. Building on ideas of a globally and digitally connected society, and the changing role of the organization in this society, it is argued that organizations can create social capital with stakeholders, and engage this capital to create global health networks in which the organization acts as the link between a community of citizen-stakeholders, nonprofit community partners, and capital-deficient communities. Additionally, they can create bridging social capital with the strong ties of their stakeholders, by getting stakeholders to engage their friends and acquaintances via social media. The desired result is global health networks in which citizens participate, act, and engage.

DISCUSSION QUESTIONS

1. Although for-profit organizations can "do great good" in the world by lending bridging capital and supporting nonprofits and global communities, is it problematic to, as Coleman (1988, p. 117) says: "substitute formal organizations for the spontaneous social organization that has, in the past, been a major source of social capital?"
2. What are some of the problems inherent to conceptualizing online citizenship?
3. Is it more important the stakeholder identifies with the organization or the cause when engaging in an organization's health initiative? How can organizational communication accommodate this?

Suggested Reading

Lin, N. (2001). Building a network theory of social capital. In N. Lin, K. S. Cook, & R. S. Burt (Eds.), *Social capital: Theory and research.* New York, NY: Aldine De Gruyter.
Taylor, M. & Kent, M. L. (2014). Dialogic engagement: Clarifying foundational concepts. *Journal of Public Relations Research, 26*, 384–398.

References

Bowen, H. R. (1953). *Social responsibilities of the businessman.* New York, NY: Harper & Row.
Braithwaite, D. O., Waldron, V. R., & Finn, J. (1999). Communication of social support in computer-mediated for people with disabilities. *Health Communication, 11*(2), 123–151.
Burt, R. (2000). The network structure of social capital. *Research in Organizational Behavior, 22*, 345–423.

Cattell, V. (2001). Poor people, poor places, and poor health: The mediating role of social networks and social capital. *Social Science and Medicine, 52*(10), 1501–16.

Change Heroes (2014). How it works. Retrieved from http://www.changeheroes.com/howitworks/.

Cobb, S. (1976). Social support as a moderator of life stress. *Psychosomatic Medicine, 38*, 300–314.

Coleman, J. S. (1988). Social capital in the creation of human capital. *The American Journal of Sociology* (Suppl.) Organizations and Institutions: Sociological and Economic Approaches to the Analysis of Social Structure, *94*, S95–S120.

Coombs, W. T. & Holladay, S. J. (2010). *PR Strategy and Application*. West Sussex, UK: Wiley-Blackwell.

Crane, A., Matten, D., & Moon, J. (2004). Stakeholders as citizens? Rethinking rights, participation, and democracy. *Journal of Business Ethics, 53*(1–2), 107–122.

Doerfel, M. L., Lai, C-H, & Chewning, L. V. (2010). The evolutionary role of inter-organizational communication: Modeling social capital in disaster contexts. *Human Communication Research, 36*, 125–162.

Eisenegger, M. (2009). Trust and reputation in the age of globalization. In J. Klewes & R. Wreschniok (Eds.). *Reputation capital: Building and maintaining trust in the 21st century* (pp. 11–22). Berlin: Springer.

Etzioni, A. (1995). *The spirit of community: Rights, responsibilities, and the communitarian agenda*. London: Fontana Press.

Folland, S. (2007). Does "community social capital" contribute to population health? *Social Science and Medicine, 64*, 2342–2354.

Gregory, A. (2010). *Planning and managing public relations campaigns: A strategic approach*. Philadelphia, PA: Kogan Page.

Hutchby, I. (2001). Technologies, texts, and affordances. *Sociology, 35*(2), 441–456.

Jackson, K. T. (2004). *Building reputational capital*. New York, NY: Oxford University Press.

Jeffres, L. W., Jian, G., & Yoon, S. (2013). Conceptualizing communication capital for a changing environment. *Communication Quarterly, 61*(5), 539–563.

Krishna, A. (2002). Active social capital: Tracing the roots of development and democracy. New York, NY: Columbia University Press.

Lee, J. & Lee, H. (2010). The computer mediated communication network: Exploring the linkage between online community and social capital. *New Media & Society 12*(5), 711–727.

Lin, N. (1999). Building a network theory of social capital. *Connections, 22*(1), 28–51. Retrieved from http://www.insna.org/PDF/Keynote/1999.pdf.

Lin, N. (2001a). Building a network theory of social capital. In N. Lin, K. S. Cook, & R. S. Burt (Eds.), *Social capital: Theory and research* (pp. 3–30). New York, NY: Aldine De Gruyter.

Lin, N. (2001b). *Social capital: A theory of social structure and action*. New York, NY: Cambridge University Press.

Loane. S. S. & D'Allesandro, S. (2013). Communication that changes lives: Social support in an online health community with ALS. *Communication Quarterly, 61*(2), 236–251.

Luoma-Aho. V. (2009). On Putnam: bowling together: Applying Putnam's theories of community and social capital to public relations. In O. Ihlen, G. van Ruler, & M. Fredriksson (Eds.), *Public relations and social theory: Key figures and concepts*. New York, NY: Routledge.

Marino, J. & Starfield, B. (2001). The utility of social capital in research on health determinants. *The Milbank Quarterly, 79* (3), 387–427.

Marsden, C. (2000). The new corporate citizenship of big business: Part of the solution to sustainability. *Business and Society Review, 105*(1), 9–25.

Morozov, E. (2011). The net delusion: The dark side of Internet freedom. New York, NY: Public Affairs.

Putnam, R. D. (1993). The prosperous community: Social capital and public life. *The American Prospect, 4*(13), 36–42.

Putnam, R. D. (1995). Bowling alone: America's declining social capital. *Journal of Democracy, 6,* 65–78.

Putnam, R. D. (2000). Bowling alone: The collapse and revival of American community. New York, NY: Simon & Schuster.

Putnam, R. D., Feldstein, L., & Cohen, D. (2003). *Better together: Restoring the American community.* New York, NY: Simon & Schuster.

Putnam, R. D., Leonardi, R., & Nanetti, R. (1993). *Making democracy work: Civic traditions in modern Italy.* Princeton, NJ: Princeton University Press.

Resnick, P. (2001). Beyond bowling together: Sociotechnical capital. *HCI in the New Milennium, 77,* 247–272.

Rocco, L. & Suhrcke, M. (2012). Is social capital good for health? A European Perspective. (ISBN 978 92 890 0273 8). Copenhagen, WHO Regional Office for Europe.

Solis, B. & Breakenridge, D. K. (2009). Putting the public back in public relations: How social media is reinventing the age of business in PR. Upper Saddle River, NJ: Pearson Education.

Stephens, K. K., Rimal, R. N., & Flora, J. A. (2004). Expanding the reach of health campaigns: Community organizations as meta-channels for the dissemination of health information. *Journal of Health Communication, 9*(1), 97–111.

Szreter, S. & Woolcock, M. (2004). Health by association? Social capital, social theory, and the political economy of public health. *International Journal of Epidemiology, 33*, 650–667.

Taylor, M. (2009). Civil society as a rhetorical public relations process. In R. Heath, E. L. Toth, & D. Waymer (Eds.), *Rhetorical and critical approaches to public relations III* (pp. 76–91). Mahwah, NJ: Lawrence Erlbaum.

Taylor, M. (2011). Building social capital through rhetoric and public relations. *Management Communication Quarterly, 25*(3), 436–454.

Taylor, M. & Kent, M. L. (2014). Dialogic engagement: Clarifying foundational concepts. *Journal of Public Relations Research, 26,* 384–398.

Unilver (2014). *What is project sunlight?* Retrieved from https://brightfuture.unilever.com/stories/396909/What-is-Project-Sunlight—See-the-possibilities-and-get-involved.aspx.

Wallack, L. (2001). The role of mass media in creating social capital: A new direction for public health. In D. S. Smedley & S. L. Syme (Eds.), *Promoting health: Intervention strategies from social and behavioral research.* Washington, DC: National Academies Press.

Wellman, B. & Gulia, M. (1999). Net surfers don't ride alone: Virtual communities as communities. In M. A. Smith and P. Kollack (Eds.), *Communities in cyberspace.* New York, NY: Routledge.

Wellman, B., Haase, A. Q., Witte, J., & Hampton, K. (2001). Does the Internet increase, decrease, or supplement social capital? Social networks, participation, and community commitment. *American Behavioral Scientist, 45,* 436–455.

Willis, P. (2012). Engaging communities: Ostrom's economic commons, social capital, and public relations. *Public Relations Review, 38,* 116–122.

22

NETWORKED FORMS OF ORGANIZING, DISASTER-RELATED DISRUPTIONS, AND PUBLIC HEALTH

Marya L. Doerfel

Interpersonal, persuasion and campaign, and information theories have been foundational in health communication with recent trends showing a surge in applied interventions by scholars collaborating with community organizations. Meanwhile, the already-existing interorganizational relationships (IORs) among community organizations that researchers enter into are simultaneously a vital component of the health of the community. IORs form networks across the community and the ways these networks are configured has implications for the community's resilience (Doerfel, Lai, & Chewning, 2010) and in terms of public health and wellness. After disaster, recovery of the public health is inextricably intertwined with the recovery of the organizations that serve and provide resources to the community. The social networks that such organizations, businesses, and agencies make up embody the social infrastructure of the community (Doerfel et al., 2010) and therefore undergird public health. The community's rebuilding involves hierarchies (e.g., government agencies) while local efforts involve more informal, networked forms of organizing (Bryson, Crosby, & Stone, 2006; Simo & Bies, 2007).

Related, inherent in any interdependent relationships are opportunities and challenges afforded by networks in terms of power and control. Networked forms of organizing involve communication processes that are distinguished from hierarchical forms of power and control, yet the two forms—networked and hierarchical—coexist. This chapter highlights ways organizations may use—but also recognize the challenges associated with—networked and hierarchical forms of organizing and how individual actions and communication by organizations within an interorganizational network support community-level initiatives. In doing so, this chapter reflects an asset approach to health, which points to positive aspects of supporting community health, including connections, capacity, and social capital (Burns, 2013; Glasgow Centre for Population Health, 2011). This chapter begins with an overview of community resilience as a form of community health, then explains networked and hierarchical forms of organizing, which often are simultaneously present yet have been compared as oppositional ways to coordinate work. Underlying both approaches are concerns with where power and control are located and related, and the ways in which individual actions constitute the broader social structures. Examples from post-Hurricane Katrina New Orleans illustrate these frameworks.

Contexts That Benefit From Networked Forms

Individual-level resilience is viewed as an ability to maintain stability despite traumatic perturbations like family death or localized incidents like disasters cause (Bonanno, 2004). Resilience has also been linked to individuals' health (Bonanno, 2004), with generally optimistic views linked to both psychological and physical health (Taylor, Kemeny, Reed, Bower, & Gruenewald, 2000). Linking individual health to the role of organizations, disaster response involves facilitating citizens' and the broader community's resilience, response, and recovery and is supported by organizations coordinating across sectors (nonprofit, government, business) (Bryson et al., 2006; Simo & Bies, 2007). Thus, the very act of disaster response involves health at multiple levels—for individuals, the organizations where they work and seek services, and the broader community. Resilient communities create the necessary stable backdrop for individuals to retain their own resilience and health. Beyond disasters, healthy communities are conceived, focus on, or provide resources that contribute to public health (i.e., fresh fruit and vegetables, green spaces, social ties, etc.) and have been identified as health assets (Burns, 2013; see also Aakhus & Harrison, this volume).

Like resilient individuals who maintain some level of stability despite traumatic events, organization-level resilience is also about maintaining balance despite chaos. Resilient organizations improvise and engage in creative problem solving, have shared views of the focal system with other members, recognize when new information is needed, and respect partners jointly managing the problem at hand (Weick & Sutcliffe, 2001). Features of resilience can be seen at the community level as devastated areas progress through disaster and recovery. Resilient communities have features that align with resilient organizations' features, including *robustness* (the ability of all elements of a system to withstand a given level of stress without degradation or loss of function), *resourcefulness* (the capacity to identify problems, establish priorities, and mobilize resources when disruption occurs), *redundancy* (elements of a system can be substitutable), and *rapidity* (the capacity to meet priorities and achieve goals in a timely manner) (Chewning, Lai, & Doerfel, 2013; Doerfel, Chewning, & Lai, 2013; Kendra &

Wachtendorf, 2003). Resilience involves organizations communicating through networks to gain and share information and resources. Thus, while much of Weick and others' work on resilience is about organizations, resilient processes extend to communities as organizing spaces. Moreover, community resilience is tantamount to community and public health. A social network view models the ways community organizations support resilience and health through networks that facilitate and constrain communication flows, norms of trust, and information and resource sharing.

For individuals and organizations alike, resilience is a matter of stability and rests in the ability to communicate and reorganize out of chaos. Across studies about organizations coping after disasters, resilience is less about a preconceived disaster plan and more as a way to use resources, non-technological and technological alike, in context to adapt to volatile and changing conditions (Chewning et al. 2012). Resilience, then, is about communicating through networks with an open and flexible orientation, recognizing when to hold old or create new communication routines and partnerships.

Networked Forms of Organizing

A social network framework on interorganizational relationships (IORs) is about opting-in and self-organized collaboration, where shared ownership of problems and their solutions, decentralized decision-making (actors are autonomous yet interdependent in designing procedures and solutions), and cross-functional teams (e.g., experts from different backgrounds, like information technology, marketing, health care) are the recognizable organizing structures. Networked IORs range from casual arrangements to formal, legally negotiated or mandated ones (see Silk & Smith chapter). The more formal the arrangement, the more the IOR may have qualities akin to traditionally bureaucratic forms of organizing (Doerfel, Atouba, & Harris, 2014). Ideally, networked forms are more flexible, in that, as goals and specific problems change, so, too, can those who coordinate related activities. Joint ownership of problems and their solutions relate to the idea that interdependence is highly valued. Autonomous partners are interdependent in that the work they do as particular experts is meant to be coordinated and thus networked to optimize results.

Network members' decisions can impact the overall goals and the abilities of others, which necessitate coordinating and complementing work processes. Having access to greater resources through partners' extended networks leverages otherwise untapped information, financial, and material resources (Baker, 1994; Burt, 1992). In IORs, organizations have resource dependent relationships with funders, clients, regulating bodies, and strategic alliance partners. Through these relationships, organizations communicate as a way to leverage information sharing, information and resource access and protect themselves from environmental threats (Benson, 1975; Pfeffer & Salancik, 1978; Van de Ven, 1976).

Interorganizational collaboration is nothing new (e.g., Barley, Freeman, & Hybels, 1992; Kogut, Shan, & Walker, 1992; Powell & Brantley, 1992), with consortia and networked organizations having emerged as the modern way of getting work done: strategically managing scarce resources, turbulent environments, and intractable problems.

The nature of relationships evolve, too, as shown in communication-centered research that tracked networks over time to reveal periods of high cooperation (e.g., Doerfel & Taylor, 2004; Flanagin, Monge, & Fulk, 2001; Taylor & Doerfel, 2003) followed by periods of intense competition among organizations (e.g., Bryant & Monge, 2008). The networked form has also been center to understanding collective actions (Bimber, Flanagin, & Stohl, 2012; Olson, 1965) like managing HIV prevention in Africa (Shumate, 2012) and power as relational and temporary interorganizational strategic alliances (Walker & Stohl, 2012). Communication-centered research underscores the value of building IORs for fostering advantages like innovation, advancing knowledge, and engaging a community for resolving complex problems. It can thus be extended to thinking about health and the ways community organizations build relationships that then provide a social infrastructure to various public health needs, which, in turn, sets the stage for community resilience as a buffer to anticipated and unanticipated problems. A complicating factor, however, is that, like disaster, public health problems involve organizations across sectors (e.g., government agencies; nonprofits) and efforts come from local and nonlocal entities (e.g., local and federal agencies). The way communication is viewed in different organizational forms (hierarchies and networks) complicates the ways in which joint efforts can be navigated.

The Clash of Networks and Hierarchies

Organizations develop social networks that have implications for power, influence, and other organizing processes like joint decision-making and resource control. It is in this context that decades of research have attempted to understand the broader political economy that unfolds (Benson, 1975; Miles & Snow, 1986; Van de Ven, 1976). For the purposes of this chapter, the networked form is discussed more generally as a framework for understanding the network of relationships that organizations enter into to address complex and community-wide problems.

Social networks have been predominantly viewed as self-directed and emergent organizing processes; however, tensions of emergence and being controlled arise when community organizations attempt to work together and across sectors (e.g., nonprofit with corporate or government agencies). Clashes of emergence and control are partly a result of hierarchical structures existing alongside networks, despite fundamentally different assumptions (see Table 22.1 for a comparison of traditional views versus networked forms of organizing). In traditionally

TABLE 22.1 Managing and Organizing Working Relationships

Organizing Features	Hierarchies	Social Networks
Reporting structures	Managers/supervisors	Partners
Decision-making; job design	Centralized	Decentralized
Policy	Legal	Negotiated
Power and authority	Management	Gatekeepers
Orientation towards communication and meaning	Clarity is valued; information is transferred	Presume ambiguity; co-constructed and negotiated
Structure	Constant; predictable; rigid	Dynamic; strategic; flows

structured organizations, control and authority are paramount, idealizing communication flows that follow lines of authority. While organizing through hierarchies was originally designed to maximize efficiency and effectiveness of work processes (Weber, 1964), practitioners and scholars alike came to realize that the way communication *actually* flows is not up and down the hierarchy nor necessarily involving traditionally recognized power structures. Talk flows in and around the system, and the underlying communication networks have come to be known as the informal structure inside organizations. As organizations coordinate work across boundaries with other organizations, these traditional structures are not typically viewed as a way to guide IORs; however, some of the same underlying assumptions about power and resource control are present.

Power and Networked Forms

Comparing hierarchies (the essence of bureaucratic forms) with networks implies an either–or structural arrangement, when in fact networks coexist alongside hierarchies. Internally, there are still organizational charts and articulated management structures (e.g., management roles; policy). At the community level, regulating bodies and funding agencies embody hierarchical forms of power (Rodriguez, Langley, Beland, & Denis, 2007). Two ways that traditionally hierarchical power structures coexist alongside networked organizations are noteworthy. First, power and authority are present in hierarchies. Bureaucratic organizations hold hierarchical status as governing bodies or because of their control over resources. Second, when more central in social networks, power and influence can be reified through brokering or gatekeeping information through the network.

Hierarchies and Power

While a foundational presence in disaster recovery, government agencies like FEMA and large nonprofits like the Red Cross have specific lines of decision-making authority with official responsibilities that impact their flexibility in the field and in partnership with local and state Office of Emergency Management (OEM) organizations. In addition to the public's views about the leadership role such agencies have in disaster relief, each agency is structured within a network of organizations that are overseen by the OEM. OEM is hierarchically structured with local offices nested within regional ones that are under the direction of the national level OEM. While personnel in the field are afforded certain autonomy, there are specific operating procedures with reporting structures to ensure resource allocation and disaster relief processes align with protocols laid out by local, state, and national OEM. When these agencies are criticized for failing, it can be seen as a clash between their limits as hierarchies despite the opportunities that such ascribed power should afford them—they are so big they are prone to fail. These structural arrangements extend to nonprofit sectors where funding agencies mete out financial resources and set policy regarding how the money is deployed (Rodriguez et al., 2007), and regulating bodies that mandate how resources are allocated. Similarly for the profit sector, strategic alliances can be highly controlled through legal arrangements and hierarchical power can also be seen in regulating bodies that sanction, certify, or affirm accreditation of field-specific practices.

Networks and Power

Hierarchies can be seen alongside networked forms when what might begin as power through holding resources, deferential treatment of those resource holders echoes notions of cultural hegemony. Social positions become dominant because deeply rooted beliefs and ideologies evolve through the elite's control of financial and information-based resources (Castells, 2011; Deetz, 1992; Gramsci, 1971; Mumby, 1997). Deference to people in positions of power and the ideals they value may seem so natural that it is done subconsciously. The result is an underlying ideology that privileges the resource-holders, who are, by association, elite, whereby even those not served by the underlying principles of the ideology value it. Meanwhile, a long-recognized pattern in social networks is the idea that resource holders and early entrants into the network come to be more central (Pfeffer & Salancik, 1978) and therefore more influential and powerful (Astley & Sachdeva, 1984; Taylor & Doerfel, 2003). Through becoming more central, organizations are given control by their partners who turn to them, which, in turn means those central organizations further control information flows in the networked system (Astley & Sachdeva, 1984; Castells, 2013). Central organizations can become gatekeepers by facilitating or becoming roadblocks to resource and communication flows. Gatekeepers can also exert their power when they broker connections by facilitating an introduction or by using their influence on one partner to support another.

The resource holders come to have power, then, through controlling resources, having the ability to control information flows in the networks, and also through an underlying view that such powerful entities are vital. Through networks and through more subtle presumptions about these power-laden positions, an organization that holds a central, gatekeeping role in a community's network comes to be treated as if it holds legitimate power and control in the system. Organizations that hold central roles can be treated in similar ways that those who are appointed to positions of hierarchically powerful positions are treated: deferentially. In short, the idea of hierarchical power can be (a) obvious because of assigned roles in bureaucratic arrangements; and (b) subtle because of underlying forces that are communicatively (in the network) and socially (through culturally constructed beliefs) ascribed through deference to particular organizations and their representatives. This is especially true from a network view when gatekeepers exert power by controlling network flows. Simply, networked forms, while ideally grassroots and emergent, are not "hierarchy-free."

The Flexibility of Networks

The ideal is that communication evolves as networks work around problems at hand with appropriate partners rather than following lines of hierarchical authority. The reality is that networks can work around hierarchies, through them, or can be constrained by them. Different organizations enter and exit the networked system as time from the disaster passes, as the problems and perceived solutions evolve, and as resources wane or grow. In addition to these dynamic qualities, networked forms span organizational boundaries where flexible relationships are negotiated over time to accomplish shared goals, and are integrated vertically, horizontally, and spatially (Baker, 1994; Miles & Snow, 1986). Such interorganizational networks can be populated by like organizations, such as consortia of competitors, or more diverse, involving cross-sector IORs as part of a larger functioning system (Doerfel et al. 2010). At the heart of the network's flexibility is the relationship (i.e., network tie) sustained through communication. Thus, in working through or around hierarchies, communication in unofficial networks (below the "radar" of hierarchies) is strategic.

For example, in post-Katrina New Orleans, a friendship tie between representatives in a shipping industry business and a Washington DC government agency facilitated work-arounds that would have otherwise been tasks rife with time-consuming paperwork and official approvals. Even simple challenges, like sneaking back into New Orleans during the mandatory evacuation involved other network partners pointing to streets not policed by the National Guard (which holds hierarchical power). Such deceptively simple work-arounds require that organizations or their representatives know and trust others' information. Each organization's rebuilding activities are social in that organizations reconnect to other organizations (suppliers, agencies, clients, and partners) located within, across, and outside the community and reveal interdependence among organizations. They thus also simultaneously fortify community resilience:

interorganizational networks that support organizations' needs are also the very source of community resilience. In this way, communication networking plays a fundamental role in survival, which is discussed next.

Networking to Manage Resilience and Survival

An interorganizational network view constitutes community by considering populations of organizations that share a common resource space (Hawley, 1986; Monge, Heiss, & Margolin, 2008) and work together towards self-serving goals ("get my business back") that end up supporting common goals ("get our community back"). A community ecology framework concerns itself with "survival" by examining variation–selection–retention (VSR) mechanisms that drive change (Monge & Contractor, 2003; Monge et al., 2008). For IORs, VSR mechanisms are considered communicative processes of *variation* (trying/testing different relationships), *selection* (environmental influences that lead to particular relationships selected), and *retention* (attachment to particular selections). Specific types of relationships are organizing mechanisms for organizational survival in general and community rebuilding in particular (Doerfel et al., 2013).

Shumate, Fulk and Monge (2012) showed that shared similar experiences among non-governmental organizations, because they were in the same cohort, geographical proximity, and shared common relationships, predicted subsequent alliances. Similarly, other communication network findings show former relationships are a strong predictor of future ones (Doerfel et al., 2010; Doerfel & Taylor, 2004; Flanagin et al., 2001; Stohl & Stohl, 2005). In disaster response, network ties strengthen through heightened needs to collaborate and thus ties become even more enduring (Doerfel et al., 2013). Monge et al. (2008) proposed that VSR processes are carried out through the formation and maintenance of an organization's communication networks. Organizations initiate communication to explore opportunities for obtaining resources (e.g., advice, information). Development of selection processes for certain partners may then follow these trial-and-error processes. Eventually, these communication practices and partners become routine in an organization's operation. In New Orleans, for instance, of value was advice from known ties, where trust and mutual understanding were established long before Katrina hit (Doerfel et al., 2013; see also chapters in this volume by Chewning; Silk & Smith). These supportive ties were vital but, over time, they can come at a cost. Such stable relationships bring more redundant than unique information and can also exert pressure in terms of loyalty and conformity. In disaster contexts, however, strong tie benefits can far outweigh potential costs.

On the other hand, post-Katrina relationships that did not survive fitness tests failed for a variety of reasons, including due to tensions between hierarchies and networks. The Small Business Administration (SBA) had loans available; however, businesses complained about SBA as "a joke." As a photography studio owner explained, "[the SBA] required my house for collateral. What house?" For this and other businesses, a link to the SBA failed the fitness test. Meanwhile, a nonprofit that brokers grants for entrepreneurs and was embedded in the community prior to the storm provided one-time grants without requiring paperwork, collateral, or arguments about neediness. Pre-storm connections to the community allowed this grantor to extend grants based on prior knowledge. Those relationships passed the fitness test prior to the storm and took minimal but worthwhile effort to sustain them afterward. These particular networking events aggregate to create a community-level network from which SBA is isolated and the nonprofit grantor emerged as a central gatekeeper. As a gatekeeper, that nonprofit facilitated resource and information flows across the network.

Networked relationships change over time as community needs evolve. As a sector develops, initially cooperative IORs (during early phases of community development) evolve into competitive ones (Bryant & Monge, 2008; Monge et al., 2008). Eventually, some networks dissolve as others build up as the nature of the community, itself, changes. After disasters, ebbs and flows of partnering and holding particular relationships can change with organizations' needs and with the progression of recovery. This reflects one of the ideals of networked forms—that they are flexible and dynamic. For many organizations in New Orleans, early stages involved organizations receiving advice and material resources from what would normally be their competitors (Doerfel, Lai, & Chewning, 2010). A restaurant owner brokered vegetables from farmers (who could not immediately do deliveries) to other restaurants along with deliveries to his restaurant. Museums helped other museums in advising how to populate and prioritize rebuilding strategies. These initial survival patterns aligned with the VSR processes. The organizations engaged in cooperative partnering with their organizational peers (competitors) to accomplish goals. In early phases, competitors empathized and shared insider knowledge about business needs. Over time, these ties dissipated as organizations turned their energies to different IORs as recovery challenges evolved.

Two aspects of networked forms are evident in identifying fit ties and their relevance to current needs. First, link quality is fundamental to the overall network configuration. Engaging in relationships that earn reciprocal, in-kind attention builds up social support, cohesion, and system stability, all of which are important health assets for the community. Tit-for-tat relationships that begin with small favors can evolve into enduring positive relationships (Axelrod, 1984; Vangen & Huxham, 2003). Second, past networks are vital but, also, tie fitness can be influenced by broader environmental conditions where past ties lie dormant until circumstances warrant their activation. New Orleans organizations rebuilt their former networks and, for many, expanded them (Doerfel & Haseki, 2015). Previous links predicted subsequent ones and competitive partners were eventually less involved than complementary partners like suppliers and alliances. Networked cooperative-competitors eventually broke apart and returned to dormancy as traditional supply chain, coalition, and alliance networks reactivated.

From a network view, these organizations' particular survival activities are the micro-level actions that collectively constitute an evolving community.

An advantage of networked organizing and viewing communities this way is to recognize what Milgram (1967) first termed the "small-world problem." An organization's network is made up of direct contacts that then also have networks made up of their own direct contacts. The ways in which contacts are willing to share their networks suggests the quality of those particular relationships (fitness) as well as a way to gauge the ability for information to flow around the system. Milgram's "problem" has transformed into multidisciplinary knowledge about strategic networks (Baker, 1994) that hold opportunities yet also constrain organizational autonomy (Burt, 1992; Gargiulo & Benassi, 2000).

Networks as Opportunities and Constraints

The ways organizations are linked in their networks and the general network configurations can have both benefits and drawbacks. For organizations, advantages stem from information access while disadvantages come from information overload or information transfer blockages due to a lack of connections. For the community, networks rich with strong ties that are interconnected indicate social capital (see Chewning, this volume) while also exerting normative social pressures. Likewise, a loosely connected structure held together through weak ties supports unique ideas and information flows, albeit among less loyal partnerships or simply less familiar and less open ones. These tensions are seen at organization and community levels.

Organization-Level Opportunities and Constraints

An organization can be *central* relative to other organizations because of the number of ties it has (a popularity dimension) and/or through being in a position that connects parts of the network that would otherwise not be connected (a gatekeeping dimension). Figure 22.1 illustrates an example of a network in the immediate aftermath of hurricane Katrina. The business (left in the figure) has a client organization that occupies the center of this network. The client has networks to various forms of government (city, federal, and a government agency) and to ties to the professional association, higher education, a bank, etc. The client is a gatekeeper and can share its network by facilitating information flows, withholding information, or by deciding what information or introductions are worthy of brokering. The strategy for the focal business is knowing when ties actually share their networks and are willing to act as brokers. Likewise, when an organization is the gatekeeper because it connects otherwise disconnected network components, that organization can be seen as an important leader because of its gatekeeping activities (Burt, 1992; Doerfel & Taylor, 2004). A gatekeeper has the power to make introductions and, where multiple gatekeepers' bridge

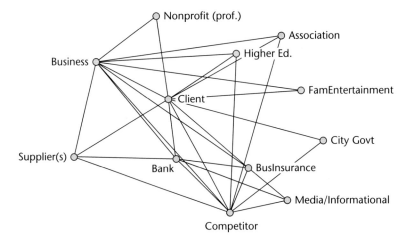

FIGURE 22.1 Post-Katrina Music Industry Organization.

networks. to networks, the world becomes smaller if those central members facilitate the flows of information.

On the other hand, a pressure on the key client in Figure 22.1 is that it is also popular—this client does not just bridge different parts of its network, it also has the most ties (n=9; equal to the competitor shown at the lower right). Central organizations may not have the capacity to treat all of their relationships equally (more relationships require more time and attention). Privileging a few relationships over others can be a reputational risk, where partners may feel neglected and thus view the popular organization as less cooperative (Doerfel & Taylor, 2004). For example, the business (Figure 22.1, left) was part of the New Orleans music industry and connected to the local bank. The business owner criticized the bank for its non-responsiveness and, considering the bank was a former relationship he deemed to be strong (fit), he thus felt slighted by it. The business owner turned to his network and leveraged influence by asking his key client (Figure 22.1, center) to talk to the bank. The client helped through personally contacting the bank manager, who then orchestrated work-arounds through the red tape. Through its gatekeeper-client, the business used its network to transcend the hierarchical component (bank forms) that constrained resource flows. The client activated its central role by brokering influence on behalf of the music business owner.

Community-Level Opportunities and Constraints

Communication flowing in and around the community can be supported through the way the overall network is configured. Networks with select-few gatekeepers can mimic organizational hierarchies where select-few managers control resource and information flows. Gatekeepers' central roles, especially when they remain central over time, mean they have social control and power in the community as a whole, much the way appointed managers inside an organization are deemed powerful because of their hierarchical status (Hales, 2002). The overall network becomes highly centralized when information flows are dependent on gatekeepers who have the prerogative to be liaisons of information, or become bottlenecks that slow the information flows, or roadblocks by withholding or hoarding information and introductions from one part of the network to another.

On the other hand, gatekeepers can be helpful to the whole network while they also benefit from being information brokers. This can be seen when gatekeepers share knowledge and information from relationships in one part of their network with other parts of their network; they facilitate expansive or radiating networks. In this way, the structure supports diverse information flowing through the networks made up of relatively weak but reliable ties (Burt, 1992; Granovetter, 1973). For example, a performing arts center president reached out to the Louisiana Philharmonic Orchestra (LPO) and brokered his network. Through that, various forms of resources poured in to help the LPO thrive (Kaiser, 2010; field interviews). Through new contacts, the LPO's resilience was supported by a broker who created opportunities around which flexible networks could mold. Through that broker, the LPO's network radiated out, enabling access to a variety of information and resources from a diverse and expanding network.

Alternatively, a highly dense network can be observed when all of its members communicate with each other (Figure 22.2). Strong social capital is the signature of these decentralized networks which tend to be made up of relationships that are homophilous and highly cohesive, and have strong normative influences (Brass & Krackhardt, 2012; Gargiulo & Benassi, 2000). A social cost comes with a highly connected and dense network—members tend to know each other well enough, meaning innovation is not as likely as it can be in loosely connected networks that facilitate unique information flowing into the system. In crises and post-disaster, however, this type of redundancy in the network reassures a sense of community through knowing social bonds are intact (Chewning & Doerfel, 2013; Doerfel & Haseki, 2015; Doerfel, Lai, & Chewning, 2010; Powley, 2003). Opportunities and constraints, then, depend on needs for creativity and innovativeness or support and trust.

Networking Through Disruptions

In disaster management, a good deal of successes stem from the flexibility of networked organizations coordinating through and around problems. Indeed, public–private partnerships have emerged in disaster response and are now recognized as a way to improve community resilience (Boyne, 2002; Busch & Givens, 2013; Feeney & Rainey, 2010). The flexibility of private firms enables community support while government agencies manage around more rigid structures stemming from hierarchies and regulatory policy/mandates. Yet not all public–private partnerships are alike, with some public–private partnerships being somewhat nominal with parallel work as opposed to integrated and interdependent work (Robinson & Gaddis, 2012).

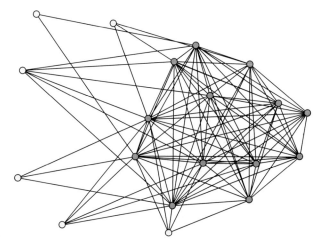

FIGURE 22.2   Hypothetical Dense and Decentralized Network. (Gate keeping relatively dispersed.) Solid-fill circles represent organizations that make up the relatively dense component of the network.

The above sections addressed core social networks concepts that are simultaneously individual and collective, having structures that speak to individual-organization's activities and their roles in the network level that facilitate communication flows and influence. Complicating network-level flows are power and control dynamics embedded in networks, as well as in hierarchies that are both designed (official agencies like OEM) and cultural (through deferential treatment of statuses). While it may appear that OEM is at the center of disaster management (hierarchical organizing), grassroots organizations emerge alongside other organizations and businesses that are already embedded and rebuilding the community in their own ways (an approach that mirrors that of Sir Harry Burns of community-driven approaches to wellness, as presented in Aakhus and Harrison, this volume). Distinct government and grassroots networks can result in a clash between hierarchies and networked forms. Table 22.2 lists levels of focus and hierarchies and networked forms' joint roles in recovery and resilience. Organizational theory asserts that resilience is in the networks but, indeed, community-level resilience and recovery are both hierarchical and networked. Thus, Table 22.2 shows organizational examples that can be found at the intersection of the level of focus and type of organizing form, with implications for the degree to which the network is flexible and able to change over time.

Networking Community Health

A complicating factor of building up resilience to thwart the worst consequences of disaster is that potential problems are pervasive across communities, necessitating

TABLE 22.2   The Clash of Organizing Forms

Level of Focus	Organizing Form	
	Networks	Hierarchies
Organization	Homophilous organizations (e.g., competitors), professional associations, suppliers, clients	Small Business Administration, US Department of Housing and Urban Development, banks, insurance companies
Community	- Grassroots organizations, nonprofits, local businesses, faith-based groups, and the structure formed by their information flows. - Information flows controlled by gatekeepers - Striking balance of dense relations and weak tie networks is an ongoing challenge to manage complex, and ambiguous information	- Office of Emergency Management (OEM) (relationships with other relief organizations like FEMA, Red Cross, National Guard) - Information flows controlled by officials/management - Optimizes efficiencies and uncertainty reduction

broad involvement, from local and national, nonprofit and profit, along with media and government agencies. Similarly, other community health problems are well known to be complex, tackled by various partners across public and private sectors spanning from local to national sources. These contexts involve networks and hierarchies, with emergent and designed structures working together and clashing. The emergent aspects are seen in the power of central and gatekeeping members to facilitate information flows, connecting networks of networks. The top-down/designed aspects are seen in hierarchies that hold resources and control the ways in which those resources get meted out. Grassroots organizations that work together on more non-disaster community health (see Feeley & O'Mally, this volume) could glean lessons from the post-disaster organizations that become tasked with (re)building the very relationships across levels and sectors that make up the pre-disaster community and, therefore, public health.

For example, one legal nonprofit that specializes in working for underprivileged families reported in a post-Katrina interview with me:

The Department of Housing and Urban Development initially threatened to cut funding for all homeless services in New Orleans claiming that we no longer had homeless people because they were all evacuated. We actually wound up having to meet with an Undersecretary and bring the media in and raise a stink before they reinstated our funding. So it varied with the grant sources. HUD was horrible.

This roadblock in their network was due to HUD's bureaucracy. Despite having the tie, the organization had to leverage its other network ties to improve the tie fitness with HUD and advocate for those resources which were vital to restoring health to the community.

Other Considerations: When Bureaucracies Network

Complicating networked forms is that they require flexibility and the ability for representatives to make decisions on behalf of their organizations while simultaneously coordinating those decisions with other partners' efforts. Organizations in the network vary—some are locally owned and operated, some are nonprofit entities, while others might be larger corporations or local offices of larger government agencies. The different types of organizations can face their own "macro"-level clash of organizing forms. The form of a small business or nonprofit might be one of autonomous employees who can make decisions on the fly or promise deliverables because the representative has the power to do so. On the other hand, representatives from larger entities might have more internal approval policies and practices (i.e., they have to take it "up the chain"). Organizational forms clash when some of the organizations in the network feel held back while others might be bottlenecks to information flows, work processes, or sharing and acquiring resources. It is no surprise that SBA failed to become a key partner after Katrina while the grant-giving nonprofit was a key partner. SBA was isolated from having fit ties in the disaster-struck business networks—its relationships were bureaucratic. It had inflexible policy while the nonprofit accessed pre-Katrina networks. As Table 22.2 shows, the SBA ends up disconnected from the grassroots networks with limited capacity—SBA maintains only hierarchical relations.

Pitfalls to Avoid

Most organizations still hold traditional organizing structures, like reporting and authority structures and hierarchies. So a networked form has to find some way to coexist with the hierarchical mentality that remains embedded in underlying assumptions about power and authority (Castells, 2011; Deetz, 1992; Mumby, 1997). Meanwhile, organizations that have flexibility for unplanned events despite more formal aspects of their organization will be more resilient, which, in turn, aggregates to a more resilient community with implications for public health. Networks must also be flexible as needed. Tried and true partners take time to build up (Vangen & Huxham, 2003) but settling into the same partnerships brings constraints. A stable network can become so rigid as to mimic power and control constraints deemed problematic in hierarchies (Hales, 2002). Finally, organizations that demand stricter adherence to policies and procedures will encounter ongoing challenges due to the clash of forms: hierarchies versus networks.

Lessons for Community Health

When tackling intractable problems like public health, a networked approach's value is its flexibility. If networks become overly stable, ideas and creativity can be stale and central members come to be seen as hierarchically controlling and powerful as opposed to emergent and sharing leadership (see Williams, this volume for discussion on leadership). Such networks become more rigid, then, undermining their ability to change as the problems change. Impediments could come from a difficult-to-penetrate dense in-group where support and loyalty dominate. Rigid networks can be avoided when partners agree about values like flexibility in terms of work arrangements and membership. Networks, indeed, have been the way work gets done despite hierarchies when networks remain flexible through fit relationships that support information flows through the overall network over time.

Conclusion

An important feature of successfully managing public health and the general health of the community is the underlying social infrastructure created through cross-sector interorganizational communication. Understanding organizing forms that community partnerships embody includes recognizing the intersection of networks and hierarchies, the power dynamics they both produce, and the implications for facilitating information flows that facilitate partnering. Likewise, such networks fortify the health of a community itself by building the health assets of a community.

DISCUSSION QUESTIONS

1. Considering organizations and their leaders often suffer from information overload, they have to make tough choices about allocating their time. Where is their time best spent in terms of building their network? Why?

2. Organizations with resources often emerge as highly central. What are the costs and benefits to such centrality? Think of an organization in your community that is highly central. What is their reputation? Are they seen as a community leader or roadblock?

3. In what ways can a community's local Office of Emergency Management ensure the community organizations are networking to build up their own and the broader community's resilience? Given the types of power discussed in this chapter, what opportunities or problems could emerge?

4. Building up interorganizational trust takes time and effort. What are the costs and benefits for the organizations and the broader network of organizations investing in building relationships that are well known and trusted?

Suggested Reading

Doerfel, M. L., Chewning, L. V., & Lai, C.-H. (2013). The evolution of networks and the resilience of interorganizational relationships after disaster. *Communication Monographs, 80,* 553–559.

Vangen, S. & Huxham, C. (2003). Nurturing collaborative relations: Building trust in interorganizational collaboration. *The Journal of Applied Behavioral Science, 39,* 5–31.

References

Astley, W. G. & Sachdeva, P. S. (1984). Structural sources of interorganizational power: A theoretical synthesis. *Academy of Management Review, 9,* 104–113.

Axelrod, R. (1984). *The evolution of cooperation.* Cambridge, MA: Basic Books.

Baker, W. E. (1994). *Networking smart: How to build relationships for personal and organizational success.* New York, NY: McGraw-Hill, Inc.

Barley, S. R., Freeman, J., & Hybels, R. C. (1992). Strategic alliances in commercial biotechnology. In N. Nohria & R. G. Eccles (Eds.), *Networks and organizations: Structure, form, and action* (pp. 311–347). Boston, MA: Harvard Business School Press.

Benson, J. K. (1975). The interorganizational network as a political economy. *Administrative Science Quarterly, 20,* 229–249.

Bimber, B., Flanagin, A. J., & Stohl, C. (2012). *Collective action in organizations: Interaction and engagement in an era of technological change.* New York, NY: Cambridge University Press.

Bonanno, G. A. (2004). Loss, trauma, and human resilience: Have we underestimated the human capacity to thrive after extremely aversive events? *American Psychologist, 59,* 20–28.

Boyne, G. (2002). Public and private management: What's the difference? *Journal of Management Studies, 39,* 97–122.

Brass, D. J. & Krackhardt, D. M. (2012). Power, politics, and social networks in organizations. In G. R. Ferris & D. C. Treadway (Eds.), *Politics in organizations: Theory and research considerations* (pp. 355–375). New York, NY: Routledge.

Bryant, J. A. & Monge, P. R. (2008). The evolution of the children's television community, 1953–2003. *International Journal of Communication, 2,* 160–192.

Bryson, J. M., Crosby, B. C., & Stone, M. M. (2006). The design and implementation of cross-sector collaborations: Propositions from the literature. *Public Administration Review, 66,* 44–55.

Burns, H. (2013). Assets for health. In E. Loeffler, G. Power, T. Bovaird, & F. Hine-Hughes (Eds.), *Co-production of health and wellbeing in Scotland* (pp. 28–33). Scotland: Governance, International.

Burt, R. S. (1992). *Structural holes: The social structure of competition.* Cambridge, MA: Harvard University Press.

Busch, N. E. & Givens, A. D. (2013). Achieving resilience in disaster management: The role of public-private partnerships. *Journal of Strategic Security, 6,* 1–19.

Castells, M. (2011). A network theory of power. *International Journal of Communication, 5,* 773–787.

Castells, M. (2013). *Communication power.* Oxford, UK: Oxford University Press.

Chewning, L. V. & Doerfel, M. L. (2013). Integrating crisis into the organizational lifecycle through transitional networks. *International Journal of Humanities and Social Science, 3,* 39–52.

Chewning, L. V., Lai, C.-H., & Doerfel, M. L. (2013). Organizational resilience and using information and communication technologies to rebuild communication structures. *Management Communication Quarterly, 27*, 237–263. Doi: 10.1177/0893318912465815.

Deetz, S. A. (1992). *Democracy in an age of corporate colonization: Developments in communciation and the politics of everyday life*. Albany, NY: State University of New York Press.

Doerfel, M. L., Atouba, Y., & Harris, J. (2014, November). *Bureaucratic control in emergent communication networks*. Paper presented at the annual meetings of the National Communication Association, Chicago, IL.

Doerfel, M. L., Chewning, L. V., & Lai, C.-H. (2013). The evolution of networks and the resilience of interorganizational relationships after disaster. *Communication Monographs, 80*, 533–559.

Doerfel, M. L. & Haseki, M. (2015). Networks, disrupted: Media use as an organizing mechanism for rebuilding. *New Media & Society, 17*, 432–452.

Doerfel, M. L., Lai, C.-H., & Chewning, L. V. (2010). The evolutionary role of interorganizational communication: Modeling social capital in disaster contexts. *Human Communication Research, 36*, 125–162.

Doerfel, M. L. & Taylor, M. (2004). Network dynamics of inter organizational cooperation: The Croatian civil society movement. *Communication Monographs, 71*, 373–394.

Feeney, M. K. & Rainey, H. G. (2010). Personnel flexibility and red tape in public and nonprofit organizations: Distinctions due to institutional and political accountability. *Journal of Public Administration Research & Theory, 20*, 801–826.

Flanagin, A. J., Monge, P., & Fulk, J. (2001). The value of formative investment in organizational federations. *Human Communication Research, 27*, 69–93.

Gargiulo, M. & Benassi, M. (2000). Trapped in your own net? Network cohesion, structural holes, and the adaptation of social capital. *Organization Science, 11*, 183–196.

Glasgow Centre for Population Health. (2011). *Asset-based approaches for health improvement: Redressing the balance* (Briefing paper). Glasgow, Scotland. Retrieved from http://www.gcph.co.uk/.

Gramsci, A. (1971). *Selections from the prison notebooks*. (Q. Hoare & G. N. Smith, Trans.). New York, NY: International Publishers.

Granovetter, M. S. (1973). The strength of weak ties. *The American Journal of Sociology, 78*, 1360–1380.

Hales, C. (2002). "Bureaucracy-lite" and continuities in managerial work. *British Journal of Management, 13*, 51–66.

Hawley, A. H. (1986). *Human ecology: A theoretical essay*. Chicago, IL: University of Chicago Press.

Kaiser, M. (2010, April 24). My arts management hero: Babs Mollere. *Huffington Post*. US. Retrieved from http://www.huffingtonpost.com/michael-kaiser/my-arts-management-hero-b_b_471211.html.

Kendra, J. & Wachtendorf, T. (2003). Elements of resilience after the World Trade Center disaster: Reconstituting New York City's Emergency Operations Centre. *Disasters, 27*, 37–53.

Kogut, B., Shan, W., & Walker, G. (1992). The make-or-cooperate decision in the context of an industry network. In N. Nohria & R. G. Eccles (Eds.), *Networks and organizations: Structure, form, and action* (pp. 348–365). Boston, MA: Harvard Business School Press.

Miles, R. E. & Snow, C. C. (1986). Organizations: New concepts for new forms. *California Management Review, 28*, 62–73.

Milgram, S. (1967). The small world problem. *Psychology Today, 1,* 60–67.

Monge, P. R. & Contractor, N. S. (2003). *Theories of communication networks.* New York, NY: Oxford University Press.

Monge, P. R., Heiss, B. M., & Margolin, D. B. (2008). Communication network evolution in organizational communities. *Communication Theory, 18,* 449–477.

Mumby, D. K. (1997). The problem of hegemony: Rereading Gramsci for organizational communication. *Western Journal of Communication, 61,* 343–375.

Olson, M. (1965). *The logic of collective action: Public goods and the theory of groups.* Cambridge, MA: Harvard University Press.

Pfeffer, J. & Salancik, G. R. (1978). *The external control of organizations.* New York: Harper & Row.

Powell, W. W. & Brantley, P. (1992). Competitive cooperation in biotechnology: Learning through networks? In N. Nohria & R. G. Eccles (Eds.), *Networks and organizations: Structure, form, and action* (pp. 366–394). Boston, MA: Harvard Business School Press.

Powley, E. H. (2003). Reclaiming resilience and safety: Resilience activation in the critical period of crisis. *Human Relations, 62,* 1289–1326.

Robinson, S. E. & Gaddis, B. S. (2012). Seeing past parallel play: Survey measures of collaboration in disaster situations. *The Policy Studies Journal, 40,* 256–273.

Rodriguez, C., Langley, A., Beland, F., & Denis, J.-L. (2007). Governance, power, and manadated colalboration in an interorganizational network. *Administration & Society, 39,* 150–193.

Shumate, M. (2012). The evolution of the HIV/AIDS NGO hyperlnik network. *Journal of Computer Mediated Communication, 17,* 120–134.

Shumate, M., Fulk, J., & Monge, P. (2005). Predictors of the international HIV-AIDS INGO network over time. *Human Communication Research, 31,* 482–510.

Simo, G. & Bies, A. L. (2007). The role of nonprofits in disaster response: An expanded model of cross-sector collaboration. *Public Administration Review, 67,* 125–142.

Stohl, M. & Stohl, C. (2005). Human rights, nation states, and NGOs: Structural holes and the emergence of global regimes. *Communication Monographs, 72,* 442–467. Doi: 10.1080/03637750500322610.

Taylor, M. & Doerfel, M. L. (2003). Building interorganizational relationships that build nations. *Human Communication Research, 29,* 153–181.

Taylor, S. E., Kemeny, M. E., Reed, G. M., Bower, J. E., & Gruenewald, T. L. (2000). Psychological resources, positive illusions, and health. *American Psychologist, 55,* 99–109.

Van de Ven, A. H. (1976). On the nature, formation, and maintenance of relations among organizations. *Academy of Management Review, 1,* 24–36.

Vangen, S. & Huxham, C. (2003). Nurturing collaborative relations: Building trust in interorganizational collaboration. *The Journal of Applied Behavioral Science, 39,* 5–31.

Walker, K. & Stohl, C. (2012). Communicating in collaborating groups: A longitudinal network analysis. *Communication Monographs, 79,* 448–474.

Weber, M. (1964). *The theory of economic and social organization.* New York, NY: Free Press.

Weick, K. E. & Sutcliffe, K. M. (2001). *Managing the unexpected: Assuring high performance in an age of complexity.* San Francisco, CA: Jossey-Bass.

23

COMMUNITY ACCEPTANCE THEORY IN THE SHADOW OF EBOLA

Building Health and Empowerment Networks

Maureen Taylor and Michael L. Kent

The questions asked in a health crisis and the answers provided by government, medical institutions, and citizens, tell us much more than just how to understand sickness or health; they encapsulate larger questions about a society. Health crises often prompt questions about health policies and practices, health-focused organizations, individual and community behaviors, and societal norms, processes and structures. Health is positioned at the intersection of the individual, group, organization, community, and society.

When people mobilize to address a health crisis, suffering is decreased (e.g., polio, smallpox, and guinea worm eradication), and communities emerge stronger and more fully functioning (Heath, 2006). Conversely, when the various levels of societal processes and structures (individual, group, organizational, community, governmental) are too weak to be mobilized, health crises grow and the repercussions are long-lasting. Separating individual behaviors from the collective behaviors in many health contexts is difficult. Tradition, cultural, values and practices, geography, economic and political development, interpersonal and familial relationships, and other contexts all influence health. Indeed, an individual's health often mirrors the community in which s/he lives.

This chapter explores the framework of the community acceptance approach as a theory of health organizing. The chapter identifies the components of the theory and illustrates the theory through the story of how a civil society organization, the YMCA (Young Men's Christian Association) of Liberia, is building a grassroots advocacy network around neglected health issues. The *Peer Education in Neglected Health Issues Project* (PENHIP) was created in 2012 to educate youth about health issues in the poorest areas of Liberia. The project leaders believed that, once young people had accurate and correct health information, they would be able to educate their peers and elders in their community. Moreover, individual health empowerment can eventually lead to social empowerment as youths who have learned how to conduct basic research, talk to others about health issues, and advocate for or against community health practices can use their skills to enact a larger role in community decision-making (see also Doerfel, and Aakhus and Harrison, this volume, for discussion of health assets as a similar approach).

There are many different kinds of capacities required in health contexts (Fawcett, 2002; Fawcett et al., 1995; Fawcett et al., 1996). Capacity is a development concept that refers to individuals in a community or region possessing the knowledge, skills, and training, in management, communication, research, and other areas, needed to achieve some programmatic or campaign goal (Fawcett et al., 1995; Roussos & Fawcett, 2000). The premise of the chapter is that much of the research in the development literature proceeds from an implicit assumption that *community infrastructure* and *capacity* are built first. The infrastructure is important because it provides the tangible building blocks of a community: schools, hospitals, clinics, health systems, and economic development. Community capacity is also viewed as important because it includes the leaders, history, local knowledge, networks of relationships and values of the community. Infrastructure and community capacity are viewed as the means through which communities can tackle issues such as health.

In the PENHIP project, the development premise is reversed. The community acceptance approach suggests that young people develop individual capacities during health training and meetings, such as the ability to conduct research, public speaking, accurate health information, persuasion, and behavior change. Individual levels of health information and self-efficacy are invoked to tackle neglected issues such as hygiene, depression, sexually transmitted infections and substance abuse, and communication skills are developed further. When individuals are empowered to be healthy and have the skills to share their knowledge about health with others, then the other individual skills learned within the health context can be applied to social advocacy at the community level.

The Theoretical Framework

The PENHIP is based on a *community acceptance approach* (the term used by the YMCA to describe its theory of change) that takes a systems approach to interventions. Systems theory describes relationships in complex system (Bertalanffy, 1969). A system can exist at the group, organization, community or even a nation-state level. Systems theory examines relationships, processes and structures among sub-systems. Closed systems resist change and limit the influx of new information and ideas, while open systems are adaptive and open to new information, change, and progress. Systems theory provides a lens to understand the different levels of the community acceptance approach because it sees communities as dynamic, complex systems with varying information needs and dependencies.

The community acceptance approach currently exists as a "lay theory." Lay theories are community sense making strategies that develop organically to explain personal, group, and social experiences. Lay theories also are used to socialize, explain and control the behavior of community members. The community acceptance approach acknowledges the powerful role that community values and leaders play in sense making about new or divergent messages (see Williams, this volume, for discussion of the importance of leader communication). The idea of community-based theories is not new (cf., community power, communitarianism, etc.). The idea of communitarianism, for example, is that people take responsibility for themselves, and for the people in the communities around themselves. This chapter seeks to systematize the community acceptance approach and conceptualize it as a theory for health organizing.

Theories are valuable because they address specific research problems and provide instruction in how to achieve complex goals. The problem that the community acceptance approach addresses is the relationship between individual health empowerment and community empowerment. *We posit that as individuals (youth) become more knowledgeable and empowered in their own health, they will also become more empowered in their communities.* Currently, five variables of interest comprise the community acceptance theory as it applies to health: (a) level of interaction, (b) sensemaking, (c) communication channels, (d) health information, and (e) relational change. Below we explore each variable in depth. The features of the theoretical framework include the people who enact the information and change, the health messages themselves that need to be interpreted, explained, and extended in ways that resonate with local citizens, the community context which includes a ladder of effects from health empowerment (young people's knowledge of, and ability to address neglected health issues) to social empowerment (youth participation in community issues) (see Figure 23.1).

Variable I: Level of Interaction

The first variable is the level of interaction (individual, group/organizational, community and society). This variable identifies the location of communication interaction about health and social empowerment. Interactions can take place at many levels and range from interpersonal interactions to publically shared messages. Interaction can also take place between individuals of similar or dissimilar social, economic, age, gender, and status backgrounds and along several levels and relationships: Individual–Individual, Individual–Group/Organization, Individual–Community, Individual–Society.

Communities include both networked and hierarchical relationships (See Doerfel, this volume). The community acceptance theory recognizes that individuals interact with other individuals (family, friends, coworkers, elders etc.) at

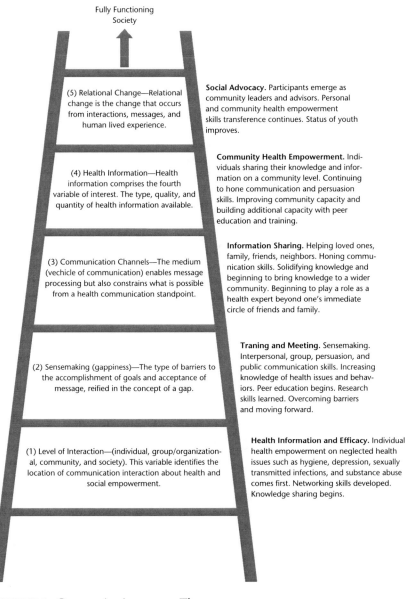

FIGURE 23.1 Community Acceptance Theory.

various social levels, as well as in group and public settings. The enactment of the community acceptance theory takes place at various levels.

Peer education programs that facilitate interpersonal relationships characterize one level. Peer educational programs are undertaken by organizations like the YMCA, as well as public clinics, and community health care workers. A second level of relationship building can also occur between individuals and groups/ organizations such as between individuals and health educators, formally in hospitals, and by civil society organizations and non-governmental organizations. And a third level of interactions focuses on individual–societal level interactions where individual citizens enact their civic duty as a member in a fully functioning society with both rights and responsibilities (examples of this include advising community, political, and social leaders, collaborating with NGOs, seeking or holding official and unofficial public positions, acting as information sources to local, state, and national media outlets, etc.). Finally, groups and organizations also have a role to play at the societal level. Organizations such as the YMCA or hospitals facilitate information flow and help or hinder communication about health.

Variable II: Sensemaking

The second variable of interest in the community acceptance approach is the type of barriers to the accomplishment of goals and acceptance of messages, reified in the concept of a gap (Dervin, 1991, 1998). Gappiness is a metaphor that describes the psychic gulf or chasm that exists between where a person is in his/her life, and where s/he wants to be or go. Gaps are influenced by lived experience, culture, education, communication competence, and other factors. Gappiness also informs the process of sensemaking, which refers to the means by which people make sense of the world around them. According to Dervin and Frenette (2001), this metaphor "rests on a discontinuity assumption—that gappiness is pervasive both in and between moments in time and space and in and between people" (p. 73).

Sensemaking has its roots in both critical research areas as well as mainstream social science areas that focus on the study of human cognitive processes. Sensemaking as it pertains to health-seeking behaviors can be understood by its sophistication or "gappiness" (Dervin, 1989). The gap comprises the barriers to moving forward (i.e., information seeking or questioning behaviors, trust, fear, confusion, source credibility, memories, stories, etc.).

The term gap-defining and gap-bridging explains cognitive strategies used for answering questions—in the context of this chapter, health questions. We know how individuals interpret information, and how information can be derived internally from an individual's own thinking or is derived externally from friends, peers, or health professionals. Often, however, there is something impeding the sensemaking process. Gap-defining and gap-bridging activities are influenced by both individual and situational variables.

Variable III: Communication Channels

The channels of communication are a third variable of interest. As McLuhan (1964) noted over half a century ago, "the medium is the message." The medium (vehicle of communication) can enable message processing but it can also constrain what is possible.

Channels may include face-to-face communication, print and broadcast information, mediated and mass communication channels, social media communication, etc. Channels offer both opportunities and challenges for health messages. For instance, face-to-face communication provides the richest and most immediate type of communication. Interpersonal health information from peers and trusted sources may be the most powerful for knowledge, attitude formation and behavior change. However, information from non-experts is often erroneous.

Broadcast sources such as television, radio, and print also carry health and information campaign messages, and have the potential to reach wider groups, but are also subject to bias and manipulation by government officials, biased talk-show hosts, and uninformed or ill informed media professionals (Kent & Taylor, 2011a).

Finally, social media in the form of blogs, Facebook, Twitter, Wechat, and other localized social media provide hybrid communication channels that enable individuals and groups to share information and reach technologically connected stakeholders and publics. Social media provide a rich source for information and public access, and provide the ability to distribute, textual, audio, video, and other content quickly and inexpensively. Social media can transcend traditional relationship boundaries, and link people who are otherwise not connected (see also Stephens and Zhu, and Harrison, this volume for more on message channels and message diffusion processes).

Variable IV: Health Information

Health information comprises the fourth variable of interest. The type, quality and quantity of health information available to individuals and communities matters a great deal.

Type

Health information exists in both formal and informal types. There is informal health information, much like a lay theory, that guides behavior. This type of information is often culture bound with anecdotes and stories providing guidance to members of a community. The type of health information will influence acceptance and health decision-making.

Quality

Health information quality also matters. The concept of quality can be understood as the credibility of the source and the currency and relevance of the information. Quality varies as different groups will expect different levels of quality. Is the information supported by facts or merely opinion? Is the information from a credible source? Is the information relevant or valuable to the recipient?

Quantity

Health information must compete for attention with many other communication messages. Messages that only appear once or a few times have a smaller chance of being effective. Repetition matters and repeated messages, especially when adding cumulative information each time, create more well-rounded health information.

Variable V: Relational Change

Relational change is the change that occurs from interactions, messages, and human lived experience. Relational change can occur at the individual, group, organizational, community and societal level, and relational change is not only limited to health contexts. Indeed, changes in one context, such as the economy or political system, may create changes in other contexts. The idea of relational change goes back millennia and essentially refers to objects and people experiencing change over time (Lombard, 1978). The most basic premise of relational change is that everything and everybody changes, sometimes in subtle, almost imperceptible ways, and sometimes change occurs in dramatic ways. Moreover, as systems theory suggests, change is inevitable and beyond individual control.

What is within our control, however, is how we respond to change. Relational change does not have to be a powerless withdrawal from external events, or passive acceptance of the inevitable. By becoming informed about health issues and taking that knowledge to one's friends, colleagues, and peer networks, individuals are empowered to enact social and cultural change themselves, enabling individual health empowerment and community health empowerment.

Assumptions of Health and Community Empowerment

A systems approach allows us to place health organizing at various levels. *Individual health empowerment* recognizes that youth often fail to understand all of the health risks facing them. However, when youth obtain individual health empowerment knowledge and skills, they are more likely to be engaged in their communities and are able to help family, friends, and peers make better decisions about their own health. *Community health empowerment* recognizes that communities may also fail to understand all of the health risks facing them. Just as a lack of knowledge harms individuals and prevents everyday citizens from making good health decisions, communities that hide behind misinformation, social mores, and prejudicial values, do harm to the entire collective. Recognizing both individual and community health empowerment, there are four assumptions of the theoretical framework. Each assumption is explained below.

Assumption 1: Elders' and Influentials' Role in Community Change

In the developing world, especially in rural areas, people have access to very few services. In such an environment, people turn to networks of friends, family members, elders, and community leaders for information and advice.

Community elders and influential opinion leaders are the entry point to community level change. The importance of opinion leaders and influential community members to enacting change has been known for decades. Indeed, one of the ways that the Diffusion of Innovation process works is because of the role played by "innovators" and "opinion leaders" (cf., Rogers, 1995). When members of an individual's immediate network or community leaders have erroneous information or are ill informed, everyone suffers. Conversely, well-informed or accurately informed network members allow communities to thrive.

Essentially, the PENHIP is a community power theory (cf., Domhoff, 2014; Mill, 1956) that assumes that people get information from friends, elders and other influential members of the community. The difference in PENHIP is that the education and information is first collected and shared among young people, challenging the paternalistic Western top-down model of health communication. The second assumption of the community acceptance approach is that health messages pass through filters of community values and culture.

Assumption 2: Health Messages Filtered by Community Values

The idea that health messages are filtered through a community's values and experiences is not something new. Community values are shaped by a number of factors including history, religion, intercommunal relations, war and conflict, and power, political, and social relations that have emerged over time. Sometimes ideas based on superstition, or erroneous or inaccurate information, are taken at face value. Scientific health messages often clash with traditional knowledge about health. In many parts of the world, mental illness is highly stigmatized. Mental illness is not viewed through a scientific or medical lens but as a personal deficiency or defect. Communities still ostracize individuals who display symptoms of mental illness, even after an assortment of governmental public information campaigns about post traumatic stress and depression.

Assumption 3: Neglected Issues and Taboo Topics Create Tensions but Provide Opportunities

Many health issues are taboo topics in isolated and closed communities. Moreover, in communities with limited social capital and trust, becoming sick often means being isolated and shunned by neighbors and friends. Illnesses that attack the body such as tuberculosis, HIV/AIDs, malaria, cholera, and hepatitis are often suffered in isolation from the rest of the community.

The idea that problems and opportunities go hand in hand is a basic assumption of crisis, risk, and communication campaign planning. By educating people about taboos or feared topics citizens are empowered to enact change and take different courses of personal, social, and community action. The new actions may not have been possible before the new information. Superstition, fear, and misinformation about taboo topics are not a new phenomenon. Indeed, every culture has its own stockpile of topics and issues that everyday people ignore or refuse to confront, be it prejudice, poverty, race, or disease.

Assumption 4: Health Empowerment Is a Gateway to Social Empowerment

Youth who learn about and advocate for the open discussion of and education on neglected heath issues can join a network of others as they apply their knowledge and skills to health, social education, and social justice contexts. They see new opportunities. Their empowerment makes their communities stronger and better equipped to cope with future health and social problems. Knowledge and education have long been pathways to change in society, especially an understanding of health and wellness issues. Additionally, the rhetorical, persuasive, interpersonal, and group communicative skills needed to engage other people in discussions about important social issues are skills that are transferable to contexts such as health, economics, politics, and individual success.

The first steps involve education about the health issues and providing people with the skills needed to communicate or share that knowledge (Kent & Taylor, 2011a, p. 3). As suggested earlier, barriers like cultural and linguistic differences make it difficult to talk about complicated health issues. People who are empowered to take charge of their own health and welfare issues in terms of threats from Ebola or AIDS are eventually able to shift their focus to other intractable social issues. The PENHIP approach relies on empowering local community workers to build community acceptance (learning informational and persuasive skills) as a precursor to change.

Health Empowerment

Health empowerment is a desired outcome of the community acceptance approach. Health empowerment is twofold. First, it means that people have the information and know what to do with it. Second, it means that people are allowed to pursue health options even if they go against traditional values. Eventually, once a tipping point is reached, choosing mainstream medicine over traditional medicine becomes a routine decision, not subject to social or community sanction.

Social Empowerment

Social empowerment is the highest-level outcome from the community acceptance approach. At this point in a project, youth who began their advocacy as peer mentors are now fully trained and ready to tackle other societal issues and activities. The peer mentors are comfortable speaking in public, engaging people across different age and status levels, and they have the confidence to participate in community discussions on topics that would have been impossible just a few months earlier. Moreover, they have also learned an assortment of interpersonal communication skills and a repertoire of strategies to enable dialogue rather than violence. Full social empowerment will result as a cadre of younger community members shift to becoming community leaders.

The community acceptance framework is important for understanding organizing around health-related issues because it helps to show the connection between health efficacy and societal efficacy. It also helps us to understand how societies can become more fully functioning as civil society processes build relationships among community members (Taylor, 2010) and create social capital (see Chewning, this volume).

The best way to illustrate the community acceptance approach is through a case study of how the YMCA in Liberia mobilized its peer mentors to educate people about the Ebola virus in 2014 and 2015. The community acceptance approach created a form of organizing that both helped to save lives and continue the fragile peace in communities across Liberia. The next section of the chapter presents the PENHIP campaign through the lens of the community acceptance approach.

Community Acceptance Theory in Action: In the Shadow of Ebola

Even in the most advanced economic and educated societies, health information and health literacy are low. In many rural or traditional communities, health information is passed down from parents to youth. The community acceptance theory posits that communities need accurate health information even if it contradicts local knowledge.

For instance, in Liberia, individuals experiencing forms of mental illness are rarely brought to qualified medical experts. Instead, they are brought to traditional healers. "The reliance on traditional medicine to address health needs requiring modern medicine is a concern in a country with a high disease burden" (Kruk, Rockers, Varpilah, & Macauley, 2011, p. 585). Government and civil society information campaigns attempt to build awareness about health information, but local knowledge often trumps complex, technical, and sometimes difficult to understand health information.

In Liberia, relations within communities are strained because formal institutions are weak, property disputes are endemic, youth lack opportunity and access to community resources, and violence is often used to resolve disputes. During the civil war, youth–elder disputes often ended in violence. Blair, Blattman, and Hartman (2014) noted that both informal and formal community structures overtly favored certain groups over others. For instance, "youth–elder disputes stem from struggles over power in the community, such as having a voice in decisions about collective agriculture or community fines and taxes" (p. 8). In a community acceptance approach, different groups have to work together for the good of the community. Relationships need to be built where they do not exist and they need to be sustained and enhanced where they already exist.

Health has emerged as a topic for civil society in Liberia. The YMCA, founded in 1881, is one of the oldest civil society organizations in Liberia. The YMCA developed a peer education program to promote health information and behavior change among the most vulnerable youth populations including teenage mothers, street kids, ethnic minorities and "phen phen" drivers (poor, often orphaned or former child soldiers, who provide motorbike taxi services). Neglected health issues include topics that no one wants to talk about such as hygiene, depression, sexually transmitted diseases and infections, and substance abuse. The YMCA's program has a rural focus seeking to reach those living in remote areas with restricted access to services (YMCA 2014 a, b).

In fall 2012, the YMCA set ambitious goals to train 500 enumerators to conduct a baseline survey of youth health literacy and then, based on the findings, train 5,000 vulnerable youth in Liberia on healthy living. Additional training topics included public speaking, instruction about health topics, training in how to participate in community decision-making, and advocacy. The goal was to create an empowered network from vulnerable youth who then could take their empowerment to the community level.

Organizing for Health and Social Empowerment

The PENHIP originally had two objectives. The short-term objective was to raise awareness about neglected health issues. Health, however, serves only as the initial building block for the long-term objective: to actively engage young people in community advocacy. The long-term objectives treat health knowledge and empowerment as a precursor to political and economic empowerment. The peer education program provides a unique opportunity to study how health empowerment builds a foundation for political and economic empowerment. By building the capacity of local community youth to serve as peer educators, the YMCA hopes to create a cadre of people skilled in communication, organizing, and advocacy. The peer educator network will become the cornerstone of other types of empowerment programs that help to improve the economic and political well-being of marginalized youth in Liberia.

The YMCA team identifies influential persons in the poorest communities in rural and urban Liberia, informs the community at large about the peer education activities, explains how many peer educators will be trained, and shows how this process will benefit the larger community. The final step of the program develops a youth advocacy strategy with the support of policy and decision-makers that extends beyond health issues.

For the first 18 months, the project proceeded according to the plan. The 500 enumerators collected data in four counties and training for vulnerable youth took place in the poorest urban and rural communities in Liberia. YMCA project managers tracked progress.

The network was tested by events that occurred in Guinea in December 2013 when a two-year-old child died from Ebola. Borders in West Africa are porous with people moving easily between countries. In March 2014, Ebola appeared in rural Lofa County, in the northwest corner of Liberia that borders Guinea. By July, the disease had spread through Lofa as the failures in both the health system and the government's capacity to treat those affected by the virus exacerbated the situation. By August, the first cases appeared in the capital of Monrovia as people from the rural areas, hoping to escape the disease, brought it with them and infected family and friends.

No government agency, health organization or civil society group in Liberia was prepared for the Ebola virus. The 14-year Liberian civil war (1989–2003) had weakened Liberia's social, economic and political systems. There was always the chance that civil war would return because many of the militants who created the violence were still living in the country, or had bases nearby in Cote D'Ivoire or Sierra Leone. But the spread of Ebola was made worse by a pervasive lack of trust between citizens and the government.

Yet, local civil society groups emerged to disseminate information about the virus and more importantly deescalate tensions between the people, the police, the military, and the government. Liberian civil society groups played an important role in both the health of communities and the sustainment of peace. It is within this background that the reminder of this chapter explores health organizing. This next section explores the community acceptance approach framework, organizing processes, and outcomes of how the YMCA of Liberia mobilized for health and community peace.

Mobilizing the Network for Ebola

The PENHIP was originally scheduled for six communities in three counties, but full implementation has been delayed because of the outbreak of Ebola. The PENHIP started before the Ebola virus hit Liberia but its actions during the Ebola outbreak provide a timely and highly relevant context to study the intersection of health organizing and community empowerment.

It would be an understatement to say that Liberia was unprepared for the Ebola outbreak. Liberia's medical system is weak, and the cultural practices noted earlier exacerbated the spread of the disease. Additionally, low trust in government information messages meant that individuals and communities were on their own to cope with the disease.

But they were not alone, the YMCA peer mentors, originally trained under PENHIP, were joined by 100 new mentors. Reflecting the sensemaking and health information variables, all mentors were trained in Ebola facts and prevention methods. They mobilized and moved into vulnerable communities to communicate Ebola messages. Just as they had been trained to talk about STIs and drug abuse, the PENHIP volunteers were now ready to talk about Ebola prevention and treatment. Reflecting a nimble and very adaptive organizational structure, the peer mentors implemented a broader nationwide prevention and response strategy to on-going Ebola outbreaks (instead of the previously planned three counties).

There were multiple levels of interaction in this effort. The volunteers began as planned with introductions, meetings, and interactions with the community leaders. The PENHIP teams were flexible and worked to increase awareness about the spread and dangers of Ebola, particularly targeting youth and adolescents in the concerned communities through the training of staff and volunteers, radio programming, and other outreach activities. The volunteers engaged both urban and rural communities, urging them to be more proactive in their response to preventing the spread of Ebola. This community-based campaign embodies what Feeley and O'Mally (this volume) suggest for health outreach.

One of the success stories of the PENHIP is the way that the YMCA mobilized in West Point. The West Point community is the poorest and most marginalized slum in the capital, Monrovia. The West Point community is often a flash point in the capital as residents react violently to unpopular government or police initiatives. When Ebola first arrived in Monrovia in August 2014, the Liberian President Ellen Johnson Sirleaf followed the advice of the military to impose emergency measures including the community quarantine and a "cordon sanitaire." West Point was cordoned off from the rest of the capital by the military. This action essentially isolated the most vulnerable people in an already vulnerable country from health, sanitation, schools, and jobs. The residents protested and rushed the barricades. During the protests against the blockade, the military fired on the demonstrators, killing a 15-year old boy and wounding others. The community was at risk for even more widespread violence as food prices soared and social services disappeared.

The YMCA had been involved in the West Point community for many years and it had built a network of relationships with youth, community leaders and other civil society groups. In September, after the blockade was lifted, members of the PENHIP surveyed young people living in West Point to gather a clear understanding of their situation. Members who had been trained under the PENHIP conducted focus groups and key informant interviews. Based on the findings, the YMCA designed a short-term emergency response project which addressed both health and social issues. To improve community health, the YMCA conducted an information campaign through various communication channels to educate people about the Ebola virus. The campaign included door-to-door visits, radio and televisions PSA jingles in local languages, and posters and fliers outlining the do's and don'ts of Ebola prevention. It also opened public hand washing facilities to minimize the spread of the virus.

At the social empowerment level, YMCA members facilitated social advocacy, outreach and community engagement activities to help diffuse the tensions in the community. Here we see the relational change variable at work. The YMCA helped facilitate town hall meetings and public forums fostering relational change. What makes the process so uplifting is that the most vulnerable people in West Point—the marginalized youth—undertook the steps. These were not doctors or nurses or even health workers communicating the Ebola messages; they were teenagers who six months earlier had been ostracized by the very people, structures and hierarchies that they now worked to save.

The community acceptance approach provided the foundation for creating a cadre of young people who have the skills and confidence to enact both individual and community change. We see the five variables of interest—level of interaction, sensemaking, communication channels, health information, and relational change—come to life.

Unique Contributions of the Theory and Practice to Health Organizing

The community acceptance approach is not yet well established in the health and development literature. Work by Fawcett (2002), and Boothroyd, Fawcett, and Foster-Fishman (2003), appears to come the closest to conceptualizing a community acceptance approach as a theory. Interviews with YMCA staff suggest that the framework is more descriptive than theoretical. Yet, we believe the framework has heuristic value for addressing health-related issues and organizing processes in a variety of contexts. The community acceptance theory positions health messages and behavior change within a larger community system and the outcome is not just healthy youth, but healthy youth who can apply the skills they learned by being peer health advocates to other community advocacy areas.

The unique contribution of the community acceptance theory is that most of the health research in the development literature proceeds from an implicit assumption that community capacity is built first and then the capacity is applied to contexts such as health, youth, gender and conflict management. In this project, the process is reversed. Health information and efficacy on neglected issues come first. The communities in which the information is delivered suffer from low or no capacity. Information about health is the first step in the intervention and then training and meetings move up the ladder of behavior change to finally focus on social advocacy at the community level.

We treat the community acceptance theory as different than the theory of reasoned action, the theory of planned behavior, and other behavior change theories (typically based on gaining support from influentials), because it starts with a community focus on informing those at the bottom, and through those individuals, organizational and community efficacy is achieved through a ladder effect (illustrated in Figure 23.1). This chapter scales up the community acceptance approach framework by operationalizing messages, message features, interactions, and other organizing and communication constructs.

Factors to Be Considered

The community acceptance approach is based on the concept of community engagement. Community engagement is the process of working collaboratively with and through groups. The groups can be geographic (a neighborhood, village, town or city) or a collective with shared special interests or similar situations (cultural community or membership community). A community acceptance approach recognizes that partnerships and coalitions within a community help to mobilize resources and influence systems, change relationships among partners, and serve as catalysts for changing policies, programs, and practices (Fawcett et al., 1995).

Avoiding the Pitfalls

There are of course limitations and pitfalls to the community acceptance approach discussed in this chapter. The theoretical framework is not yet a codified organizational, health or persuasion theory. Because the community acceptance approach is a community- or system-based theory, there are many factors that need to be accounted for as the theory develops. Each community will have its own unique history, culture, values, rituals and control mechanisms—something true of every theory. Accounting for each of these complex factors requires multiple theoretical frameworks and methodologies—something true of every system.

Additionally, for the community acceptance approach to become a codified theory, scholars and researchers may eventually want to stipulate the kinds of skills that are necessary for the community acceptance approach to succeed. In dialogic theory, for example, principles such as risk and trust are prerequisites to successful dialogue (e.g., Kent & Taylor, 2002), but the theory never actually stipulates *how* those relational features should be achieved. Similarly, in the community acceptance approach skills such as conflict management, decision-making, group communication, persuasion, and public communication skills are needed, but how to enumerate the skills and knowledge that is needed will vary from community to community and still needs to be determined.

Also, training in intercultural communication (Kent & Taylor, 2011b) might usefully accompany other communication PENHIP training. Communities are diverse in Liberia and each town and region often has distinctive patterns of social and cultural relations. By understanding the communicative aspects of culture more fully, youth volunteers will be better prepared to succeed. The context for this case study illustrating community acceptance theory is very narrow and there are challenges to collecting reliable data, and testing theory, in places like Liberia. The challenge is accentuated as the Ebola crisis continues in Liberia and other nations.

Future Theorizing

This chapter described how the enactment of local knowledge and lay theories can be systematized into valuable theories and better interventions. The next step in fully conceptualizing and operationalizing the community acceptance theory is to continue to study the Liberian context and revise the lay theory so that is can become a theoretical framework. The case study of the PENHIP provides an opportunity to explore the intersection of organizing and health in new ways. The community-level approach recognizes the systems that individuals live in, and acknowledges that community practices and values influence health as much as mental and physical diseases.

Moreover, this approach is valuable because in places where the community structure and values play such an important role in the lives of the people, a bottom-up, systems-based approach that combines the strengths of the least empowered members of society with the most powerful has the potential to transform everyday life. One of the principles of systems theory is a concept called "equifinality," which suggests that there are many paths to solving the same problem. The community acceptance approach is organic and adaptive. Every community and group is different, requiring not rule-bound structures, such as we see in capacity building efforts, but bottom-up organizing and persuasion skills. By building relationships among community members, the community acceptance approach builds social capital and has the potential to lead to a more fully functioning society.

DISCUSSION QUESTIONS

1. How are health and social empowerment linked?
2. What are the roles for communication as a meaning making process in the community acceptance approach?
3. What is the difference between a lay theory and a scientific theory?
4. What other variables might be included in the model? What other theories or concepts might be added to make the theory more comprehensive?
5. How would you study a community acceptance approach? Explain the method(s) that you might use to collect data.

Suggested Reading

Dervin, B. (1998). Sense-making theory and practice: An overview of user interests in knowledge seeking and use. *Journal of Knowledge Management, 2*(2), 36–46.

Kent, M. L. & Taylor, M. (2011, July). *Ethiopian dialogue: Merging theory and praxis in journalism training.* Competitive Paper delivered to The Annual Conference of The International Association for Media and Communication Research (IAMCR), Journalism Research and Education Section, Istanbul Turkey.

Roussos, S. T. & Fawcett, S. B. (2000). A review of collaborative partnerships as a strategy for improving community health. *Annual Review of Public Health, 21,* 369–402.

References

Bertalanffy, L. (1969). *General system theory.* New York, NY: George Braziller.

Blair, R. A., Blattman, C., & Hartman, A. (2014). Predicting local violence. Available at SSRN: http://ssrn.com/abstract=2497153 or http://dx.doi.org/10.2139/ssrn.2497153.

Boothroyd, R. I., Fawcett, S. B., & Foster-Fishman, P. G. (2003). Community development: Enhancing the knowledge base through participatory action research. In L. A. Jason, C. B. Keys, Y. Suarez-Balcazar, R. R. Taylor, M. I. Davis, J. A. Durlak, et al. (Eds.), *Participatory community research: Theories and methods in action* (pp. 32–57). Washington, DC: American Psychological Association.

Dervin, B. (1991). Comparative theory reconceptualized: From entities and states to processes and dynamics. *Communication Theory, 1,* 59–69

Dervin, B. (1998). Sense-making theory and practice: An overview of user interests in knowledgeseeking and use. *Journal of Knowledge Management, 2,* 36–46.

Dervin, B. & Frenette, M. (2001). Sensemaking methodology: Communicating communicatively with campaign audiences. In R. E. Rice & C. K. Atkins (Eds.), *Public communication campaigns* (3rd ed.) (pp. 69–87). Thousand Oaks, CA: Sage.

Domhoff, G. W. (2014). Power structure research and the hope for democracy. Retrieved from www2.ucsc.edu/whorulesamerica/methods/power_structure_research.html.

Fawcett, S. B. (2002). Evaluating comprehensive community initiatives: A bill of rights and responsibilities. In S. Isaacs (Ed.), *Improving population health: The California Wellness Foundation's Health Improvement Initiative* (pp. 229–233). San Francisco, CA: Social Policy Press.

Fawcett, S. B., Paine-Andrews, A., Francisco, V. T., Schultz, J. A., Richter, K. P., Lewis, R. K, Harris, K. J., Williams, E. L., Berkley, J. Y., Fisher, J. L., Lopez, C. M. (1995). Using empowerment theory in collaborative partnerships for community health. *American Journal of Community Psychology, 23,* 677–697.

Fawcett, S. B., Paine-Andrews, A., Francisco, V. T., Schultz, J. A., Richter, K. P., Lewis, R. K, Harris, K. J., Williams, E. L., Berkley, J. Y., Lopez, C. M., Fisher, J. L. (1996). Empowering community health initiatives through evaluation. In D. M. Fetterman, S. J. Kaftarian, & A. Wandersman (Eds.), *Empowerment evaluation: Knowledge and tools for self-assessment & accountability* (pp. 161–187). Thousand Oaks, CA: Sage.

Heath, R. L. (2006). Onward into more fog: Thoughts on public relations' research directions. *Journal of Public Relations Research, 18,* 93–114.

Kent, M. L. & Taylor, M. (2002). Toward a dialogic theory of public relations. *Public Relations Review, 28,* 21–37.

Kent, M. L. & Taylor, M. (2011a, July). *Ethiopian dialogue: Merging theory and praxis in journalism training.* Competitive Paper delivered to The Annual Conference of The

International Association for Media and Communication Research (IAMCR), Journalism Research and Education Section, Istanbul Turkey.

Kent, M. L. & Taylor, M. (2011b). How intercultural communication theory informs global public relations practice. In N. Bardhan & K. Weaver (Eds.), *Public relations in global public relations contexts: Multiparadigmatic perspectives* (pp. 50–76). New York, NY: Routledge

Kruk, M., Rockers, P., Varpilah, T., & Macauley, R. (2011) Which doctor? Determinants of utilization of formal and informal health care in Postconflict Liberia. *Medical Care, 49*(6), 585–591.

Lombard, L. B. (1978). Relational change and relational changes. *Philosophical studies: An international journal for philosophy in the analytic tradition, 34*, 63–79.

McLuhan, M. (1964/1999). *Understanding media: The extensions of man.* Cambridge, MA: The MIT Press.

Mills, C. W. (1956). *The power elite.* New York, NY: Oxford University Press.

Rogers, E. M. (1995). *Diffusion of innovations* (4th ed.). New York, NY: The Free Press.

Roussos, S. T. & Fawcett, S. B. (2000). A review of collaborative partnerships as a strategy for improving community health. *Annual Review of Public Health, 21*, 369–402.

Taylor, M. (2010). Public relations in the enactment of civil society. In R. L. Heath (Ed.), *Handbook of public relations II* (pp. 5-12). Thousand Oaks, CA: Sage.

YMCA-Liberia (2014a). Liberia YMCA ACT 2 Live on neglected health issues. Retrievedfromhttp://www.ymcaliberia.org/index.php?option=com_content&view=article&id=93:-ymcan-act-2-live-on-neglected-health-issues&catid=9:education&Itemid=4.

YMCA-Liberia (2014b). YMCA holds forum. Retrieved from http://www.ymcali beria.org/index.php?option=com_content&view=article&id=91:-liberia-ymca-holds-community-forum&catid=9:education&Itemid=4.

24

DESIGN THINKING ABOUT COMMUNICATION IN HEALTH SYSTEM INNOVATION

Orchestrating Interaction and Participation for Wellness

Mark Aakhus and Tyler R. Harrison

Health systems are quintessentially communicative phenomena; these systems are entangled in how people relate to each other and the world around them. Health systems are consequential for how individuals' health is understood, valued, and acted upon. Brawley and Goldberg (2012) capture this point well in the case description of Edna, a patient who suffered an automastectomy (where her breast had fallen off from advanced untreated cancer).

> She knew it was breast cancer, and in her experience, everyone who got breast cancer died quickly, painfully. Insurance problems kept her away from the doctor, as did fear of dying. She knew she would die after going to the doctor. Several of her friends had. [. . .] Edna tells me that she feared the disease, but she also feared the system. Would the doctors scold her? Would they experiment on her? Would they give her drugs that caused nausea, vomiting, hair loss? Would the hospital kill her? Edna's decision to stay out of the medical system was about fear: fear of breast cancer, fear of the medical profession, fear of losing the roof over her kids' heads. Fear intensified after her employer started to require copayments from workers who wanted to be insured. This extra $3,000 a year made health insurance too expensive to keep.
>
> *(p. 9)*

Edna's fear was tied to sensemaking processes that resulted from interactions with friends and family as well as her encounters with structural barriers designed into the system. Indeed, Farmer (2004) has been strident in his assertions about the ways in which social, political, and economic arrangements put individuals and populations in harm's way and how this "structural violence" (where social structures or social systems preclude individuals from meeting their basic needs, causing them harm) is not adequately understood or addressed even within medical professions. Others have documented dysfunctions of global governance to reveal how the multiple causes of health inequalities are "rooted in how the world is organized" (Ottersen et al., 2014). At the heart of these medical practitioners' insights is the central importance of the ways in which we construct health practices (the built environment) and their consequences for the health of individuals.

A challenge for communication theory and its application is whether it has anything to offer in understanding these built environments for health practice. The built environment stands in contrast to the natural environment—it depends on the natural environment but is artificial in its adaptation of the natural world toward human goals and purposes (Simon, 1996). For example, where a kidney is natural, a dialysis machine is artificial. The built environment is a mix of the natural with human ideas that vary in their efficacy and legitimacy. At a system level, we might see health organizations, professional practices, insurance policies, and health information systems, as part of the built environment for health. Built environments are not just empirical creations, but are also normative ones that call for reflective engagement on their consequences and their potential for redesign.

We argue that communication theory can realize its potential for improved understanding of health practice by embracing a design stance toward the built environment. The first step is recognition of the built environment as meta-communicative in the way it brings people into relation with each other and the world around them by defining possible and preferable roles and actions. The second is to see the built environment as designed but, following Lyytinen (2004), to see design "not as a singular technical activity, but as a joint weaving of the tapestries of thinking, communication, and acting supported by the diverse technologies that inscribe our behaviors" (p. 226). A design stance is a shift in perspective important for expanding our understanding about how communication matters for health practice—to see how communication is entangled in the biophysical, social, and political determinants of disease (e.g., Farmer, Nizeye, Stulac, and Keshavjee, 2006; Ottersen et al., 2014) but also in wellness.

This chapter takes a design stance in its treatment of health systems as communicative phenomena and highlights the potential role of communication design practice for the reinvention of health practice. First, the concept of design is introduced as an important contemporary movement for addressing social problems, including health issues. Second, we position communication in terms of design and point out how it can realize its potential for contributing to the practice and theory of organizations and health communication. Third, we illustrate this potential by reconstructing the communication design practice evident in the work of two health entrepreneurs seeking open, social innovation for health systems by redesigning health practice. In conclusion, we consider the implications of communication as design for theory about organizations, health, and communication.

Design and Health

Design has gained traction as a basis from which to understand organization, management, and business (e.g., Jelinek, Romme, & Boland, 2008; Boland & Collopy, 2004; Martin, 2009). It has been popularized by people such as Brown (2008) who argue for a revitalized approach to business grounded in design thinking that pursues innovation with a human-centered focus. While design is often understood as a downstream activity in the innovation process that involves packaging an innovation for a customer, Brown (2008) highlights the opposite: "it is a discipline that uses the designer's sensibility and methods to match people's needs with what is technologically feasible and what a viable business strategy can convert into customer value and market opportunity" (p. 2). Brown further argues that as economies shift toward knowledge and service, the realms for design have shifted toward innovation in "processes, services, IT-powered interactions, entertainments, and ways of communicating and collaborating—exactly the kind of human-centered activities in which design thinking can make a decisive difference" (p. 2).

Design is not simply about products but about the services and contexts required to make something new and useful. The movement toward "design thinking" highlights "design's ability to deal with integrative treatment of ill-defined problems" (Devitt & Robbins, 2013, p. 39). This movement has caught on in the world of health as an approach to handling the complexities and challenges in making products, services, and systems more human centered. Design firms such as frog (frogdesign.com) have been engaged by UNICEF and MDG Health Alliance to develop tools and services for frontline public health workers; the influential company IDEO has dedicated a whole branch of their firm to health and wellness. Some hospitals, including the Mayo Clinic, have reconfigured their technology transfer and commercialization operations into innovation centers premised on human centered design.

Design thinking as an organizational practice emphasizes the involvement of diverse stakeholders in the design of a product or service, pays great attention to the details of the setting and the everyday experience of people in relation to other people, artifacts, and systems, and makes a commitment to experimentation by prototyping and tracking what happens in order to provide input into redesign. As Brown and Wyatt (2010) point out:

> One of the biggest impediments to adopting design thinking is simply fear of failure. The notion that there is nothing wrong with experimentation or failure, as long as they happen early and act as a source of learning, can be difficult to accept.
>
> *(p. 35)*

Design thinking is a way of attending to the built environment and its consequences by seeing opportunities for improvement.

While Brown and other design theorists argue for human-centered design, they have generally taken communication for granted as a matter of design (Jackson & Aakhus, 2014). Greater attention can be given to *designs for communication* by investigating how the built environment is a communicative phenomena that is constructed, at least in part, through *communication design work* that makes specifications about how communication works and how it ought to work (Aakhus, 2007). Such activity can be deeply empirical, as it is very concerned with the way things are and how things work, but it also deeply normative, as it is concerned with consequences and what current practice values (or not). It is in that interplay between what is and what ought to be where designers discover what is possible. It is in this arena of discovery and normative concern that we see the importance of a design stance for health practice.

Design, Communication, and Health

Along with our colleagues we have endeavored to bring design to the field of communication as a mode of inquiry and knowledge generation grounded in understanding communication design practice (see Jackson & Aakhus, 2014). A design stance appreciates the role of communication in shaping the world around us but takes a particular interest in the designability of interaction and the ways in which people constitute communication—that is, to shape and discipline communication so that certain kinds of activity are more possible than other kinds (Aakhus & Jackson, 2005). Examples of this include when a dispute mediator uses questions and summaries to change a quarrel into a negotiation or when social media is implemented within an organization to shift from messaging across the enterprise to a culture of idea generation. Design involves knowledge about how to orchestrate interactivity to generate particular forms and qualities of communication. It is "communicative imagination," which is a "capacity to recognize how mundane aspects of human interaction are consequential for the content, direction, and outcomes" of activity and the purposeful use of that knowledge to construct particular communicative and argumentative possibilities (e.g., Aakhus, 2007, p. 33; 2001, p. 364). Design is focused on theory in practice and, like practical theory more generally, is more interested in the cultivation of practice than in the application of abstract theory for the purpose of proving the theory (Barge & Craig, 2009). As Craig and Tracy (2014) have pointed out, communication as design is not so much about *praxis* as it is about *techne* due to its emphasis on direct intervention, outcomes, and the designability of practice.

Brown (2008) offers the following rich example of the potential for a more thorough commitment to examining design in communication. The staff at Kaiser Permanente noticed a problem in shift changes where information exchanges between nurses took up to 45 minutes, often missed key details of patient treatment and status, and left patients and families feeling like there were holes in their care. To help remedy this (and encourage other innovations), Kaiser taught design thinking to nurses, doctors, and administrators. A core team composed of a nurse, organizational development specialist, a process designer, a union representative, and a technology expert worked with designers to identify problems in shift changes and design a new process to alleviate these issues. A few simple changes to the system, such as passing on patient information in front of the patient rather than at the nursing station and creating the ability to input patient information into a notes system throughout the shift, rather than at the end, cut shift time exchanges in half, and increased both job satisfaction and patient satisfaction.

While Brown's (2008) example highlights the potential for focusing on communication in design, recent work in health communication has expanded on this potential by focusing more definitively on the communicative implications of design as it relates to health. For example, Harrison (2014) illustrates how design can be used to situate campaigns and health messages to specific sites of intervention. In their organ donation campaign in drivers' license bureaus in Michigan, Harrison and colleagues (2010, 2011) addressed the communicative problem of creating a dialogue space about organ donation where none previously existed. Clerks were responsible for registering individuals who wished to be donors, but they were not allowed to ask customers if they wished to become organ donors, placing the burden on customers to be proactive about their registration decision without knowing that this was an expectation of the system. The researchers were able to redesign the process after exploring how customers actually interacted with clerks and utilized the spaces of driver's license facilities. Based on this formative research, Harrison et al. (2010, 2011) created prompts and messages to overcome structural barriers such that a dialogic space to register as a donor was created without adding burden to the clerks. While similar to Brown's (2008) change in communication protocols, this example also stands in contrast to Brown as the design thinking about communication explicitly incorporated communication theories, such as media priming (e.g., Cappella, Fishbein, Hornik, Ahern, & Sayeed, 2000), to redesign features of the setting with the aim of changing the *given* communication to the *preferred* communication. Harrison and colleagues' studies hold in common an attention to how interventions and inventions conceptualize communication and subsequently lead to insights for designing improved communication (see also Barbour, Gill, & Dean; Harrison; and Morgan & Mouton, this volume). They engage in theory-driven interventions, which mean that theory is treated as a resource for innovations in practice. Thus, they aim to produce better health practices by attending to communication.

Research in health communication has long attended to communication's designability by giving primacy to health messaging in campaigns, doctor–patient interaction, information seeking, and social support and health networks. While health communication research makes valuable contributions to the understanding of the effects of messages on behavior, these contributions tend to be limited to micro or meso levels of analysis. This is a particularly poignant issue when the built environment, and its consequences for health, are taken into account. Health practice is not simply located in any one message, campaign, information system, hospital, clinical practice, medical technology, or physician–patient interaction. Many challenging problems tend to be systemic products of the built environment that flow from health practice in society, as medical practitioners, such as Brawley and Goldberg (2012), Farmer (2004), and Ottersen et al. (2014), repeatedly point out. The challenge these real-world practitioners have put forward for communication research is the daunting task of understanding how the complex relationships among health organizations, individuals, social and economic systems, and the environment are mediated by health systems that resist technical-expert resolution and often buckle under the pursuit of self-interest. Indeed, while we have a few good examples of communication design at micro and macro levels, inspired by particular communication theories, we may be lacking good examples of communication design at the interorganizational and system level and, moreover, communication theory to demonstrate the effects of the built environment on health and wellness as a communicative phenomenon. There is a need to become more reflective about the role of design in communication by treating both the process and outcome of designs for communication as knowledge about communication; this type of reflection can inspire better design and deeper understanding of communication (Jackson and Aakhus, 2014).

Communication Design Practice in Health Practice Innovation

In this section we explore communication design thinking in the work performed to change the built environment of health practice at the more macro level of health systems. We highlight a complementary approach to other chapters in this volume concerned with design by focusing on the communication design thinking of experts and innovators intervening to redesign health practice. Here we reflect upon the work of Sir Harry Burns, former Chief Medical Officer of Scotland, and Dr. Jeffery Brenner, a New Jersey physician. The goal of Burns' approach to is to fundamentally redesign health practice in the Scottish Health System by treating the health of individuals as a collectively developed community asset. Brenner recently won the MacArthur Genius award for his work on "Hot Spotting" which is challenging the way health care organizations approach the care of the most costly patients. The aim for this section is to cultivate an understanding of how excellence in communication design practice can transform health and wellness systems.

We examine Burns and Brenner's work to better understand the intuitions these expert practitioners have honed about communication in making sense of complex, often perverse, systems and circumstances; how they reason from these intuitions, concepts, and the evidence at hand helps us to reconceptualize what is possible in health practice through the redesign of communication. What is noteworthy is their attention to changing health practice by changing communication practice—in particular, their design thinking about arranging interactivity to realize particular forms and qualities of communication among those with a stake in creating health and wellness across levels of the health system.

We illustrate a reconstruction of the communication design practice evident in the work of these expert practitioners by using four key concepts from grounded practical theory (GPT) following Craig and Tracy (1995) and communication as design (CAD) following Aakhus (2001, 2002): (a) exigency: the societal need or demand that is at stake; (b) problem: what is taken to be the key recurring communicative issues to be addressed in the context of the exigency; (c) solution: the principles and techniques for reflection or design used for resolving the communicative problems and addressing the exigency; and (d) rationale: the empirical and normative justifications for the effectiveness and legitimacy of the solutions to the communicative problem. We base our reconstruction on publicly available materials including speeches, news reports, websites, and other documents where Burns, Brenner, and others describe what they do. Our interpretations are also informed by our first-hand encounters with these health entrepreneurs through an international collaborative focused on Health as an Asset.

Burns: Redesigning Health Practice Toward Salutogenesis

Exigency

Burns asserts that societal exigency regarding health practice is grounded in an imbalanced understanding of the relationship between disease, medicine, social context and health. In a speech he explains, that:

> I never once wrote a death certificate saying the cause of death was living in a horrible house or unemployment. People die of molecular deaths, such as proteins coagulating in arteries and causing heart attacks and strokes. Yet we know that poor [social] conditions lead to poor health and premature deaths.
>
> *(Burns, 2012, p. 2)*

Burns highlights what he sees as an obsession with the cause of disease (pathogenesis) rather than attention to the causes of wellness (salutogenesis). The consequence is an overburdened medical system asked to do more than it can or is meant to do. The focus on disease obscures the ways that social inequalities perpetuate disease across generations because people and communities acquire and transmit incompetencies for managing stress and staying well.

Burns takes salutogenesis to be the fundamental principle for redesigning health practice. Health practice, from this vantage point, must start with the goal of helping individuals attain a sense of coherence in their relations with others and the world around them—that is, following the work of Antonovsky (1987), rendering the world as comprehensible, manageable, and meaningful. When systems undermine the natural connections among people as families, friends, and communities, or disrupt the ways in which people learn how to give order to their lives, such as through good parenting, then the system diminishes the capacity for wellness and contributes to illness.

Burns' perspective has evolved along with his understanding of Glasgow's social history of de-industrialization and research on human development, which point to the dual effects of the loss of social context on human development and their susceptibility to disease (Linklater, 2013). Burns sums up the situation:

> People who do not feel in control over their lives struggle because the system does things to them—it doesn't work with them and help them create 'wellness' for themselves . . . when things happen that alienate people, they lose that sense of control and a whole range of biological, as well as psychological, things occur.
>
> *(Hetherington, 2014)*

Burns' analysis of the societal exigency for health practice suggests that communication is significant to the nature of the exigence and its resolution. Key to changing health practice is the redesign of interactivity, and its support through systems, to achieve forms of communication that have otherwise been difficult, impossible, or unimagined for cultivating relationships, purpose, and meaning as the fundamental in promoting health.

Communicative Problems

A recurring problem for health practice is that decision-making is too often unnecessarily top-down. As Burns explains in an interview:

> The idea that you have one person at the top saying "You will do this" and everyone will jump just doesn't work in our society. So it's about communities, third sector organizations, health service, central government, co-producing the interventions that are needed. But the co-production requires the active collaboration of the people . . . the phrase I use nowadays is "Do things with people, not to people."
>
> *(Linklater, 2013, pp. 32–33)*

The problem, according to Burns, occurs when institutions for communication do not engender radical involvement where users and providers of services work together to create the service that is needed. This follows from his general perspective of salutogenesis for the individual, which emphasizes the need for people to learn how to give meaning to their world and to exercise self-control within it. Burns extends this principle to communities and society at large—thus developing health assets for themselves and the community.

Bottom-up, participative decision-making is not automatic and introduces the recurring problems to be addressed that Burns labels as "will-ideas-methods." Will refers to the need for persuasive, evidence-based arguments and compelling narratives that generate motives to act and the need for ideas. Action requires ideas (albeit there is the recurring problem of sourcing these ideas). Method refers to the challenges of implementation and assessment. Using a bottom-up approach requires work and resources to bring together those with will with those with ideas with those with methods.

Communicative Solution

Solving the communicative demands of participative decision-making communication for co-producing new health practice focuses on two strategies. Intervention is aimed at findings ways for people to take some control over the meaning and direction of their life quality, not just as individuals but as communities and as society. First, Burns orchestrates interaction among stakeholders so that they attend to the little things in the system that are problematic and focus on them as opportunities for invention (*Idea*). Burns highlights the participative design principle of the Early Years Collaborative, which is an initiative involving a coalition of community planning partners in the areas of health, education, social services, police, and other parties to reduce inequalities for Scotland's vulnerable children:

> Small changes in a lot of areas deliver a big change in overall performance . . . [I]ncremental changes will lead to a big change in infant mortality. This kind of improvement science is catching people's attention.
>
> *(Wade, 2014)*

While the aim is for big change, the approach changes the communication about system problems by keeping participants focused on locally relevant and comprehensible matters and by promoting experimentation with solutions and relevant risk taking.

Second, communication is orchestrated to promote participatory evidence-based discovery of what works. Burns is convinced of this approach from his experience as a doctor and in his role as a government official where he found that policy makers are persuaded by evidence. Thus, the will to do something is tightly linked to proof that it can work in preferred ways. So, when participants experiment with the little things they must also figure out how to track whether the experiment is working and find ways to convey that information (*Will*). It can be simple but it must be done.

The bedtime story initiative illustrates the communicative solution. Members of the collaborative noticed that bedtime stories could be a place to advance meaningful, supportive engagement for children: more bedtime stories, more connection between child and significant adult. They tracked the percentage of preschoolers receiving stories. They devised different interventions to increase the percentage, such as by giving preschoolers bedtime bears that needed bedtime stories. They kept what worked and shared their results with other preschools (*Method*).

The Early Years collaborative highlights several ways that various kinds of meetings can be used to convene people from multiple constituencies to discuss health and to figure out small meaningful experiments they could try and develop to foster salutogenesis. The power of the experimentations comes from its replication over time and across places by participants developing the solutions they have created. The creators and users must convince themselves that their new solution works and that then becomes the basis for changing practice. Unlike empirical, academic research, the participants are not looking for full explanations about the causes of their situations but instead are working with their best understanding to devise solutions that work in advancing salutogenesis.

Communicative Rationale

Within Burns' analysis of the societal exigency, communication is an expression of the broader communitarian ethos. As Burns would point out, if the problem is alienation, then the answer is community. The efficacy and legitimacy of the design thinking is grounded in the fact that communication within the community becomes an antidote to a lack of coherence; participation aims to facilitate comprehension, manageability, or meaning for individuals and the community. Proponents of this approach view communities as the experts and express a motto of "Nothing about this community without this community," which represents a fundamental shift in thinking that recognizes how systems are communicative phenomena. The systems are the routine ways through which health is understood and must shift focus away from needs-based assessments that only look for deficiencies, provide fragmented responses, and drive top-down approaches (Lewis, n.d.). Instead, the system should be treated as an instrument for engagement that must avoid putting people into unhealthy relations with each other and their world and instead put them into relations that promote health.

There is a profound pragmatism in Burns' approach that resembles Dewey's community of inquirers working together to understand their circumstances and formulate a course of action based on the exchange of evidence-based reasons. The approach for bending health practice toward salutogenesis does not aim for a grand idea of a solution but instead, like any good design, works with the materials at hand with an eye toward what is possible.

Brenner: Redesigning Health Practice to Address Invisible Problems

Exigency

Brenner's conceptualization of the societal exigency for health is very similar to Burns' salutogenesis but with increased attention to how systems can generate information for building knowledge to change and improve the quality and efficacy of health care. A key insight Brenner pursues is that health systems deal in averages and typical cases but this renders important factors for wellness invisible. Brenner highlights the point by explaining what a doctor may face when prescribing treatment:

> You might decide to increase [a patient's] insulin dose and change his blood-pressure medicine. But you wouldn't grasp what the real problem was until you walked up the cracked concrete steps of the two-story brownstone where he lives with his mother, waited for him to shove aside the old newspapers and unopened mail blocking the door, noticed Cordero's shake of the head warning you not to take the rumpled seat he's offering because of the ant trail running across it, and took in the stack of dead computer monitors, the barking mutt chained to an inner doorway, and the rotten fruit on a newspaper-covered tabletop. According to a state evaluation, he was capable of handling his medications, and, besides, he lived with his mother, who could help. But one look made it clear that they were both incapable.
>
> *(Gawande, 2011, p. 44)*

Fundamental to this perspective is that medical treatment is in a complex relationship with social context and that given systems for health often cannot see that relationship, let alone appreciate it, because health systems cater to the average or the typical patient. One consequence is that, when a patient violates the norm of a prototypical case, they are in danger of falling outside of the health system or between its cracks. Another consequence is that the health system treats repeated cases as single events instead of looking at the larger pattern for clues to why the pattern exists.

So, rather than thinking of patients as fitting an average or preconceived prototype, Brenner began to looking for patterns of health system utilization in terms of where health care resources were expended. Medical billing records provided a key source of information for understanding how the health system is used. Brenner used this data to build block-by-block, color-coded maps of Camden, New Jersey, based on the costs obtained from the medical billing data. He found that one building in the city, for instance, accounted for more serious falls than any other with a cost of three million dollars in health bills. Similarly, one nursing home and one low-income housing tower had over four thousand visits to the emergency room, resulting in nearly two hundred million dollars in health bills over a six-year period (Gawande, 2011). Using these medical billing records, Brenner identified what he called "hot spots" of expenditure and struck upon the idea of identifying high utilizers as opportunities for reducing overall costs by improving the efficacy of their medical treatment and the quality of their health care. That is, rather than looking for overall incremental improvement at the margins of average cases, he saw the most opportunity for improvement in those cases requiring the most from the system. By doing this, the overall cost of health in the city could go down through smarter use of health resources to care for people.

The hotspotting approach reframes the relationship between medicine and social context by envisioning a new practice for health care organizations that promotes health by changing how health care organizations attend to their environments. In particular, attention must be paid to how health care organizations categorize cases and make sense of them in terms of resource allocation. The basic strategy for redesigning health practice is to "look for the most expensive patients in the system and then direct resources and brainpower toward helping them" (Gawande, 2011). As Brenner puts it, "emergency-room visits and hospital admissions should be considered failures of the health-care system until proven otherwise" (Gawande, 2011). The realization of this strategy entails ideas about how communication ought to be designed to realize this new practice.

Communicative Problem

A fundamental communicative problem for the hotspotting strategy is how to make the invisible visible, a problem which presents itself at the immediate level of service but also in the management and innovation of services. One aspect of the problem lies in the way high utilizers and medical professionals engage each other in the design of treatment and provision of services, specifically of finding ways to integrate the technical medical matters and the social context matters into a health promotion. Understanding the patient's circumstance is crucial to developing treatment. As Brenner's first high utilizer patient said, "[Brenner's] whole premise was 'I'm here for you. I'm not here to be a part of the medical system. I'm here to get you back on your feet'" (Gawande, 2011). The ongoing communicative challenge is about building a relationship between the medical provider and the patients as people, not just their roles in the broader system. Patient trust enables clinicians to gain a deeper understanding of the patient's situation and to personalize treatment while simultaneously enabling the patient to develop confidence that the system can work for them, and thus facilitating treatment. As Brenner puts it, "high-utilizer work is about building relationships with people who are in crisis. The ones you build a relationship with, you can change behavior. Half we can build a relationship with. Half we can't" (Gawande, 2011).

The other communicative aspect of the problem lies at the organizational level; organization members must maintain a reflective awareness about the utilization of treatments and services to determine whether quality and efficacy are achieved overall as well as in individual cases. In other words, the problem focuses on the need to design the system based on the environment within which it is situated in order to devise effective medical services.

Communicative Solution

The strategy for addressing recurrent communicative problems that arise from making the invisible visible is evident in the engagement and deep participation designed into Brenner's approaches to managing health care resources. At the level of direct treatment and service, providing attention to the sickest is an opportunity to develop teams and networks of care providers focused on helping high utilizers find ways to make effective use of the resources for health and wellness. As Brenner explained, this includes embedding nurses in high-cost buildings and primary care practices charged with coordinating care and developing outreach teams to find and support high utilizers (Brenner, 2012). This changes the way the health system engages with the patient and can include a social worker who can help the patient find disability insurance, encourage the person to find other kinds of stability such as joining a community group, or help the patient find someone in the community to make vital repairs to their home. The development of these teams and a redefinition of health care provider roles open up ongoing conversations with the high utilizers aimed at helping them find reasons and means to be well within their social contexts, thus creating the conditions for their medical treatment to work. This process of embedding interaction, support, and information into the spaces and daily patterns of high utilizers is similar to the approach used by Harrison and colleagues (2010, 2011) in embedding new interaction patterns in the drivers' license bureaus to promote organ donation registries.

Brenner's design thinking is also seen at the organizational and interorganizational level of service. Brenner assembled a team within the hospital to build and manage a new kind of health information process based on the hotspotting strategy focused on just-in-time information about utilization trends (Brenner, 2012). These systems for sensing the environment are critical to deep participation by health care providers as they identify triggers or conditions of high utilizers, allowing them to intervene before emergencies occur. Brenner also recognizes the importance of interogranizational cooperation and engagement in helping high utilizers achieve wellness—the hospital and primary care providers are only individual parts of a broader system. Resolving high-utilizer issues involves many kinds of specialists and services from across the city that can also be further coordinated. This involves organizing regular interagency meetings for sensemaking as well as the coordination of care and wellness. Finally, and crucially, this approach to deep participation involves incorporating local residents into decision-making about resource usage. Community involvement necessitates training for the local residents so they can participate in the health care system more effectively through awareness of their health care utilization, its costs, and choices they could make, based on using cost savings, in order to further improve their health resources.

Communicative Rationale

Building collaborative teams, engaging the high utilizer, and developing the high utilizers' social relationships and resources are an expression of a commitment to deep participation in evidence-based decision-making. It focuses on changing the way the high utilizer relates to others in their social and environmental context and to the health system and encourages high utilizers to engage in self-help while simultaneously creating the conditions where the utilizers can find the resources to do so. In many ways, the intervention is not complicated so much as it is persistent; as Brenner says, "My philosophy about primary care is that the only person who has changed anyone's life is their mother. The reason is that she cares about them, and she says the same simple thing over and over and over" (Gawande, 2011). The effectiveness and legitimacy of the approach is grounded in the development of learning through evidence and discovery of strategy. The Camden Coalition of Health Care Providers sums up the rationale in their statement of core values: servant leadership, communication and collaboration, compassion and respect, innovation, and being data driven. The approach is Edisonian in the sense that technologies (such as medical equipment and therapies) are not deterministic but conditions for their effectiveness must be created; this is somewhat akin to the usefulness of a light bulb depending on the presence of an electrical system to light it.

Discussion and Conclusion

Both Burns and Brenner are innovators committed to a principle that systems for health and wellness are not limited to those that are required to treat disease or illness. Indeed, health care systems must be understood as part of a system for the co-creation of health and wellness. Burns and Brenner are each committed to changing health practice in a particular context where current health practice undermines the very possibilities for promoting health and generating wellness. They both see health practice as a built environment that, while a recalcitrant reality, can be changed. Their respective analyses attend to what others refer to as structural violence by recognizing a given health practice as a profoundly communicative problem where change must be grounded in altering how people relate to each other and the world around them and where people participate in altering those relations. Burns and Brenner are latter-day pragmatists in that the truth and the value of the arrangement of human relations must be discovered through experience and disciplined reflection on consequences of conduct, habits, and customs of action. They do not advocate a specific theory about the arrangement of human relations for all contexts but instead they offer a way for communities of diverse participants to figure out the arrangements for their context. The work of Brenner and Burns and their colleagues points to a communication design practice concerned with "making communication possible that is otherwise difficult, impossible, or unimagined" (Aakhus, 2007) by "weaving the tapestries of thinking, communication, and acting supported by the diverse technologies that inscribe behavior" (Lyytinen, 2004).

The present chapter can only scratch the surface of the work performed by Burns and Brenner but has done so with the aspiration of motivating further inquiry into communication design practice for health and wellness. This includes at least three directions that attention to communication design work can contribute to better understanding organizations, communication, and health, and how that understanding can contribute to engaging the built environment for health practice. First, more meaningful attention must be given to organizations and systems as communicative phenomena. Rather than simply seeing organizations as platforms where people perform or viewing systems as conduits for messages or actions, organizations and systems need to be deeply implicated in the nature of communication. It is popular in organizational communication to claim that organization emerges in communication. Taking that as a premise, the question remains as to how that happens. This chapter has focused on the work of two practitioners who are concerned with the constitution of communication—that is, how to shape and discipline communication in order to ground the practices of acting and knowing by communities of diverse participants. Second, deeper attention must be given to the practical theories people and practitioners devise to frame communication problems and solutions. Vocabularies and habits of thought are an important resource of invention and intervention on communication and for understanding design thinking. As these are reconstructed, theories in practice are uncovered and available for reflection and refinement of the specifications about how communication works and ought to work. Third, more significant attention must be given to design practice as both hypothetical and theoretical. The practitioner work here illustrates careful attention to devising disciplined reflection on the consequences of the inventions and interventions devised by the community. They do not pursue evidence and evaluation as an end, but as a means for generating common ground and objectivity for a community of diverse participants to see what works and to come to some agreement about the effectiveness and legitimacy of an intervention or invention. There is much to learn from practice, especially from those who are gifted at bending health systems by creating the communication needed to manage the biophysical, social, and political determinants of ill health into assets for generating health and wellness.

DISCUSSION QUESTIONS

1. What assets does your community or organization hold that could contribute to wellness?
2. Identify a problem in health care. How can design thinking help you address the problem is a different way?
3. Sir Harry Burns believes that human connection and support is critical for well-being. How can we redesign and orchestrate interaction and participation in to support wellness?
4. One of the key approaches Brenner and Burns use involves interorganizational cooperation to bring together multiple stakeholders to help solve problems. What types of problems are likely to arise when bringing these stakeholders together? How can we engage participants to focus on design thinking?

Suggested Reading and Viewing Materials

Jackson, S. & Aakhus, M. (2014). Becoming more reflective about the role of design in communication, *Journal of Applied Communication Research, 42*, 125–134.
Dr. Jeffery Brenner: http://tedxtalks.ted.com/video/TEDxBigApple-Jeffrey-Brenner-Be.
Sir Harry Burns: https://www.youtube.com/watch?v=yEh3JG74C6s.

References

Aakhus, M. (2001). Technocratic and design stances toward communication expertise: how GDSS facilitators understand their work. *Journal of Applied Communication Research, 29*(4), 341–371.
Aakhus, M. (2002). Modeling reconstruction in groupware technology. In F. H. van Eemeren (Ed.), *Advances in pragma-dialectics* (pp. 121–126). Newport News, VA: Vale Press.
Aakhus, M. (2007). Communication as design. *Communication Monographs, 74*, 112–117.
Aakhus, M. & Jackson, S. (2005). Technology, interaction and design. In K. Fitch & B. Sanders (Eds.), *Handbook of language and social interaction* (pp. 411–435). Mahwah, NJ: Lawrence Erlbaum.
Antonovsky, A. (1987). *Unraveling the mystery of health: How people manage stress and stay well.* San Francisco, CA: Jossey-Bass
Barge, J. K. & Craig, R. T. (2009). Practical theory in applied communication scholarship. In L. Frey & K. N. Cissna (Eds.), *Routledge handbook of applied communication research* (pp. 55–78). New York, NY: Routledge.
Boland, J. R. & Collopy, F. (Eds.) (2004). *Managing as designing.* Stanford, CA: Stanford University Press.
Brawley, O. W. & Goldberg, P. (2012). *How we do harm: A doctor breaks ranks about being sick in America.* New York, NY: St. Martins Press.
Brenner, J. (2012, March 14). Jeffrey Brenner: Bending the cost curve in healthcare. [Video File]. Retrieved from http://tedxtalks.ted.com/video/TEDxBigApple-Jeffrey-Brenner-Be.

Brown, T. (2008). Design thinking. *Harvard Business Review*, June, p. 1–10.

Brown, T. & Wyatt, J. (2010). Design thinking for social innovation. *Development Outreach, 12*, 29–43.

Burns, S. H. (2012). *Kilbrandon's Vision - Healthier lives: Better futures. The Tenth Kilbrandon Lecture, Sir Harry Burns, Chief Medical Officer for Scotland.* The Scottish Government. Retrieved from http://www.scotland.gov.uk/Resource/0040/00403544.pdf).

Cappella, J. N., Fishbein, M., Hornik, R., Ahern, R. K., & Sayeed, S. (2000). Using theory to select messages in antidrug media campaigns: Reasoned action and media priming. In R. Rice & C. K. Atkin (Eds.), *Public communication campaigns* (pp. 214–230). Thousand Oaks, CA: Sage.

Craig, R. T. & Tracy, K. (2014). Building grounded practical theory in applied communication research: Introduction to the special issue. *Journal of Applied Communication Research, 42*, 229–243.

Devitt, F. & Robbins, P. (2013). Design, thinking and science. In M. Helfert & B. Donnellan (Eds.), *Design science: Perspectives from Europe* (pp. 38–48). Switzerland: Springer International Publishing.

Farmer, P. (2004). Anthropology of structural violence. *Current Anthropology, 45*, 305–326.

Farmer, P. E., Nizeye, B., Stulac, S., & Keshavjee, S. (2006). Structural violence and clinical medicine. *PLoS Medicine, 3*, E449

Gawande, A. (2011, January 24). The hot spotters: Can we lower medical costs by giving the neediest patients better care? *New Yorker*, 40–51.

Harrison, T. R. (2014). Enhancing communication interventions and evaluations through communication design. *Journal of Applied Communication Research, 42*, 135–149.

Harrison, T. R., Morgan, S. E., King, A. J., DiCorcia, M. J., Williams, E. A., Ivic, R. K., & Hopeck, P. (2010). Promoting the Michigan Organ Donor Registry: Evaluating the impact of a multi-faceted intervention utilizing media priming and communication design. *Health Communication, 25*, 700–708.

Harrison, T. R., Morgan, S. E., King A. J., & Williams, E. A. (2011). Saving lives branch by branch: The effectiveness of driver licensing bureau campaigns to promote organ donor registry sign-ups to African Americans in Michigan. *Journal of Health Communication, 16*, 805–819.

Hetherington, P. (2014, March 12). Harry Burns: 'We need compassion, not judgments about poor people'. *The Guardian*. Retrieved from http://www.theguardian.com/society/2014/mar/12/harry-burns-scotland-chief-medical-officer-health.

Jackson, S. & Aakhus, M. (2014). Becoming more reflective about the role of design in communication, *Journal of Applied Communication Research, 42*, 125–134.

Jelinek, M., Romme, A. G. L., & Boland, R. J. (2008). Introduction to the special issue organization studies as a science for design: Creating collaborative artifacts and research. *Organization Studies, 29*, 317–32.

Lewis, N. (n.d) *Early years collaborative: Mapping community assets.* Institute for Healthcare Improvement. Retrieved from http://www.scotland.gov.uk/Resource/0041/00413571.pdf.

Linklater, M. (2013, January 12). Sir Harry Burns: 'I say do things with people, not to people'. *The Times Scotland*. Retrieved from http://www.thetimes.co.uk/tto/news/uk/scotland/article3655700.ece.

Lytinnen, K. (2004). Designing of what? What is the design stuff made of? In R. J. Boland, Jr. & F. Collopy (Eds.), *Managing as design* (pp. 221–226). Stanford, CA: Stanford University Press.

Martin, R. (2009). *The design of business: Why design thinking is the next competitive advantage.* Cambridge, MA: Harvard Business Press.

Ottersen, O. P., Dasgupta, J., Blouin, C., Buss, P., Chongsuvivatwong, V., Frenk, J., . . . Scheel, I. B. (2014). The political origins of health inequity: Prospectus for change. *Lancet, 383,* 630–667.

Simon, H. A. (1996). *The sciences of the artificial* (3rd ed.). Cambridge, MA: MIT Press.

Wade, M. (2014, January 23). Scotland's poor health a myth, says medical chief. *The Times* (United Kingdom). Retrieved from RU database.

INDEX